3 800   D0238447

LANCHESTER LIBRARY, Coventry University
Gosford Street, Coventry CVI 5DD Telephone 024 7688 7555

ONE WEEK LOAN COLLECTION

3 1 MAR 2009		
2 2 JUN 2009		

This book is due to be returned not later than the date and
time stamped above. Fines are charged on overdue books

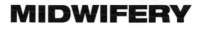

SURVIVAL GUIDE TO
MIDWIFERY

Commissioning Editor: *Mairi McCubbin*
Development Editor: *Sheila Black*
Project Manager: *Anne Dickie*
Designer: *Charles Gray*
Illustration Manager: *Merlyn Harvey*
Illustrator: *Ian Ramsden*

SURVIVAL GUIDE TO

MIDWIFERY

Edited by

Diane M. Fraser BEd MPhil PhD MTD RN RM

Professor of Midwifery and Head of the Academic Division
of Midwifery, School of Human Development,
Faculty of Medicine and Health Sciences,
University of Nottingham, Nottingham, UK

Margaret A. Cooper BA MTD RGN RM

Director of Pre-Registration Midwifery Programmes and
Associate Professor, School of Human Development,
Faculty of Medicine and Health Sciences,
University of Nottingham, Nottingham, UK

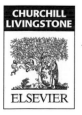

CHURCHILL
LIVINGSTONE

ELSEVIER

Edinburgh   London   New York   Oxford   Philadelphia   St Louis   Sydney   Toronto 2008

CHURCHILL
LIVINGSTONE
ELSEVIER

An imprint of Elsevier Limited

© 2008, Elsevier Limited. All rights reserved.

The right of Diane M. Fraser and Margaret A. Cooper to be identified as authors of this work has been asserted by them in accordance with the Copyright, Designs and Patents Act 1988

No part of this publication may be reproduced, stored in a retrieval system, or transmitted in any form or by any means, electronic, mechanical, photocopying, recording or otherwise, without the prior permission of the Publishers. Permissions may be sought directly from Elsevier's Health Sciences Rights Department, 1600 John F. Kennedy Boulevard, Suite 1800, Philadelphia, PA 19103-2899, USA: phone: (+1) 215 239 3804; fax: (+1) 215 239 3805; or, e-mail: *healthpermissions@elsevier.com*. You may also complete your request on-line via the Elsevier homepage (http://www.elsevier.com), by selecting 'Support and contact' and then 'Copyright and Permission'.

ISBN: 978-0-443-10388-9

British Library Cataloguing in Publication Data
A catalogue record for this book is available from the British Library

Library of Congress Cataloging in Publication Data
A catalog record for this book is available from the Library of Congress

Note
Knowledge and best practice in this field are constantly changing. As new research and experience broaden our knowledge, changes in practice, treatment and drug therapy may become necessary or appropriate. Readers are advised to check the most current information provided (i) on procedures featured or (ii) by the manufacturer of each product to be administered, to verify the recommended dose or formula, the method and duration of administration, and contraindications. It is the responsibility of the practitioner, relying on their own experience and knowledge of the patient, to make diagnoses, to determine dosages and the best treatment for each individual patient, and to take all appropriate safety precautions. To the fullest extent of the law, neither the Publisher nor the Authors assume any liability for any injury and/or damage to persons or property arising out or related to any use of the material contained in this book.

The Publisher

**your source for books,
journals and multimedia
in the health sciences**
www.elsevierhealth.com

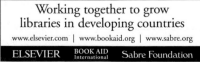

Working together to grow
libraries in developing countries
www.elsevier.com | www.bookaid.org | www.sabre.org

ELSEVIER   BOOK AID International   Sabre Foundation

The Publisher's policy is to use **paper manufactured from sustainable forests**

Printed in China

Coventry University Library

Contents

Contents

Preface

This *Survival Guide* has been developed in response to requests from midwives and student midwives. Whilst there are excellent textbooks for midwives, size precludes them from being carried around in clinical practice. This pocket-sized reference text has therefore been designed so that it can be drawn upon to advance knowledge and understanding during practice, as well as providing a useful revision text for examinations and assessments.

No attempt has been made to replace full textbooks, as more detail, especially on psycho-social issues, and evidence sources continue to be essential and can only be provided in a larger and more comprehensive book. To allow easy reading, no references have been included in this *Survival Guide* and readers are directed to textbooks for this purpose and to explore wider practice issues.

The strategy for the development of this *Survival Guide* has been to summarise information considered to be key for quick reference during practice. In addition, a list of common abbreviations, medications, terms and normal values have been included as an easily accessible source of information.

Nottingham, 2007

Diane M. Fraser
Margaret A. Cooper

Acknowledgements

These must be given to the *Myles Textbook for Midwives* authors on whose chapters this *Survival Guide* has been based. They are: Jean Bains, Diane Barrowclough, Ruth Bennett, Eileen Brayshaw, Linda Brown, Terri Coates, Helen Crafter, Susan and Victor Dapaah, Margie Davies, Soo Downe, Jean Duerden, Carole England, Phil Farrell, Alison Gibbs, Claire Greig, Adela Hamilton, Sally Inch, Carmel Lloyd, Sally Marchant, Carol McCormick, Sue McDonald, Irene Murray, Margaret Oates, Patricia Percival, Maureen Raynor, Jane Rutherford, Christine Shiers, Norma Sittlington, Amanda Sullivan, Denise Tiran, Tom Turner, Anne Viccars and Stephen Wardle.

In addition, thanks are extended to consultant obstetrician Margaret Ramsay and midwife teachers at the University of Nottingham for sharing their expertise, and to Lesley Dingley for her typing, reformatting and administrative support.

Common Abbreviations

Use with caution, as some may have more than one meaning.

ACTH	Adrenocorticotrophic hormone
AFP	Alpha fetoprotein
AID	Artificial insemination by donor
AIH	Artificial insemination by husband
AIMS	Association for Improvements in the Maternity Services
ALT	Alanine transaminase
ANC	Antenatal clinic
APH	Antepartum haemorrhage
ARM	Artificial rupture of membranes
BBA	Born before arrival
BFI	Baby-Friendly Initiative
BMI	Body mass index
BMR	Basal metabolic rate
BP	Blood pressure
BPD	Biparietal diameter
BPM	Beats per minute
BTS	Blood Transfusion Service
CCT	Controlled cord traction
CDH	Congenital dislocation of hips
CEMACH	Confidential Enquiry into Maternal and Child Health
CF	Cystic fibrosis
CMV	Cytomegalovirus
CNS	Central nervous system
CNST	Clinical negligence scheme for Trusts
CPAP	Continuous positive airways pressure
CPR	Cardiopulmonary resuscitation
CSF	Cerebrospinal fluid
CTG	Cardiotocograph
CVP	Central venous pressure
CVS	Chorionic villus sampling

D&C	Dilatation and curettage
DIC	Disseminated intravascular coagulation
DVT	Deep vein thrombosis
EBM	Expressed breast milk
ECG	Electrocardiogram
ECV	External cephalic version
EDD	Expected date of delivery
EEG	Electroencephalogram
EFM	Electronic fetal monitoring
EUA	Examination under anaesthetic
FACH	Forceps to aftercoming head
FAS	Fetal alcohol syndrome
FBC	Full blood count
FBS	Fetal blood sampling
FDPs	Fibrin degradation products
FGM	Female genital mutilation
FH	Fetal heart
FHH	Fetal heart heard
FIGO	International Federation of Gynaecologists and Obstetricians
FSE	Fetal scalp electrode
FSH	Follicle-stimulating hormone
GA	General anaesthetic
GBS	Group B haemolytic streptococcus
GI	Gastrointestinal
GIFT	Gamete intrafallopian transfer
G6PD	Glucose 6-phosphate dehydrogenase
G&S	Group and save serum
GTT	Glucose tolerance test
GU	Genitourinary
Hb	Haemoglobin
HBV	Hepatitis B virus
HCC	Healthcare Commission
HCG	Human chorionic gonadotrophin
HDN	Haemolytic disease of the newborn
HDU	High-dependency unit

HELLP	Haemolysis, elevated liver enzymes, low platelets
HIV	Human immunodeficiency virus
HPL	Human placental lactogen
HPV	Human papillomavirus
HVS	High vaginal swab
ICM	International Confederation of Midwives
ICSI	Intracytoplasmic sperm injection
ICU	Intensive care unit
IG	Immunoglobulin
IM	Intramuscular
IOL	Induction of labour
IUCD	Intrauterine contraceptive device
IU(F)D	Intrauterine (fetal) death
IUGR	Intrauterine growth restriction
IV	Intravenous
LAM	Lactational amenorrhoea method
LFT	Liver function tests
LGA	Large for gestational age
LH	Luteinising hormone
LMP	Last menstrual period
L:S	Lecithin:sphyngomyelin
LSA	Local Supervising Authority
LSCS	Lower segment caesarean section
MAP	Mean arterial pressure
MSU	Midstream specimen of urine
NEC	Necrotising enterocolitis
NICE	National Institute for Health and Clinical Excellence
NICU	Neonatal intensive care unit
NMC	Nursing and Midwifery Council
NND	Neonatal death
NSF	National Service Framework
NT	Nuchal translucency
NTD	Neural tube defect
PE	Pulmonary embolism (care — may also be used for pre-eclampsia)
PGD	Patient group direction

PIH	Pregnancy-induced hypertension
PKU	Phenylketonuria
PPH	Postpartum haemorrhage
PROM	Premature rupture of membranes
PV	Per vaginam
RBC	Red blood cell
RCM	Royal College of Midwives
RCOG	Royal College of Obstetricians and Gynaecologists
RCT	Randomised controlled trial
RDS	Respiratory distress syndrome
Rh	Rhesus
SB	Stillbirth
SCBU	Special care baby unit
SGA	Small for gestational age
SIDS	Sudden infant death syndrome
SLE	Systemic lupus erythematosus
SPD	Symphysis pubis dysfunction
SROM	Spontaneous rupture of membranes
STI	Sexually transmitted infection
TIA	Transient ischaemic attack
TOP	Termination of pregnancy
TPN	Total parenteral nutrition
TSH	Thyroid-stimulating hormone
U&E	Urea and electrolytes
UNICEF	United Nations Children's Fund
USS	Ultrasound scan
UTI	Urinary tract infection
VBAC	Vaginal birth after caesarean
VDRL	Venereal Disease Research Laboratory
VE	Vaginal examination
WHO	World Health Organization
ZIFT	Zygote intrafallopian transfer

Section 1

Anatomy and Reproduction

The Female Pelvis and the Reproductive Organs

The Female Pelvis

The normal pelvis is comprised of four pelvic bones:

■ two *innominate bones*

■ one *sacrum*

■ one *coccyx*.

The innominate bones (Fig. 1.1)

Each innominate bone is composed of three parts:

■ the *ilium*

■ the *ischium*

■ the *pubic bone*.

The ilium

■ At the front of the iliac crest is a bony prominence known as the *anterior superior iliac spine*; below it is the *anterior inferior iliac spine*.

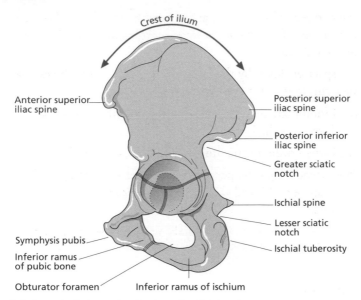

Fig. 1.1: Innominate bone showing important landmarks.

- Two similar points at the other end of the iliac crest are called the *posterior superior* and the *posterior inferior iliac spines*.
- The concave anterior surface of the ilium is the *iliac fossa*.

The ischium

The ischium is the thick lower part.

- The *ischial tuberosity* is the prominence on which the body rests when sitting.
- Behind and a little above the tuberosity is an inward projection, the *ischial spine*.

In labour the station of the fetal head is estimated in relation to the ischial spines.

The pubic bone

- This has a body and two oar-like projections: the *superior ramus* and the *inferior ramus*.

- The two pubic bones meet at the symphysis pubis and the two inferior rami form the *pubic arch*, merging into a similar ramus on the ischium.

- The space enclosed by the body of the pubic bone, the rami and the ischium is called the *obturator foramen*.

- The innominate bone contains a deep cup, the *acetabulum*, which receives the head of the femur.

On the lower border of the innominate bone are found two curves:

- One extends from the posterior inferior iliac spine up to the ischial spine and is called the *greater sciatic notch*. It is wide and rounded.

- The other lies between the ischial spine and the ischial tuberosity and is the *lesser sciatic notch*.

The sacrum

This is a wedge-shaped bone consisting of five fused vertebrae. The first sacral vertebra juts forward and is called the *sacral promontory*.

The coccyx

The coccyx consists of four fused vertebrae, forming a small triangular bone.

The pelvic joints

There are four pelvic joints:

- The *symphysis pubis* is formed at the junction of the two pubic bones, which are united by a pad of cartilage.

- Two *sacroiliac joints* join the sacrum to the ilium and thus connect the spine to the pelvis.

- The *sacrococcygeal joint* is formed where the base of the coccyx articulates with the tip of the sacrum.

In the non-pregnant state there is very little movement in these joints, but during pregnancy endocrine activity causes the ligaments to soften, which allows the joints to give.

The pelvic ligaments

Each of the pelvic joints is held together by ligaments:

- *interpubic* ligaments at the symphysis pubis
- *sacroiliac* ligaments
- *sacrococcygeal* ligaments.

Two other ligaments are important in midwifery:

- the *sacrotuberous* ligament
- the *sacrospinous* ligament.

The sacrotuberous ligament runs from the sacrum to the ischial tuberosity, and the sacrospinous ligament from the sacrum to the ischial spine. These two ligaments cross the sciatic notch and form the posterior wall of the pelvic outlet.

The True Pelvis

The true pelvis is the bony canal through which the fetus must pass during birth. It has a brim, a cavity and an outlet.

The pelvic brim

The fixed points on the pelvic brim are known as its landmarks (see Fig. 1.2 and Box 1.1).

Diameters of the brim

Three diameters are measured (Figs 1.3 and 1.4):

- anteroposterior
- oblique
- transverse.

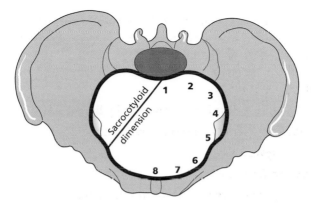

Fig. 1.2: Brim or inlet of female pelvis (see Box 1.1).

Box 1.1 Landmarks of the pelvic brim (commencing posteriorly)

See Figure 1.2 for numbers

- Sacral promontory (1)
- Sacral ala or wing (2)
- Sacroiliac joint (3)
- Iliopectineal line: the edge formed at the inward aspect of the ilium (4)
- Iliopectineal eminence: a roughened area formed where the superior ramus of the pubic bone meets the ilium (5)
- Superior ramus of the pubic bone (6)
- Upper inner border of the body of the pubic bone (7)
- Upper inner border of the symphysis pubis (8)

The anteroposterior diameter

This is a line from the sacral promontory to the upper border of the symphysis pubis.

■ When the line is taken to the uppermost point of the symphysis pubis, it is called the *anatomical conjugate* (12 cm).

■ When it is taken to the posterior border of the upper surface, it is called the *obstetrical conjugate* (11 cm).

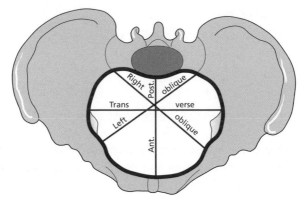

Fig. 1.3: View of pelvic inlet showing diameters.

	Anteroposterior	Oblique	Transverse
Brim	11	12	13
Cavity	12	12	12
Outlet	13	12	11

Fig. 1.4: Measurements of the pelvic canal in centimetres.

■ The *diagonal conjugate* is also measured anteroposteriorly from the lower border of the symphysis to the sacral promontory. It may be estimated on vaginal examination as part of a pelvic assessment and should measure 12–13 cm.

The oblique diameter

This is a line from one sacroiliac joint to the iliopectineal eminence on the opposite side of the pelvis (12 cm).

The transverse diameter

This is a line between the points furthest apart on the iliopectineal lines (13 cm).

Another dimension is described, the *sacrocotyloid* (Fig. 1.2). It passes from the sacral promontory to the iliopectineal eminence on each side and measures 9–9.5 cm.

The pelvic cavity

This extends from the brim above to the outlet below.

- The anterior wall is formed by the pubic bones and symphysis pubis and its depth is 4 cm.
- The posterior wall is formed by the curve of the sacrum, which is 12 cm in length.

The cavity forms a curved canal; its lateral walls are the sides of the pelvis, which are mainly covered by the obturator internus muscle.

The cavity is circular in shape, and although it is not possible to measure its diameters exactly, they are all considered to be 12 cm (Fig. 1.4).

The pelvic outlet

Two outlets are described: the anatomical and the obstetrical. The *obstetrical outlet* includes the narrow pelvic strait, through which the fetus must pass. This outlet is diamond-shaped. Its three diameters are as follows (Fig. 1.4):

- The *anteroposterior diameter* is a line from the lower border of the symphysis pubis to the sacrococcygeal joint.

- The *oblique diameter* is said to be between the obturator foramen and the sacrospinous ligament, although there are no fixed points.

- The *transverse diameter* is a line between the two ischial spines.

The false pelvis

The false pelvis is the part of the pelvis situated above the pelvic brim. It is of no significance in obstetrics.

Pelvic inclination

When a woman is standing in the upright position, her pelvis is on an incline; as can be seen in Figure 1.5, the brim is tilted and forms an angle of 60º with the horizontal floor. The angles are important to understand when women are in different positions for an abdominal examination.

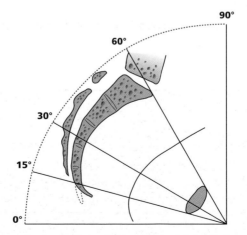

Fig. 1.5: Median section of the pelvis showing the inclination of the planes and the axis of the pelvic canal.

The pelvic planes

These are imaginary flat surfaces at the brim, cavity and outlet of the pelvic canal at the levels of the lines described above.

The axis of the pelvic canal

A line drawn exactly half-way between the anterior wall and the posterior wall of the pelvic canal would trace a curve known as the *curve of Carus*. An understanding of this is necessary when assessing progress in labour.

The four types of pelvis (Table 1.1)

Classically, the pelvis has been described according to the shape of the brim. If one of the important measurements is reduced by 1 cm or more from the normal, the pelvis is said to be contracted; this may give rise to difficulty in labour or necessitate caesarean section.

The *gynaecoid pelvis* is the ideal pelvis for childbearing. Its main features are:

- a rounded brim
- generous forepelvis (the part in front of the transverse diameter)
- straight side walls

Table 1.1 Features of the four types of pelvis

Features	Gynaecoid	Android	Anthropoid	Platypelloid
Brim	Rounded	Heart-shaped	Long oval	Kidney-shaped
Forepelvis	Generous	Narrow	Narrowed	Wide
Side walls	Straight	Convergent	Divergent	Divergent
Ischial spines	Blunt	Prominent	Blunt	Blunt
Sciatic notch	Rounded	Narrow	Wide	Wide
Subpubic angle	90°	<90°	>90°	>90°
Incidence	50%	20%	25%	5%

- a shallow cavity with a broad, well-curved sacrum, blunt ischial spines, a rounded sciatic notch and a subpubic angle of 90°.

It is found in women of average build and height with a shoe size of 4 or larger.

The pelvic floor

The pelvic floor is formed by the soft tissues that fill the outlet of the pelvis. The most important of these is the strong diaphragm of muscle slung like a hammock from the walls of the pelvis. Through it pass the urethra, the vagina and the anal canal.

The pelvic floor comprises two muscle layers:

- the superficial layer (Fig. 1.6)
- the deep layer (Fig. 1.7).

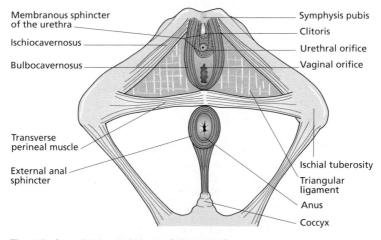

Fig. 1.6: Superficial muscle layer of the pelvic floor.

The Vulva

The term 'vulva' applies to the external female genital organs (Fig. 1.8).

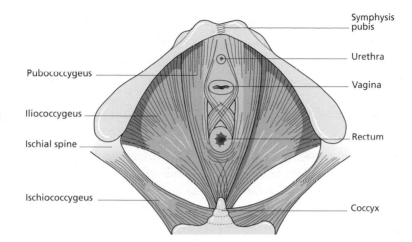

Fig. 1.7: Deep muscle layer of the pelvic floor.

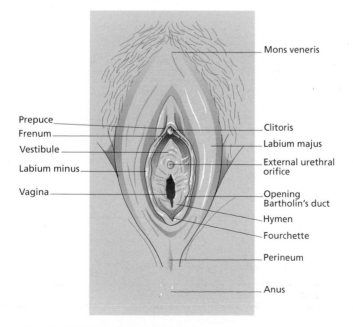

Fig. 1.8: Female external genital organs, or vulva.

The Vagina

The vagina is a canal running from the vestibule to the cervix, passing upwards and backwards into the pelvis along a line approximately parallel to the plane of the pelvic brim.

A knowledge of the relations of the vagina to other organs is essential for the accurate examination of the pregnant woman and the safe birth of her baby (see Figs 1.9 and 1.10).

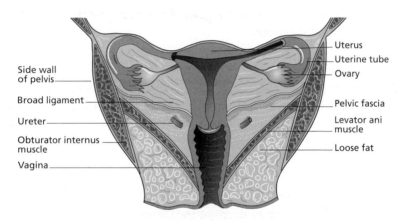

Side wall of pelvis

Broad ligament

Ureter

Obturator internus muscle

Vagina

Uterus

Uterine tube

Ovary

Pelvic fascia

Levator ani muscle

Loose fat

Fig. 1.9: Coronal section through the pelvis.

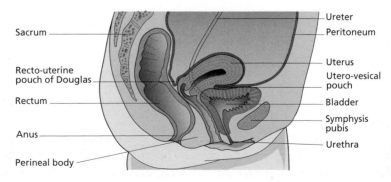

Sacrum

Recto-uterine pouch of Douglas

Rectum

Anus

Perineal body

Ureter

Peritoneum

Uterus

Utero-vesical pouch

Bladder

Symphysis pubis

Urethra

Fig. 1.10: Sagittal section of the pelvis.

The Uterus

The uterus is situated in the cavity of the true pelvis.

Relations
See Figures 1.9 and 1.10.

Supports
The uterus is supported by the pelvic floor and maintained in position by several ligaments.

Structure
The non-pregnant uterus is a hollow, muscular, pear-shaped organ. It is 7.5 cm long, 5 cm wide and 2.5 cm in depth, each wall being 1.25 cm thick. The cervix forms the lower third of the uterus and measures 2.5 cm in each direction.

The uterus consists of the following parts:

The body or corpus
This forms the upper two-thirds of the uterus.

The fundus
The fundus is the domed upper wall between the insertions of the uterine tubes.

The cornua
These are the upper outer angles of the uterus where the uterine tubes join.

The uterine tubes extend laterally from the cornua of the uterus towards the side walls of the pelvis. They arch over the ovaries, the fringed ends hovering near the ovaries in order to receive the ovum. Each tube is 10 cm long. The lumen of the tube provides an open

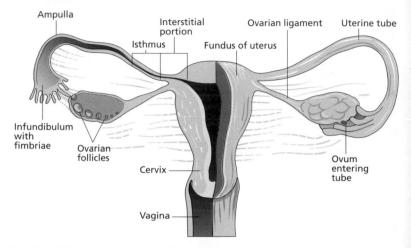

Fig. 1.11: The uterine tubes in section. Note the ovum entering the fimbriated end of one tube.

pathway from the outside to the peritoneal cavity. The uterine tube has four portions:

- the interstitial portion
- the isthmus
- the ampulla
- the infundibulum (Fig. 1.11).

The cavity

The cavity is a potential space between the anterior and posterior walls. It is triangular in shape, the base of the triangle being uppermost.

The isthmus

The isthmus is a narrow area between the cavity and the cervix, which is 7 mm long. It enlarges during pregnancy to form the lower uterine segment.

The cervix

This protrudes into the vagina.

- *The internal os* is the narrow opening between the isthmus and the cervix.
- *The external os* is a small round opening at the lower end of the cervix. After childbirth it becomes a transverse slit.
- The *cervical canal* lies between these two ora and is a continuation of the uterine cavity.

Layers

The layers of the uterus are called:

- the endometrium
- the myometrium
- the perimetrium.

The endometrium

This forms a lining of ciliated epithelium on a base of connective tissue or stroma.

In the uterine cavity this endometrium is constantly changing in thickness throughout the menstrual cycle. The basal layer does not alter, but provides the foundation from which the upper layers regenerate. The epithelial cells are cubical in shape and dip down to form glands that secrete an alkaline mucus.

The cervical endometrium does not respond to the hormonal stimuli of the menstrual cycle to the same extent. Here the epithelial cells are tall and columnar in shape and the mucus-secreting glands are branching racemose glands. The cervical endometrium is thinner than that of the body and is folded into a pattern known as the 'arbor vitae'. The portion of the cervix that protrudes into the vagina is covered with squamous epithelium similar to that lining the vagina. The point where the epithelium changes, at the external os, is termed the squamocolumnar junction.

The myometrium

This layer is thick in the upper part of the uterus but sparser in the isthmus and cervix. Its fibres run in all directions and interlace to surround the blood vessels and lymphatics that pass to and from the endometrium. The outer layer is formed of longitudinal fibres that are continuous with those of the uterine tube, the uterine ligaments and the vagina.

In the cervix the muscle fibres are embedded in collagen fibres, which enable it to stretch in labour.

The perimetrium

This is a double serous membrane, an extension of the peritoneum, which is draped over the uterus, covering all but a narrow strip on either side and the anterior wall of the supravaginal cervix, from where it is reflected up over the bladder.

Blood supply

The uterine artery arrives at the level of the cervix and is a branch of the internal iliac artery. It sends a small branch to the upper vagina, and then runs upwards in a twisted fashion to meet the ovarian artery and form an anastomosis with it near the cornu. The ovarian artery is a branch of the abdominal aorta. It supplies the ovary and uterine tube before joining the uterine artery. The blood drains through corresponding veins.

Lymphatic drainage

Lymph is drained from the uterine body to the internal iliac glands and also from the cervical area to many other pelvic lymph glands.

Nerve supply

This is mainly from the autonomic nervous system, sympathetic and parasympathetic, via the inferior hypogastric or pelvic plexus.

The Ovaries

The ovaries are situated within the peritoneal cavity. They are attached to the back of the broad ligaments but are supported from above by the ovarian ligament medially and the infundibulopelvic ligament laterally. Each ovary is composed of a medulla and cortex, covered with germinal epithelium. (See ch. 3 for changes associated with the menstrual cycle.)

Chapter 2

The Female Urinary Tract

The urinary system has an elimination function, which it fulfils via the production of urine. It also has important functions in connection with the control of water and electrolyte balance and of blood pressure.

The Kidneys

The kidneys are two bean-shaped glands that have both endocrine and exocrine secretions.

Functions

Functions of the kidneys are shown in Box 2.1.

Box 2.1 Functions of the kidneys

- Elimination of waste, particularly the breakdown products of protein, such as urea, urates, uric acid, creatinine, ammonia and sulphates
- Elimination of toxins
- Regulation of the water content of the blood and indirectly of the tissues
- Regulation of the pH of the blood
- Regulation of the osmotic pressure of the blood
- Secretion of the hormones renin and erythropoietin

Position and appearance

The kidneys are positioned at the back of the abdominal cavity, high up under the diaphragm. Each kidney is about 10 cm long, 6.5 cm wide and 3 cm thick. It weighs around 120 g and is covered with a tough, fibrous capsule.

The inner border of the organ is indented at the hilum; here the large vessels enter and leave, and the ureter is attached by its funnel-shaped upper end to channel the urine away.

Inner structure

- The glandular tissue is formed of *cortex* on the outside and *medulla* within. The cortex is dark with a rich blood supply, whereas the medulla is paler.

- A collecting area for urine merges with the upper ureter and is called the *pelvis*. It is divided into branches or calyces.

- Each calyx forms a cup over a projection of the medulla known as a *pyramid*. There are some 12 pyramids in all and they contain bundles of tubules leading from the cortex.

- The tubules create a lined appearance and these are the *medullary rays*.

- The base of each pyramid is curved and the cortex arches over it and projects downwards between the pyramids, forming columns of tissue (*columns of Bertini*).

The nephrons (Fig. 2.1)

The tissue of the kidney is made up of about 1 million nephrons, which are its functional units.

- Each nephron starts at a knot of capillaries called a *glomerulus*.

- It is fed by a branch of the renal artery, the *afferent arteriole*. (Afferent means 'carrying towards'.)

- The blood is collected up again into the *efferent arteriole*. (Efferent means 'carrying away'.)

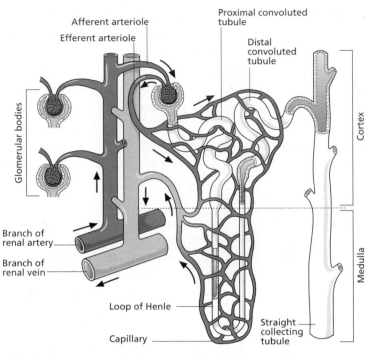

Fig. 2.1: A nephron.

■ Surrounding the glomerulus is a cup known as the *glomerular capsule*, into which fluid and solutes are exuded from the blood.

■ The glomerulus and capsule together comprise the *glomerular body*. The pressure within the glomerulus is raised because the afferent arteriole is of a wider bore than the efferent arteriole; this factor forces the filtrate out of the capillaries and into the capsule. At this stage there is no selection; any substance with a small molecular size will filter out.

■ The cup of the capsule is attached to a tubule, as a wine glass is to its stem. The tubule initially winds and twists, then forms a straight loop which dips into the medulla, rising up into the cortex again to wind and turn before joining a *straight collecting tubule*, which receives urine from several nephrons.

■ The first twisting portion of the nephron is the *proximal convoluted tubule*, the loop is termed the *loop of Henle* and the second twisting portion is the *distal convoluted tubule*.

The whole nephron is about 3 cm in length. The straight collecting tubule runs from the cortex to a medullary pyramid; it forms a medullary ray and receives urine from over 4000 nephrons along its length.

Juxtaglomerular apparatus

The distal convoluted tubule returns to pass alongside granular cells of the afferent arteriole, and this part of the tubule is called the *macula densa*. The two are known as the *juxtaglomerular apparatus*. The granular cells secrete renin, whereas the macula densa cells monitor the sodium chloride concentration of fluid passing through.

Blood supply

The renal arteries are early branches of the descending abdominal aorta and divert about a quarter of the cardiac output into the kidneys. Blood is collected up and returned via the renal vein.

The making of urine

This takes place in three stages:
■ filtration
■ reabsorption
■ secretion.

Filtration

This is the simple process whereby water and the substances dissolved in it are passed from the glomerulus into the glomerular capsule as a result of the raised intracapillary pressure. Blood components such as corpuscles and platelets, as well as plasma proteins, which are large molecules, are kept in the blood vessel; water, salts and glucose escape through the filter as the *filtrate*. A vast amount of fluid passes out in this way: about 2 ml per second or 120 ml per minute. Ninety-nine per cent of this must be recovered. Filtration is increased in pregnancy, as it helps to eliminate the additional waste substances created by maternal and fetal metabolism.

Reabsorption

The body selects from the filtrate those substances that it needs: water, salts and glucose.

Normally, all the glucose is reabsorbed; only if there is already more than sufficient in the blood will any be excreted in the urine. The level of blood glucose at which this happens is the *renal threshold* for glucose:

- In the non-pregnant woman, the threshold is 10 mmol/l.
- In the pregnant woman, the threshold is 8.3 mmol/l.

It is more likely, therefore, that glucose will appear in the urine during pregnancy.

The water is almost all reabsorbed. The posterior pituitary gland controls the reabsorption of water by producing antidiuretic hormone (ADH). Minerals are selected according to the body's needs. The reabsorption of sodium is controlled by aldosterone, which is produced in the cortex of the adrenal gland. The interaction of aldosterone and ADH maintains water and sodium balance. The pH of the blood must be controlled and if it is tending towards acidity then acids will be excreted. However, if the opposite pertains, alkaline urine will be produced. Often this is the result of an intake of an alkaline substance.

Secretion

Certain substances, such as creatinine and toxins, are added directly to the urine in the ascending arm of the loop of Henle.

Endocrine activity

The kidney secretes two hormones:

- *Renin* is produced in the afferent arteriole and is secreted when the blood supply to the kidneys is reduced and in response to lowered sodium levels. It acts on angiotensinogen, which is present in the blood, to form angiotensin, which raises blood pressure and encourages sodium reabsorption.

- *Erythropoietin* stimulates the production of red blood cells.

The urine

An adult passes between 1 and 2 litres of urine daily, depending on fluid intake. Pregnant women secrete large amounts of urine because of the increased glomerular filtration rate. In the first day or two postpartum a major diuresis occurs and urine output is copious.

The specific gravity of urine is 1.010–1.030. It is composed of:

- 96% water
- 2% urea
- 2% other solutes.

Urea and uric acid clearance are increased in pregnancy. Urine is usually acid and contains no glucose or ketones; nor should it carry blood cells or bacteria. Women are susceptible to urinary tract infection (UTI) but this is usually an ascending infection acquired via the urethra. A low count, less than 100 000 per ml, of bacteria in the urine (bacteriuria) is treated as insignificant.

The Ureters

The ureters convey urine from the kidneys to the bladder. They assist the passage of the urine by the muscular peristaltic action of their walls. The upper end is funnel-shaped and merges into the pelvis of the kidney, where the urine is received from the renal tubules.

Each tube is about 25–30 cm long and runs from the renal hilum to the posterior wall of the bladder. In the abdomen the ureters pass down the posterior wall, remaining outside the peritoneal cavity. On reaching the pelvic brim, they descend along the side walls of the pelvis to the level of the ischial spines and then turn forwards to pass beside the uterine cervix and enter the bladder from behind. They pass through the bladder wall at an angle, so that when the bladder contracts to expel urine the ureters are closed off and reflux is prevented.

The hormones of pregnancy, particularly progesterone, relax the walls of the ureters and allow dilatation and kinking. In some women this is quite marked and it tends to result in a slowing down or stasis of urinary flow, making infection a greater possibility.

The Bladder

The bladder is the urinary reservoir, storing the urine until it is convenient for it to be voided. It is described as being pyramidal and its base is triangular. When it is full, however, it becomes more globular in shape as its walls are distended. Although it is a pelvic organ, it may rise into the abdomen when full.

Structure

- The base of the bladder is termed the *trigone*. It is situated at the back of the bladder, resting against the vagina. Its three angles are formed by the exit of the urethra below and the two slit-like openings of the ureters above. The apex of the trigone is thus at its lowest point, which is also termed the neck.

- The anterior part of the bladder lies close to the pubic symphysis and is termed the *apex* of the bladder. From it the urachus runs up the anterior abdominal wall to the umbilicus. The empty bladder is of similar size to the uterus; when full of urine, its capacity is around 600 ml but it is capable of holding more, particularly under the influence of pregnancy hormones.

The Urethra

The urethra is 4 cm long in the female and consists of a narrow tube buried in the outer layers of the anterior vaginal wall. It runs from the neck of the bladder and opens into the vestibule of the vulva as the urethral meatus. During labour the urethra becomes elongated, as the bladder is drawn up into the abdomen, and may become several centimetres longer.

Micturition

The urge to pass urine is felt when the bladder contains about 200–300 ml of urine; psychological and other external stimuli may also trigger a desire to empty the bladder. The sphincters relax, the detrusor muscle contracts and urine is passed. In summary, the bladder fills and then contracts as a reflex response. The internal sphincter opens by the action of Bell's muscles. If the urge is not resisted, the external sphincter relaxes and the bladder empties. The act of emptying may be speeded by raising intra-abdominal pressure either to initiate the process or throughout voiding. The act of micturition can be temporarily postponed.

Key points for practice are summarised in Box 2.2.

Box 2.2 Key points for practice

- Pregnant and postnatal women produce large amounts of urine
- Glucose in the urine might be due to a temporary reduced reabsorption threshold or diabetes (pre-existing or gestational)
- Protein in the urine might be due to contamination, UTI, pre-eclampsia or renal dysfunction
- A full bladder can impede progress in labour and prevent contraction of the uterus following birth

---

Chapter 3

Hormonal Cycles: Fertilisation and Early Development

The hypothalamus is the ultimate source of control, governing the anterior pituitary gland by hormonal pathways. The anterior pituitary gland in turn governs the ovary via hormones. Finally, the ovary produces hormones that control changes in the uterus. All these changes occur simultaneously and in harmony. A woman's moods may change along with the cycle, and emotional influences can alter the cycle because of the close relationship between the hypothalamus and the cerebral cortex.

The Ovarian Cycle

- Under the influence of follicle-stimulating hormone (FSH) and, later, luteinising hormone (LH) the Graafian follicle matures and moves to the surface of the ovary. At the same time it swells and becomes tense, finally rupturing to release the ovum into the fimbriated end of the uterine tube; this is *ovulation*.

- The empty follicle, known as the *corpus luteum*, collapses, the granulosa cells enlarge and proliferate over the next 14 days, and the whole structure becomes irregular in outline and yellow in colour.

- Unless pregnancy occurs, the corpus luteum will then atrophy and become the *corpus albicans*.

Ovarian hormones

Oestrogen

This is produced under the influence of FSH by the granulosa cells and the theca in increasing amounts until the degeneration of the corpus luteum, when the level falls.

The effects of oestrogen are as follows:

- It is responsible for the secondary female sex characteristics.
- It influences the production of cervical mucus and the structure of the vaginal epithelium.
- During the cycle, it causes the proliferation of the uterine endometrium.
- It inhibits FSH and encourages fluid retention.

Progesterone

This, with related compounds, is produced by the corpus luteum under the influence of LH. They act only on tissues that have previously been affected by oestrogen.

The effects of progesterone are mainly evident during the second half of the cycle:

- It causes secretory changes in the lining of the uterus, when the endometrium develops tortuous glands and an enriched blood supply in readiness for the possible arrival of a fertilised ovum.
- It causes the body temperature to rise by 0.5°C after ovulation and gives rise to tingling and a sense of fullness in the breasts prior to menstruation.

Relaxin

This hormone is at its maximum level between weeks 38 and 42 of pregnancy. It originates in the corpus luteum.

Relaxin is thought to relax the pelvic girdle, to soften the cervix and to suppress uterine contractions.

Pituitary Control

Under the influence of the hypothalamus, which produces gonadotrophin-releasing hormone (GnRH), the anterior pituitary gland secretes two gonadotrophins: FSH and LH. The gonadotrophic activity of the hypothalamus and the pituitary is influenced by positive and negative feedback mechanisms from ovarian hormones.

FSH

This hormone causes several Graafian follicles to develop and enlarge, one of them more prominently than all the others. FSH stimulates the secretion of oestrogen. The level of FSH rises during the first half of the cycle and when the oestrogen level reaches a certain point its production is stopped.

LH

This is first produced a few days after the anterior pituitary starts producing FSH. Rising oestrogen causes a surge in both FSH and LH levels, the ripened follicle ruptures and ovulation occurs. Levels of both gonadotrophins then fall rapidly. Progesterone inhibits any new rise in LH in spite of high oestrogen levels, but if no pregnancy occurs, the corpus luteum degenerates after 14 days. The negative feedback effect of progesterone ceases and FSH and LH levels rise again to begin a new cycle.

Prolactin

This is also produced in the anterior pituitary gland, but it does not play a part in the control of the ovary. If produced in excessive amounts, however, it will inhibit ovulation, a phenomenon that occurs naturally during breastfeeding.

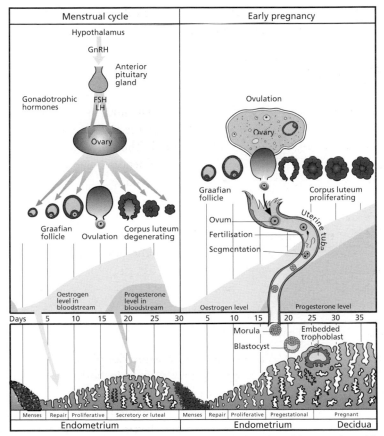

Fig. 3.1: The menstrual cycle and early pregnancy. Left: action of the gonadotrophic hormones on the ovary and of the ovarian hormones on the endometrium. Right: ovulation, fertilisation, decidual reaction and embedding of the fertilised ovum.

The Uterine Cycle or Menstrual Cycle

Although each woman has an individual cycle that varies in length, the average cycle is taken to be 28 days long. The first day of the cycle is the day on which menstruation begins (Fig. 3.1). There are three main phases and they affect the tissue structure of the endometrium, controlled by the ovarian hormones.

Fertilisation

Following ovulation, the ovum passes into the uterine tube and is moved along towards the uterus. At this time the cervix, under the influence of oestrogen, secretes a flow of alkaline mucus that attracts the spermatozoa. Sperm that reach the loose cervical mucus survive to propel themselves towards the uterine tubes, while the remainder are destroyed by the acid medium of the vagina. More will die on the journey through the uterus. Those that reach the uterine tube meet the ovum, usually in the ampulla. It is only during this journey that the sperm finally become mature and capable of releasing the enzyme hyaluronidase, which allows penetration of the zona pellucida and the cell membrane surrounding the ovum. Many sperm are needed for this to take place but only one will enter the ovum. The sperm and the ovum each contribute half the complement of chromosomes to make a total of 46.

- The sperm and ovum are known as the male and female *gametes*.
- The fertilised ovum is known as the *zygote*.

Fertilisation is most likely to occur when intercourse takes place not more than 48 hours before or 24 hours after ovulation.

Development of the Fertilised Ovum

When the ovum has been fertilised, it continues its passage through the uterine tube and reaches the uterus 3 or 4 days later.

- During this time the fertilised ovum divides and subdivides to form a cluster of cells known as the *morula*.

- Next, a fluid-filled cavity appears in the morula, which now becomes known as the *blastocyst*.

- Around the outside of the blastocyst there is a single layer of cells known as the *trophoblast*.

- The remaining cells are clumped together at one end forming the *inner cell mass*.

The trophoblast will form the placenta and chorion, while the inner cell mass will become the fetus, amnion and umbilical cord.

See Chapter 9 for calculation of the expected date of delivery based on menstrual history.

The decidua

This is the name given to the endometrium during pregnancy. From the time of conception the increased secretion of oestrogens causes the endometrium to grow to four times its non-pregnant thickness. The corpus luteum also produces large amounts of progesterone, which stimulate the secretory activity of the endometrial glands and increase the size of the blood vessels. This accounts for the soft, vascular, spongy bed in which the fertilised ovum implants. Three layers are found:

- the basal layer

- the functional layer

- the compact layer.

The trophoblast

Small projections begin to appear all over the surface of the blastocyst, becoming most prolific at the area of contact. These trophoblastic cells differentiate into layers:

- the outer syncytiotrophoblast (syncytium)

- the inner cytotrophoblast

- below this, a layer of mesoderm.

The inner cell mass

While the trophoblast is developing into the placenta, the inner cell mass is forming the fetus itself. The cells differentiate into three layers, each of which will form particular parts of the fetus:

- The *ectoderm* mainly forms the skin and nervous system.
- The *mesoderm* forms bones and muscles and also the heart and blood vessels, including those in the placenta. Certain internal organs also originate in the mesoderm.
- The *endoderm* forms mucous membranes and glands.

Two cavities appear in the inner cell mass:

- The *amniotic cavity* is filled with fluid, and gradually enlarges and folds around the embryo to enclose it.
- The *yolk sac* provides nourishment for the embryo until the trophoblast is sufficiently developed to take over.

The embryo

This name is applied to the developing offspring after implantation and until 8 weeks after conception.

Problems of development are summarised in Box 3.1.

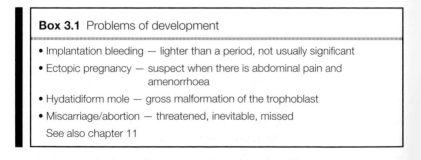

Box 3.1 Problems of development

- Implantation bleeding — lighter than a period, not usually significant
- Ectopic pregnancy — suspect when there is abdominal pain and amenorrhoea
- Hydatidiform mole — gross malformation of the trophoblast
- Miscarriage/abortion — threatened, inevitable, missed
  See also chapter 11

Chapter 4

The Placenta

Originating from the trophoblastic layer of the fertilised ovum, the placenta links closely with the mother's circulation to carry out functions that the fetus is unable to perform for itself during intrauterine life. The survival of the fetus depends upon the placenta's integrity and efficiency.

Development

Initially, the ovum appears to be covered with a fine, downy hair, which consists of the projections from the trophoblastic layer. These proliferate and branch from about 3 weeks after fertilisation, forming the *chorionic villi*. The villi become most profuse in the area where the blood supply is richest — that is, in the basal decidua.

- This part of the trophoblast is known as the *chorion frondosum* and it will eventually develop into the placenta.

- The villi under the capsular decidua, being less well nourished, gradually degenerate and form the *chorion laeve*, which is the origin of the chorionic membrane.

The villi erode the walls of maternal blood vessels as they penetrate the decidua, opening them up to form a lake of maternal blood in which they float. The maternal blood circulates slowly, enabling the villi to absorb food and oxygen and excrete waste. Each chorionic villus is a branching structure arising from one stem (Fig. 4.1). The placenta is completely formed and functioning from 10 weeks after fertilisation.

Circulation through the placenta

- Fetal blood, low in oxygen, is pumped by the fetal heart towards the placenta along the umbilical arteries and transported along their branches to the capillaries of the chorionic villi.

- Having yielded up carbon dioxide and absorbed oxygen, the blood is returned to the fetus via the umbilical vein.

- The maternal blood is delivered to the placental bed in the decidua by spiral arteries and flows into the blood spaces surrounding the villi. It is thought that the direction of flow is similar to a fountain; the blood passes upwards and bathes the villus as it circulates around it and drains back into a branch of the uterine vein.

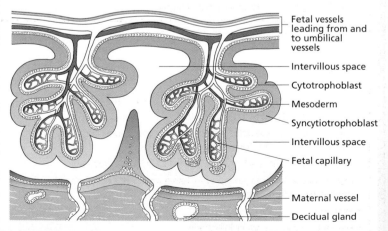

Fetal vessels
leading from and
to umbilical
vessels

Intervillous space

Cytotrophoblast

Mesoderm

Syncytiotrophoblast

Intervillous space

Fetal capillary

Maternal vessel

Decidual gland

Fig. 4.1: Chorionic villi.

It is impossible for the maternal and fetal circulations to mix unless any villi are damaged.

The Mature Placenta

Functions

The 'Green B' mnemonic (Box 4.1) can be helpful.

Appearance of the placenta at term

The placenta is a round, flat mass about 20 cm in diameter and 2.5 cm thick at its centre.

- *The maternal surface*. Maternal blood gives this surface a dark red colour and part of the basal decidua will have been separated with it. The surface is arranged in about 20 lobes, which are separated by sulci. The lobes are made up of lobules, each of which contains a single villus with its branches.

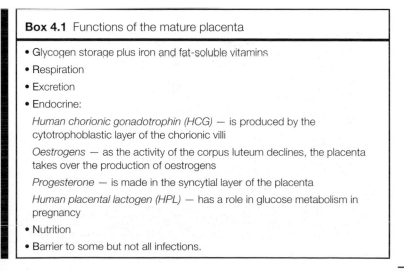

Box 4.1 Functions of the mature placenta

- Glycogen storage plus iron and fat-soluble vitamins
- Respiration
- Excretion
- Endocrine:

  Human chorionic gonadotrophin (HCG) — is produced by the cytotrophoblastic layer of the chorionic villi

  Oestrogens — as the activity of the corpus luteum declines, the placenta takes over the production of oestrogens

  Progesterone — is made in the syncytial layer of the placenta

  Human placental lactogen (HPL) — has a role in glucose metabolism in pregnancy
- Nutrition
- Barrier to some but not all infections.

■ *The fetal surface.* The amnion covering the fetal surface of the placenta gives it a white, shiny appearance. Branches of the umbilical vein and arteries are visible, spreading out from the insertion of the umbilical cord, which is normally in the centre. The amnion can be peeled off the surface, leaving the chorionic plate from which the placenta has developed and which is continuous with the chorion.

■ *The fetal sac.* The fetal sac consists of a double membrane. The outer membrane is the chorion; this is a thick, opaque, friable membrane. The inner, smooth, tough, translucent membrane is the amnion, which contains the amniotic fluid.

Amniotic Fluid

Functions

These are listed in Box 4.2.

Volume

■ The total amount of amniotic fluid increases throughout pregnancy until 38 weeks' gestation, when there is about 1 litre.

Box 4.2 Functions of the amniotic fluid

- Distends the amniotic sac and allows for the growth and movement of the fetus
- Equalises pressure and protects the fetus from jarring and injury
- Maintains a constant temperature for the fetus
- Provides small amounts of nutrients
- Protects the placenta and umbilical cord from the pressure of uterine contractions in labour, as long as the membranes remain intact, Also aids effacement of the cervix and dilatation of the uterine os, particularly where the presenting part is poorly applied

- It then diminishes slightly until term, when approximately 800 ml remains.
- If the total amount exceeds 1500 ml, the condition is known as *polyhydramnios*.
- If there is less than 300 ml, the term *oligohydramnios* is applied.

Constituents

Amniotic fluid is a clear, pale, straw-coloured fluid consisting of 99% water. The remaining 1% is dissolved solid matter, including food substances and waste products. In addition, the fetus sheds skin cells, vernix caseosa and lanugo into the fluid. Abnormal constituents of the liquor, such as meconium in the case of fetal distress, may give valuable diagnostic information about the condition of the fetus.

The Umbilical Cord

The umbilical cord extends from the fetus to the placenta and transmits the umbilical blood vessels: two arteries and one vein. These are enclosed and protected by *Wharton's jelly*. The whole cord is covered in a layer of amnion continuous with that covering the placenta. The length of the average cord is about 50 cm.

True knots should be noted on examination of the cord, but they must be distinguished from false knots, which are lumps of Wharton's jelly on the side of the cord and are not significant.

Anatomical Variations of the Placenta and the Cord

These are listed in Box 4.3. Except for the dangers noted, these varieties of conformation have no clinical significance.

See chapter 19 for inspection after birth.

Box 4.3 Anatomical variations of the placenta and the cord

Succenturiate lobe of placenta
- A small extra lobe is present, separate from the main placenta but joined to it by blood vessels that run through the membranes to reach it
- A hole in the membranes with vessels running to it is likely to indicate a retained lobe

Circumvallate placenta
- An opaque ring is seen on the fetal surface of the placenta
- It is formed by a doubling back of the chorion and amnion and may result in the membranes leaving the placenta nearer the centre instead of at the edge as is usual

Battledore insertion of the cord
- The cord is attached at the very edge of the placenta in the manner of a table-tennis bat

Velamentous insertion of the cord
- The cord is inserted into the membranes some distance from the edge of the placenta
- The umbilical vessels run through the membranes from the cord to the placenta
- If the placenta is normally situated, no harm will result to the fetus, but the cord is likely to become detached upon applying traction during active management of the third stage of labour
- If the placenta is low lying, the vessels may pass across the uterine os. The term applied to the vessels lying in this position is vasa praevia. In this case there is great danger to the fetus when the membranes rupture and even more so during artificial rupture, as the vessels may be torn, leading to rapid exsanguination of the fetus

Bipartite placenta
- Two complete and separate parts are present, each with a cord leaving it
- The bipartite cord joins a short distance from the two parts of the placenta

Tripartite placenta
- This is similar to bipartite, but with three distinct parts

Chapter 5

The Fetus

An understanding of fetal development is needed to estimate the approximate age of a baby born before term. Knowledge of organogenesis enables an appreciation of the ways in which developmental abnormalities arise.

Time Scale of Development

- For the first 3 weeks following conception the term *fertilised ovum* or *zygote* is used.
- From 3–8 weeks after conception it is known as the *embryo*.
- Following this it is called the *fetus* until birth.

Development within the uterus is summarised in Box 5.1.

Fetal Organs

Blood

The fetal haemoglobin (Hb) is of a different type from adult haemoglobin and is termed HbF. It has a much greater affinity for oxygen and is found in greater concentration (18–20 g/dl at term).

Box 5.1 Summary of development

0–4 weeks after conception

- Rapid growth
- Formation of the embryonic plate
- Primitive central nervous system forms
- Heart develops and begins to beat
- Limb buds form

4–8 weeks

- Very rapid cell division
- Head and facial features develop
- All major organs laid down in primitive form
- External genitalia present but sex not distinguishable
- Early movements
- Visible on ultrasound from 6 weeks

8–12 weeks

- Eyelids fuse
- Kidneys begin to function and fetus passes urine from 10 weeks
- Fetal circulation functioning properly
- Sucking and swallowing begin
- Sex apparent
- Moves freely (not felt by mother)
- Some primitive reflexes present

12–16 weeks

- Rapid skeletal development
- Meconium present in gut
- Lanugo appears
- Nasal septum and palate fuse

16–20 weeks

- 'Quickening' — mother feels fetal movements
- Fetal heart heard on auscultation
- Vernix caseosa appears
- Fingernails can be seen
- Skin cells begin to be renewed

Box 5.1 (Continued)

20–24 weeks
• Most organs become capable of functioning
• Periods of sleep and activity
• Responds to sound
• Skin red and wrinkled

24–28 weeks
• Survival may be expected if born
• Eyelids reopen
• Respiratory movements

28–32 weeks
• Begins to store fat and iron
• Testes descend into scrotum
• Lanugo disappears from face
• Skin becomes paler and less wrinkled

32–36 weeks
• Increased fat makes body more rounded
• Lanugo disappears from body
• Head hair lengthens
• Nails reach tips of fingers
• Ear cartilage soft
• Plantar creases visible

36–40 weeks after conception (38–42 weeks after last menstrual period, LMP)
• Term is reached and birth is due
• Contours rounded
• Skull firm

Towards the end of pregnancy the fetus begins to make adult-type haemoglobin (HbA).

In utero, the red blood cells have a shorter lifespan, this being about 90 days by the time the baby is born.

The renal tract

The kidneys begin to function and the fetus passes urine from 10 weeks' gestation. The urine is very dilute and does not constitute a route for excretion.

The adrenal glands

The fetal adrenal glands produce the precursors for placental formation of oestriols. They are also thought to play a part in the initiation of labour.

The liver

The fetal liver is comparatively large in size. From the 3rd to the 6th month of intrauterine life, it is responsible for the formation of red blood cells, after which they are mainly produced in the red bone marrow and the spleen.

Towards the end of pregnancy, iron stores are laid down in the liver.

The alimentary tract

The digestive tract is mainly non-functional before birth. Sucking and swallowing of amniotic fluid containing shed skin cells and other debris begin about 12 weeks after conception. Digestive juices are present before birth and they act on the swallowed substances and discarded intestinal cells to form meconium. This is normally retained in the gut until after birth, when it is passed as the first stool of the newborn.

The lungs

It is mainly the immaturity of the lungs that reduces the chance of survival of infants born before 24 weeks' gestation, owing to the limited alveolar surface area, the immaturity of the capillary system in the lungs and the lack of adequate surfactant. Surfactant is a lipoprotein that reduces the surface tension in the alveoli and assists gaseous exchange.

It is first produced from about 20 weeks' gestation and the amount increases until the lungs are mature at about 30–34 weeks. At term the lungs contain about 100 ml of lung fluid. About one-third of this is expelled during birth and the rest is absorbed and carried away by the lymphatics and blood vessels as air takes its place.

There is some movement of the thorax from the 3rd month of fetal life and more definite diaphragmatic movements from the 6th month.

The central nervous system

The fetus is able to perceive strong light and to hear external sounds. Periods of wakefulness and sleep occur.

The skin

- From 18 weeks after conception the fetus is covered with a white, creamy substance called *vernix caseosa*. This protects the skin from the amniotic fluid and from any friction against itself.

- At 20 weeks the fetus will be covered with a fine downy hair called *lanugo*; at the same time the head hair and eyebrows begin to form.

- Lanugo is shed from 36 weeks and a full-term infant has little left.

- Fingernails develop from about 10 weeks but the toenails do not form until about 18 weeks.

The Fetal Circulation

The key to understanding the fetal circulation (Fig. 5.1) is the fact that oxygen is derived from the placenta. At birth there is a dramatic alteration in this situation and an almost instantaneous change must occur. Several temporary structures, in addition to the placenta itself and the umbilical cord, enable the fetal circulation to function while allowing for the changes at birth (Box 5.2).

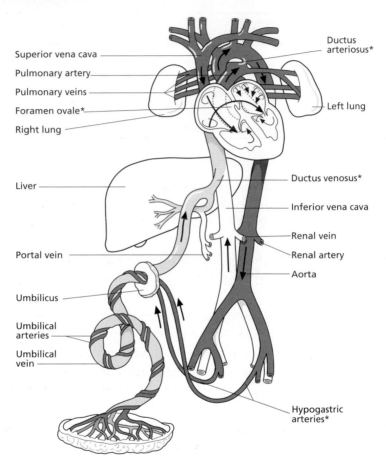

Fig. 5.1: Fetal circulation. The arrows show the course taken by the blood. The temporary structures are asterisked.

Adaptation to extrauterine life

- At birth the baby takes a breath and blood is drawn to the lungs through the pulmonary arteries.
- It is then collected and returned to the left atrium via the pulmonary veins, resulting in a sudden inflow of blood.

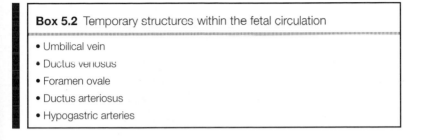

Box 5.2 Temporary structures within the fetal circulation

- Umbilical vein
- Ductus venosus
- Foramen ovale
- Ductus arteriosus
- Hypogastric arteries

■ The placental circulation ceases soon after birth and so less blood returns to the right side of the heart. In this way the pressure in the left side of the heart is greater while that in the right side of the heart lessens.

■ This results in the closure of a flap over the foramen ovale, which separates the two sides of the heart and stops the blood flowing from right to left.

■ With the establishment of pulmonary respiration the oxygen concentration in the bloodstream rises.

■ This causes the ductus arteriosus to constrict and close. For as long as the ductus remains open after birth, blood flows from the high-pressure aorta towards the lungs, in the reverse direction to that in fetal life.

■ The cessation of the placental circulation results in the collapse of the umbilical vein, the ductus venosus and the hypogastric arteries.

The Fetal Skull

The fetal skull (Fig. 5.2) contains the delicate brain, which may be subjected to great pressure as the head passes through the birth canal.

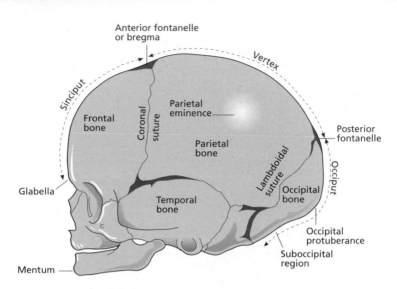

Fig. 5.2: Fetal skull showing regions and landmarks of obstetrical importance.

Ossification

The bones of the fetal head originate in two different ways:

■ The face is laid down in cartilage and is almost completely ossified at birth, the bones being fused together and firm.

■ The bones of the vault are laid down in membrane and are much flatter and more pliable. They ossify from the centre outwards and this process is incomplete at birth, leaving small gaps, which form the sutures and fontanelles. The ossification centre on each bone appears as a boss or protuberance.

Bones of the vault (Fig. 5.3)

There are five main bones in the vault of the fetal skull:

■ the *occipital bone*

■ the two *parietal bones*

■ the two *frontal bones*.

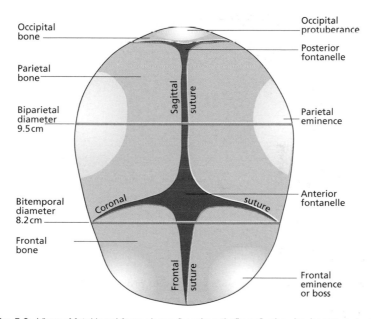

Fig. 5.3: View of fetal head from above (head partly flexed), showing bones, sutures and fontanelles.

In addition to these five, the upper part of the *temporal bone* forms a small part of the vault.

Sutures and fontanelles

Sutures are cranial joints and are formed where two bones adjoin. Where two or more sutures meet, a fontanelle is formed. There are several sutures and fontanelles in the fetal skull. Those of greatest obstetrical significance are shown in Box 5.3.

The sutures and fontanelles, because they consist of membranous spaces, allow for a degree of overlapping of the skull bones during labour and birth.

Regions and landmarks of the fetal skull

The skull is divided into the vault, the base and the face:

- The *vault* is the large, dome-shaped part above an imaginary line drawn between the orbital ridges and the nape of the neck.
- The *base* is composed of bones that are firmly united to protect the vital centres in the medulla.
- The *face* is composed of 14 small bones, which are also firmly united and non-compressible.

The regions of the skull are described as in Box 5.4.

Diameters of the fetal skull

The measurements of the skull are important because the midwife needs a practical understanding of the relationship between the fetal head and the mother's pelvis (Table 5.1 and Fig. 5.4). It will become clear that some diameters are more favourable than others for easy passage through the pelvic canal and this will depend on the attitude of the head.

Attitude of the fetal head

This term is used to describe the degree of flexion or extension of the head on the neck. The attitude of the head determines which diameters will present in labour and therefore influences the outcome.

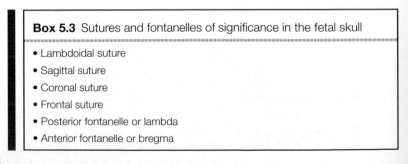

Box 5.3 Sutures and fontanelles of significance in the fetal skull

- Lambdoidal suture
- Sagittal suture
- Coronal suture
- Frontal suture
- Posterior fontanelle or lambda
- Anterior fontanelle or bregma

Box 5.4 Regions of the fetal skull

Occiput

- Lies between the foramen magnum and the posterior fontanelle.
- The part below the occipital protuberance is known as the suboccipital region

Vertex

- Bounded by the posterior fontanelle, the two parietal eminences and the anterior fontanelle

Sinciput or brow

- Extends from the anterior fontanelle and the coronal suture to the orbital ridges

Face

- Small in the newborn baby
- Extends from the orbital ridges and the root of the nose to the junction of the chin and the neck
- The point between the eyebrows is known as the glabella
- The chin is termed the mentum and is an important landmark

Table 5.1 Diameters of the fetal skull

Name of diameter	Measurement
Transverse diameters (Fig. 5.3)	
Biparietal	9.5 cm
Bitemporal	8.2 cm
Anteroposterior or longitudinal (Fig. 5.4)	
Suboccipitobregmatic (SOB)	9.5 cm
Suboccipitofrontal (SOF)	10 cm
Occipitofrontal (OF)	11.5 cm
Mentovertical (MV)	13.5 cm
Submentovertical (SMV)	11.5 cm
Submentobregmatic (SMB)	9.5 cm

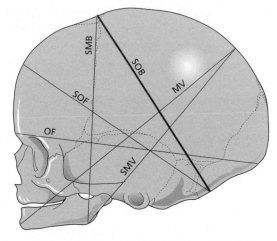

Fig. 5.4: Anteroposterior diameters of the fetal skull (see Table 5.1).

Presenting diameters

The diameters of the head, which are called the presenting diameters, are those that are at right angles to the curve of Carus. There are always two:

- an anteroposterior or longitudinal diameter
- a transverse diameter.

The diameters presenting in the individual cephalic or head presentations are as described below.

Vertex presentation

- When the head is well flexed, the suboccipitobregmatic diameter and the biparietal diameter present. As these two diameters are the same length, 9.5 cm, the presenting area is circular, which is the most favourable shape for dilating the cervix. The diameter that distends the vaginal orifice is the suboccipitofrontal diameter, 10 cm (see ch. 18).

■ When the head is not flexed but erect, the presenting diameters are the occipitofrontal, 11.5 cm, and the biparietal, 9.5 cm. This situation often arises when the occiput is in a posterior position. If it remains so, the diameter distending the vaginal orifice will be the occipitofrontal, 11.5 cm.

Brow presentation

■ When the head is partially extended, the mentovertical diameter, 13.5 cm, and the bitemporal diameter, 8.2 cm, present. If this presentation persists, vaginal birth is extremely unlikely.

Face presentation

■ When the head is completely extended, the presenting diameters are the submentobregmatic, 9.5 cm, and the bitemporal, 8.2 cm.

■ The submentovertical diameter, 11.5 cm, will distend the vaginal orifice. (See ch. 21 for mechanisms in labour.)

Moulding

This is the term applied to the change in shape of the fetal head that takes place during its passage through the birth canal. Alteration in shape is possible because the bones of the vault allow a slight degree of bending and the skull bones are able to override at the sutures. This overriding allows a considerable reduction in the size of the presenting diameters while the diameter at right angles to them is able to lengthen owing to the give of the skull bones.

In a normal vertex presentation, with the fetal head in a fully flexed attitude, the suboccipitobregmatic and the biparietal diameters will be reduced and the mentovertical will be lengthened. The shortening may amount to as much as 1.25 cm.

The intracranial membranes and sinuses (Fig. 5.5)

The skull contains delicate structures, some of which may be damaged if the head is subjected to abnormal moulding during delivery.

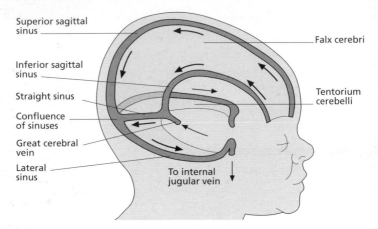

Superior sagittal sinus

Inferior sagittal sinus

Straight sinus

Confluence of sinuses

Great cerebral vein

Lateral sinus

Falx cerebri

Tentorium cerebelli

To internal jugular vein

Fig. 5.5: Intracranial membranes and venous sinuses. Arrows show direction of blood flow.

Among the most important are the folds of dura mater and the venous sinuses associated with them (Box 5.5).

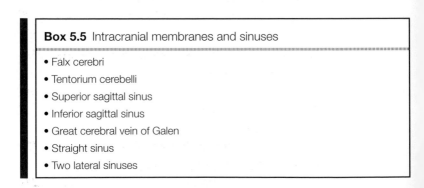

Box 5.5 Intracranial membranes and sinuses

- Falx cerebri
- Tentorium cerebelli
- Superior sagittal sinus
- Inferior sagittal sinus
- Great cerebral vein of Galen
- Straight sinus
- Two lateral sinuses

Section 2

Pregnancy

Chapter 6

Preparing for Pregnancy

Preparing for pregnancy is a positive step towards enhancing pregnancy outcome and provides prospective parents with options that may not be available once a pregnancy is confirmed. The midwife may need to support a couple as they embark on a programme that may include investigation, diagnosis and treatment in order to help them conceive, all of which may impact upon their physical, psychological and social well-being.

Preconception Care

The aims of preconception care are:

- to ensure that the woman and her partner are in an optimal state of physical and emotional health at the onset of pregnancy
- to provide prospective parents with a series of options that may not be available once a pregnancy is confirmed.

The preconception period refers to a time span of anything from 3 months to 1 year before conception.

Box 6.1 outlines the information and investigations that may be required.

Box 6.1 Information and investigations in a preconception programme

History

- Family history
- Medical history
- Menstrual history
- Obstetric history
- Method of contraception
- Medication
- Occupation
- Diet
- Smoking
- Alcohol

Observation/Investigations

- Height and weight
- Blood pressure
- Urinalysis
- Stool sample
- Blood tests:

  Haemoglobin

  Folic acid and vitamin levels

  Rubella immunity

  Venereal disease research laboratory (VDRL)

  Haemoglobinopathies

  Lead and trace elements

- Hair analysis (controversial)
- Male — semen analysis
- Female — cervical smear, high vaginal swab (HVS)

General health and fertility

Body weight

It has been well established that fertility and fatness are closely linked, with subfertility-related problems occurring in women below and above the desirable range of body weight.

- Assessment of body type is done using the Quetelet or body mass index (BMI) and is calculated by dividing the weight in kilograms by the height in metres squared.
- The desirable or healthy range is between 19.8 and 26.

A woman's nutritional status before pregnancy and during the first weeks before she realises that she is pregnant may be more important than the diet she eats once her pregnancy is confirmed. By this time much of the cell organisation, differentiation and organogenesis will have taken place. Suboptimal conditions at this time can result in fetal damage and stunted growth. Substantial evidence is accumulating that corroborates the relationship between an increased risk of pregnancy complications/adverse pregnancy outcomes and excess weight and obesity in women. The aim of preconception care is to help women achieve an appropriate BMI prior to conception to enhance pregnancy outcome. Overweight women should be encouraged to lose weight before conception; however, some caution is required, as consuming an energy-deficient diet immediately prior to conception may result in nutritional deficiencies that could disadvantage the fetus. Dietary changes and weight loss should occur at least 3–4 months before attempting conception.

Principles of a healthy diet

A simple and easy guide is to advise women to eat:

- more starchy foods, such as cereals and bread
- at least five portions of fruit and vegetables daily
- fewer fatty foods.

Folate, folic acid and neural tube defects

Folic acid is a water-soluble vitamin belonging to the B complex.

- The term 'folates' is used to describe the folic acid derivatives that are found naturally in food.
- The term 'folic acid' is used to refer to the synthetic form found in vitamin supplements and fortified foods.

The main sources of folate in the UK diet are listed in Box 6.2.

Folates are vulnerable to heat and readily dissolve in water; therefore considerable losses can occur as a result of cooking or prolonged storage. Folic acid is more stable and better absorbed than folate and is added to many brands of bread and breakfast cereal in the UK.

- To reduce the risk of first occurrence of neural tube defects (NTDs), all women should increase their daily folate and folic acid intake by an additional 400 µg prior to conception and during the first 12 weeks of pregnancy.
- Women with a history of a previous child with NTD should take a daily dose of 5 mg of folic acid to reduce the risk of recurrence.
- This dose is also recommended in women with diabetes, those taking antiepileptic medication, and those who have malabsorption syndrome.

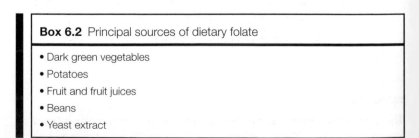

Box 6.2 Principal sources of dietary folate

- Dark green vegetables
- Potatoes
- Fruit and fruit juices
- Beans
- Yeast extract

Vitamin A

Vitamin A is essential for embryogenesis, growth and epithelial differentiation, but a high intake of the retinol form of vitamin A is known to be teratogenic.

- Women who are pregnant or planning a pregnancy should avoid eating liver and liver products such as pâté or liver sausage, as these contain large amounts of retinol.

Pre-existing Medical Conditions and Drugs

Diabetes

Infants of insulin-dependent diabetic mothers have 10 times the general population risk of congenital malformation and five times the risk of stillbirth. Diabetic complications, such as retinopathy and nephropathy, may worsen during pregnancy, particularly if associated with hypertension. Women who have severe neuropathy or cardiovascular disease may be advised against pregnancy.

- The aim of preconception care is to achieve normoglycaemia both pre- and periconception, as many of the problems seen in the insulin-dependent diabetic mother are a direct result of hyperglycaemia.

- The safety of currently available oral hypoglycaemic agents in pregnancy is not well established; therefore women with type II diabetes who are taking such treatments should be switched to insulin therapy both for the preconception period and for pregnancy.

Epilepsy

The major anticonvulsant drugs used to treat epilepsy are known to have teratogenic effects, and the newer antiepileptic drugs have not yet been sufficiently evaluated. Pregnancy is also known to alter the metabolism of antiepileptic drugs, with approximately one-third of women experiencing an increase in the number of seizures. However, this increase may be induced by deliberate non-compliance.

- The aim of preconception care for the woman with epilepsy is to help her plan her pregnancies carefully and to keep her seizure free on the lowest possible dose of anticonvulsants. For some women this may mean withdrawal of therapy and for others a reduction from polytherapy to monotherapy.

- Some anticonvulsant drugs are folate antagonists; therefore folic acid supplements are needed.

Phenylketonuria

Phenylketonuria (PKU) is an inborn error of metabolism. Some women with PKU discontinue treatment during middle childhood. However, unless they resume careful dietary control around the time of conception, the toxic effect of phenylalanine (Phe) on the developing embryo/fetus results in a high rate of fetal abnormality.

Oral contraception

Oral contraception should be stopped at least 3 months, and preferably 6 months, prior to planning a pregnancy to allow for the resumption of natural hormone regulation and ovulation. Also, the oral contraceptive pill is associated with vitamin and mineral imbalances that may need correcting.

Drug abuse

Disruption of the menstrual cycle is common among women using drugs like ecstasy, amphetamines, opiates and anabolic steroids, and heavy drug use during pregnancy is associated with miscarriage, preterm labour, low birth weight, stillbirth and abnormalities. A poor socioeconomic environment is a compounding factor. Some women may be trying to come off tranquillisers and this process can take many weeks. Drug users are unlikely to present for preconception care, as a high proportion of these women conceal their drug use.

Environmental Factors

Smoking

Fertility and pregnancy are adversely affected by smoking. In women, smoking can induce early menopause and menstrual problems; in men it can cause abnormalities in sperm morphology and motility. During pregnancy, there is an increased risk of spontaneous abortion, preterm delivery, low birth weight and perinatal mortality because of antepartum haemorrhage and placental abruption. Evidence also shows that women who smoke during pregnancy pass harmful carcinogens on to their baby. Nutritional status tends to be compromised in smokers.

- The aim of preconception care is to help the woman stop smoking, and partner involvement is known to enhance success.
- Health professionals should ask about smoking at every opportunity that advice and assistance for smoking cessation can be given, as well as enquiring about arrangements for follow-up.

Alcohol

Drinking alcohol occasionally or in moderation is a very acceptable social activity, but when consumed in large quantities alcohol can become problematic, as it is a teratogen. Fetal alcohol syndrome (FAS) is the term used to describe the congenital malformations associated with excessive maternal alcohol intake during pregnancy. High alcohol intakes in women have been associated with menstrual disorders and decreased fertility.

- Women should limit alcohol consumption in pregnancy to no more than one standard unit of alcohol per day.

- Preconception advice can be given after taking a drinking history; women with a drink problem will need specialist referral for treatment and support.

Exercise

Moderate exercise is known to be beneficial for health and the benefits of regular exercise for the healthy pregnant woman appear to outweigh the risks. However, exercise intensity should be modified according to maternal symptoms and should not continue to fatigue or exhaustion.

Workplace hazards and noxious substances

Humans are exposed to many environmental agents that may be hazardous to their reproductive capacity. Much of this exposure may occur in the workplace, even though employees are protected by the Control of Substances Hazardous to Health (COSHH) Regulations.

Exposure to solvents, ionising radiation and anaesthetic gases is known to be toxic and associated with central nervous system defects, microcephaly and an increased risk of miscarriage. Heavy metals are also known to be toxic.

There has been concern about working with visual display units (VDUs) during pregnancy and there are reports of an increased risk of miscarriages or birth defects. However, taken as a whole, the scientific studies that have been carried out to date do not show any link.

Genetic Counselling

The decision to have a baby is not always straightforward for some couples. A family history of genetic disorders, a previous baby affected with a congenital abnormality and childbearing left until later years all increase the risk of giving birth to an abnormal child. For such couples, referral for genetic counselling will help them to decide what is best.

Mendelian inheritance

Genetic disorders can occur as a result of Mendelian inheritance and are termed either dominant or recessive.

■ An *autosomal dominant* disorder occurs when the condition is present in the heterozygous state (i.e. only one gene of a pair of chromosomes need be affected). The risks associated with this inheritance pattern are relatively straightforward — there is a 1 in 2, or 50%, risk in a couple where one of them is affected with the condition.

■ An *autosomal recessive* disorder occurs only in the homozygous state (i.e. both chromosomes of a pair must be affected), which means that any offspring of an affected individual are obligatory carriers, given that the other partner is unaffected.

■ Genetic disorders can also be *X-linked*. Such disorders are inherited through the female sex chromosome; this means that females are usually carriers and any male offspring that they may have will be affected with the disorder.

Chromosome abnormalities

■ Chromosome aberrations include the *trisomies*, of which trisomy 21 (Down syndrome) is the most common; trisomy 13 and 18 are more rare. Age factors are significant, particularly in Down syndrome, for which the risk is 1% for a woman around 40 years of age.

■ *Monosomies* are usually lethal and non-viable autosomal trisomies are extremely common in spontaneous abortions. Sex chromosome abnormalities, such as Turner syndrome (XO) and Klinefelter syndrome (XXY), have a rare recurrence rate in families.

■ In *translocation*, extra chromosome material is translocated on to another chromosome; it is regarded as balanced when the total amount of chromosome material is normal but only 45 chromosomes are present. Reciprocal translocations can also occur, in which there is an exchange of chromosome material but no change in chromosome number. The recurrence risk is low if neither parent is a balanced carrier for the translocation.

Non-Mendelian disorders

The more common congenital abnormalities, such as NTDs and congenital heart disease, do not follow the Mendelian inheritance pattern, as there is no identified genetic locus; they are therefore referred to as *multifactorial*. These conditions arise as a result of a combination or interaction of environmental and genetic factors. The recurrence risk of such conditions depends upon the incidence of the disorder but is increased amongst close relatives.

Prenatal diagnosis

Prenatal diagnosis of a genetic condition usually takes place during pregnancy, but ideally, for a couple to benefit truly from the process, such diagnosis should occur before conception. Ultimately, the goal of genetic counselling is to prevent or avoid a genetic disorder. Preconception care, involving a multidisciplinary team, is the way to achieve this.

Infertility

Infertility is categorised as *primary* if there has been no prior conception and *secondary* if there has been a previous pregnancy, irrespective of the outcome.

Approximately one-third of cases of infertility involve problems with both partners, and in one-third of couples the causes of infertility remain unexplained. The most common causes are:

- ovulation failure
- sperm disorders.

Much of the initial management of the infertile couple is via primary care. The investigative process is aimed at achieving:

■ an accurate diagnosis and definition of any cause

■ an accurate estimation of the chance of conceiving without treatment

■ a full appraisal of treatment options.

Specialised investigations may need to be undertaken in a dedicated, specialist infertility clinic where there is access to appropriately trained staff and a multiprofessional team.

Assisted Reproduction Techniques

A range of assisted reproduction techniques (Box 6.3) is available to treat the infertile couple and it is important for the appropriate treatment option to be offered.

Box 6.3 Some assisted reproduction techniques

- Ovulation induction
- Intrauterine insemination (IUI)
- Donor insemination (DI) or artificial insemination by donor (AID)
- In-vitro fertilisation/embryo transfer (IVF/ET)
- Gamete intrafallopian transfer (GIFT)
- Zygote intrafallopian transfer (ZIFT)
- Intracytoplasmic sperm injection (ICSI)

Chapter 7

Change and Adaptation in Pregnancy

Physiological Changes in the Reproductive System

The body of the uterus

After conception, the uterus develops to provide a nutritive and protective environment in which the fetus will develop and grow.

Decidua

After embedding of the blastocyst there is thickening and increased vascularity of the lining of the uterus, or decidua. Decidualisation, influenced by progesterone and oestradiol, is most marked in the fundus and upper body of the uterus.

- The decidua is believed to maintain functional quiescence of the uterus during pregnancy; spontaneous labour is thought to result from the activation of the decidua with resultant prostaglandin release following withdrawal of placental hormones.
- The decidua and trophoblast also produce relaxin, which appears to promote myometrial relaxation, and may have a role to play in cervical ripening and rupture of fetal membranes.

Myometrium

Uterine growth is due to *hyperplasia* (increase in number due to division) and *hypertrophy* (increase in size) of myometrial cells under the influence of oestrogen (Table 7.1). The dimensions of the uterus vary considerably, however, depending on the age and parity of the woman.

The three layers of the myometrium become more clearly defined during pregnancy.

Muscle layers

- The outer longitudinal layer of muscle fibres is thin. It consists of a network of bundles of smooth muscles. These pass longitudinally from the front of the isthmus anteriorly over the fundus and into the vault of the vagina posteriorly, and extend into the round and transverse ligaments.

- The thicker middle layer comprises interlocked spiral myometrial fibres that are perforated in all directions by blood vessels. Each cell in this layer has a double curve so that the interlacing of any two gives the approximate form of a figure of eight. Due to this arrangement, contraction of these cells after birth causes constriction of the blood vessels, providing 'living ligatures'.

- The inner circular layer is arranged concentrically around the longitudinal axis of the uterus and bundle formation is diffuse. It forms sphincters around the openings of the uterine tubes and around the internal cervical os.

Table 7.1 Uterine growth during pregnancy

	Prior to pregnancy	**At term**
Weight of uterus	50–60 g	1000 g
Size of uterus	7.5 × 5 × 2.5 cm	30 × 22.5 × 20 cm

Uterine activity in pregnancy

The myometrium is both contractile (can lengthen and shorten) and elastic (can enlarge and stretch) to accommodate the growing fetus and allow involution following the birth.

- The contractile ability of the myometrium is dependent on the interaction between two contractile proteins, actin and myosin.

- The interaction of actin and myosin brings about contraction, whereas their separation brings about relaxation under the influence of intracellular free calcium.

- The coordination of synchronous contractions across the whole organ is due to the presence of gap junctions that connect myometrial cells and provide connections for electrical activity. Gap junctions are absent for most of the pregnancy but appear in significant numbers near term, manifesting themselves as *Braxton Hicks contractions*.

- The formation of gap junctions is promoted by oestrogens and prostaglandins.

- Progesterone, prostacyclin and relaxin, however, are all involved in inhibiting the formation of gap junctions by reducing cell excitability and cell connections and so limiting myometrial activity to small clumps of cells, thus maintaining uterine quiescence during pregnancy.

Uterine activity can be measured as early as 7 weeks' gestation, when Braxton Hicks contractions can occur every 20–30 minutes and may reach a pressure of up to 10 mmHg. These contractions facilitate uterine blood flow through the intervillous spaces of the placenta, promoting oxygen delivery to the fetus. Braxton Hicks contractions are usually painless but may cause some discomfort when their intensity exceeds 15 mmHg.

In the last few weeks of pregnancy, *prelabour* occurs:

- Further increases in myometrial contractions cause the muscle fibres of the fundus to be drawn up.

■ The actively contracting upper uterine segment becomes thicker and shorter in length and exerts a slow, steady pull on the relatively fixed cervix.

■ This causes the beginning of cervical stretching and ripening known as *effacement*, and thinning and stretching of the passive lower uterine segment.

There is little rebound between contractions, however; hence there is no cervical dilatation at this time.

Perimetrium

The perimetrium is a thin layer of peritoneum that protects the uterus. It is deflected over the bladder anteriorly to form the uterovesical pouch, and over the rectum posteriorly to form the pouch of Douglas.

■ The double folds of perimetrium (broad ligaments), hanging from the uterine tubes and extending to the lateral walls of the pelvis, become longer and wider with increasing tension exerted on them as the uterus enlarges and rises out of the pelvis.

■ The anterior and posterior folds open out so that they are no longer in apposition and can therefore accommodate the greatly enlarged uterine and ovarian arteries and veins.

■ The round ligaments (contained within the hanging folds of perimetrium) provide some anterior support for the enlarging uterus and undergo considerable hypertrophy and stretching during pregnancy, which may cause discomfort.

Blood supply

The uterine blood flow progressively increases from approximately 50 ml/min at 10 weeks' gestation to 450–700 ml/min at term.

Changes in uterine shape and size

For the first few weeks the uterus maintains its original pear shape, but as pregnancy advances the corpus and fundus assume a more globular form (Box 7.1).

Box 7.1 Changes in the pregnant uterus

10 weeks

- The uterus is about the size of an orange

12 weeks

- The uterus is about the size of a grapefruit

- It is no longer anteverted and anteflexed and has risen out of the pelvis and become upright

- The fundus may be palpated abdominally above the symphysis pubis

- The globular upper segment is sitting on an elongated stalk formed from the isthmus, which softens and which will treble in length from 7 to 25 mm between the 12th and 36th weeks

20 weeks

- The fundus of the uterus can be palpated at the level of the umbilicus

- As the uterus continues to rise in the abdomen, the uterine tubes become progressively more vertical, which causes increasing tension on the broad and round ligaments

30 weeks

- The fundus may be palpated midway between the umbilicus and the xiphisternum

38 weeks

- The uterus reaches the level of the xiphisternum

- As the upper segment muscle contractions increase in frequency and strength, the lower uterine segment develops more rapidly and is stretched radially; along with cervical effacement and softening of the tissues of the pelvic floor, this permits the fetal presentation to begin its descent into the upper pelvis

- This leads to a reduction in fundal height known as *lightening*, relieving pressure on the upper part of the abdomen but increasing pressure in the pelvis. In the majority of multiparous women, however, engagement rarely occurs prior to labour

The cervix

The cervix is composed of only about 10% muscular tissue, the remainder being collagenous tissue. During pregnancy the cervix remains firmly closed, providing a seal against external contamination and holding in the contents of the uterus. It remains 2.5 cm long throughout pregnancy but becomes softer and swollen under the influence of oestradiol and progesterone. Its increased vascularity makes it look bluish in colour. Under the influence of progesterone the mucous glands become distended and increase in complexity, resulting in the secretion of a thick, viscous, mucoid discharge. It forms a cervical plug called the *operculum*, which provides protection from ascending infection.

As uterine activity builds up during pregnancy, the cervix gradually softens, or *ripens*, and the canal dilates. *Effacement* or *taking up of the cervix* normally occurs in the primigravida during the last 2 weeks of pregnancy but does not usually take place in the multigravida until labour begins. Effacement of the cervix is a mechanism whereby:

- The connective tissue of the long firm cervix is progressively softened by prostaglandins and shortened from the top downwards.
- The softened muscular fibres at the level of the internal cervical os are pulled upwards or 'taken up' into the lower uterine segment and around the fetal presenting part and the forewaters.
- The canal that was about 2.5 cm long becomes a mere circular orifice with paper-thin edges.
- The mucus plug is expelled as effacement progresses.

The vagina

During pregnancy the muscle layer hypertrophies and oestrogen causes the vaginal epithelium to become thicker and more vascular. The altered composition of the surrounding connective tissue increases the elasticity of the vagina, making dilatation easier during the birth of the baby.

In pregnancy there is an increased rate of desquamation of the superficial vaginal mucosa cells. These epithelial cells release more glycogen, which is acted on by *Döderlein's bacilli*, a normal commensal of the vagina, producing lactic acid and hydrogen peroxide. This leads to the increased and more acidic (pH 4.5–5.0) white vaginal discharge known as *leucorrhoea*.

Changes in the Cardiovascular System

Major changes take place in the cardiovascular system. Understanding these changes is important in the care of women with normal pregnancies, as well as for the management of women with pre-existing cardiovascular disease whose health may be seriously compromised with the increased demands of pregnancy.

The heart

- The heart enlarges by about 12% between early and late pregnancy.

- The growing uterus elevates the diaphragm, the great vessels are unfolded and the heart is correspondingly displaced upwards, with the apex moved laterally to the left by about 15°.

- By mid-pregnancy more than 90% of women develop an ejection systolic murmur, which lasts until the first week postpartum. If unaccompanied by any other abnormalities, it reflects the increased stroke output.

- Twenty per cent develop a transient diastolic murmur and 10% develop continuous murmurs, heard over the base of the heart, owing to increased mammary blood flow.

- Rotational and axis changes during pregnancy cause an inverted T wave to be apparent on the electrocardiogram (ECG) — essential to note if resuscitation is required.

Cardiac output

- The increase in cardiac output ranges from 35 to 50% in pregnancy, from an average of 5 L/min before pregnancy to approximately 7 L/min by the 20th week; thereafter the changes are less dramatic.

- The increased cardiac output is due to rises in both stroke volume and heart rate.

- The increase in heart rate begins in the 7th week and by the third trimester it has increased by 10–20%.

- Heart rates are typically 10–15 beats per minute faster than those of the non-pregnant woman.

- The stroke volume increases by 10% during the first half of pregnancy, and reaches a peak at 20 weeks' gestation that is maintained until term.

Blood

Blood pressure

- Early pregnancy is associated with a marked decrease in diastolic blood pressure but little change in systolic pressure. With reduced peripheral vascular resistance the systolic blood pressure falls an average of 5–10 mmHg below baseline levels and the diastolic pressure falls 10–15 mmHg by 24 weeks' gestation.

- Thereafter blood pressure gradually rises, returning to pre-pregnant levels at term. Posture can have a major effect on blood pressure. The supine position can decrease cardiac output by as much as 25%.

- Compression of the inferior vena cava by the enlarging uterus during the late second and third trimesters results in reduced venous return, which in turn decreases stroke volume and cardiac output.

The pregnant woman may suffer from *supine hypotensive syndrome*, which consists of hypotension, bradycardia, dizziness, light-headedness, nausea and even syncope if she remains in the supine position too long. By rolling the woman on to her left side the cardiac output can be instantly restored.

Blood volume

The total maternal blood volume increases 30–50% in singleton pregnancies.

The plasma volume, which corresponds with the increase in blood volume, increases by 50% over the course of the pregnancy. In a normal first pregnancy it may increase by about 1250 ml above non-pregnant levels and in subsequent pregnancies it may increase by about 1500 ml. The increase starts in the first trimester, expands rapidly up until 32–34 weeks' gestation, and then in the last few weeks of pregnancy it plateaus with very little change. The increase in plasma volume reduces the viscosity of the blood and improves capillary flow.

Red cell mass increases during pregnancy in response to the extra oxygen requirements of maternal and placental tissue. Approximately 10–15% of women will have an increase in and reactivation of maternal fetal haemoglobin. The increase in red cell mass appears to be constant throughout pregnancy but it is most marked from about 20 weeks. In spite of the increased production of red blood cells, the marked increase in plasma volume causes dilution of many circulating factors. As a result, the red cell count, haematocrit and haemoglobin concentration all decrease (Table 7.2).

Table 7.2 Falling haemoglobin and haematocrit (PCV) in pregnancy despite rising blood volume and red cell mass

	Non-pregnant	Week of pregnancy		
		20	30	40
Plasma volume (ml)	2600	3150	3750	3850
Red cell mass (ml)	1400	1450	1550	1650
Total blood volume (ml)	4000	4600	5300	5500
Haematocrit (packed cell volume, PCV) (%)	35.0	32.0	29.0	30.0
Haemoglobin (g/dl)	13.3	11.0	10.5	11.0

In healthy women with iron stores, the mean haemoglobin concentration:

- falls from 13.3 g/dl in the non-pregnant state to 11 g/dl in early pregnancy
- is at its lowest at around 32 weeks' gestation when plasma volume expansion is maximal
- after this time rises by approximately 0.5 g/dl, returning to 11 g/dl around the 36th week of pregnancy.

Anaemia in pregnancy has been defined as a haemoglobin of less than 11 g/dl in the first and third trimesters and less than 10.5 g/dl in the second trimester.

Iron therapy is unnecessary unless:

- serial estimations show that the haemoglobin has fallen below 10 g/dl, *or*
- there is a progressive reduction in mean cell volume and low serum ferritin levels.

Iron metabolism

The increased red cell mass and the needs of the developing fetus and placenta lead to increased iron requirements in pregnancy. Iron demand increases from 2 to 4 mg daily. A healthy diet containing 10–14 mg of iron per day, 1–2 mg (5–10%) of which is absorbed, provides sufficient iron for the majority of pregnant women. Caffeine interferes with iron absorption.

Plasma protein

The total serum protein content falls within the first trimester and remains reduced throughout pregnancy. Albumin plays an important role:

- as a carrier protein for some hormones, drugs, free fatty acids and unconjugated bilirubin

- because of its influence in decreasing colloid osmotic pressure, causing physiological oedema.

Clotting factors

Major changes in the coagulation system lead to the *hypercoagulable state* of normal pregnancy. The increased tendency to clot is caused by:

- reduced plasma fibrinolytic activity
- an increase in circulating fibrin degradation products in the plasma.

White blood cells (leucocytes)

From 2 months the total white cell count rises in pregnancy and reaches a peak at 30 weeks, mainly because of the increase in numbers of neutrophil polymorphonuclear leucocytes. This enhances the blood's phagocytic and bactericidal properties.

Table 7.3 is a summary of changes in blood values in pregnancy.

Table 7.3 Summary of common blood values and their changes

	Normal range (non-pregnant)	Change in pregnancy	Timing
Protein (total)	65–85 g/L	↓10 g/L	By 20 weeks then stable
Albumin	30–48 g/L	↓10 g/L	Most by 20 weeks then gradual
Fibrinogen	1.7–4.1 g/L	↑2 g/L	Progressively from 3rd month
Platelets	150–400 × 10^9 L	Slight decrease	No significant change until 3–5 days postpartum
Clotting time	6–12 min approx.	Little change	
White cell count	4–11 × 10^9 L	9 × 10^9 L	Peaks at 30 weeks then plateaus
Red cell count	4.5 × 10^{12} L	3.8 × 10^{12} L	Declines progressively to 30–34 weeks

Immunity

Human chorionic gonadotrophin (HCG) and prolactin are known to suppress the immune response of pregnant women. Lymphocyte function is depressed. There is also decreased resistance to certain viral infections. Serum levels of immunoglobulins IgA, IgG and IgM decrease steadily from the 10th week of pregnancy, reaching their lowest level at 30 weeks and remaining at this level until term.

Changes in the Respiratory System

- Increased cardiac output in pregnancy leads to a substantial increase in pulmonary blood flow.

- The blood volume expansion and vasodilatation of pregnancy result in hyperaemia and oedema of the upper respiratory mucosa, which predispose the pregnant woman to nasal congestion, epistaxis and even changes in voice.

- As the uterus enlarges, the diaphragm is elevated by as much as 4 cm, and the rib cage is displaced upwards. Expansion of the rib cage causes the *tidal volume* to be increased by 30–40%. Although the respiratory rate is little changed in pregnancy from the normal 14 or 15 breaths per minute, breathing is deeper even at rest.

- Both the alveolar oxygen partial pressure and the arterial oxygen partial pressure (PaO_2) are increased from non-pregnant values of 98–100 mmHg to pregnant values of 101–104 mmHg.

- The rise in tidal volume and decrease in residual volume facilitates a 15–20% increase in oxygen consumption, which supports the additional metabolic requirements of mother and fetus.

- The 'hyperventilation of pregnancy' causes a 15–20% decrease in maternal arterial carbon dioxide partial pressure ($PaCO_2$) from an average of 5 kPa (35–40 mmHg) in the non-pregnant woman to 4 kPa (30 mmHg) or lower in late pregnancy. The fall in $PaCO_2$ is matched by an equivalent fall in plasma bicarbonate concentration from the non-pregnant values, resulting in mild alkalaemia.

Changes in the Urinary System

- The kidneys increase in weight and lengthen by 1 cm.
- Under the influence of progesterone the calyces and renal pelves dilate.
- The ureters also dilate and lengthen and are thrown into curves of varying sizes. The right ureter is usually more dilated than the left, owing to the dextrorotation of the uterus, and as pregnancy advances the supine or upright posture may cause partial ureteric obstruction as the enlarged uterus compresses both ureters at the pelvic brim.

All these factors can lead to urinary stasis and an increased risk of urinary tract infection in pregnancy.

- After the 4th month of pregnancy the bladder trigone is lifted and there is thickening of its intraureteric margin; this process continues until term, resulting in a deepened and widened trigone. Bladder pressure increases and may result in reduced bladder capacity. To compensate for this, the urethra lengthens and intraurethral pressure increases.
- The muscles of the internal urethral sphincter relax, which, along with pressure from the pregnant uterus on the bladder, causes a significant number of women to experience some degree of stress incontinence. Antenatal teaching of pelvic floor exercises is important for helping to resolve this troublesome feature of pregnancy.

■ Urgency of micturition and urge incontinence also increase in pregnancy, partly because of the effects of progesterone on the detrusor muscle. These all usually resolve spontaneously during the puerperium.

Numerous factors affect renal function in pregnancy, including:

■ increased plasma volume
■ increased glomerular filtration rate (GFR)
■ increased renal plasma flow
■ alterations in hormones such as adrenocorticotrophic hormone (ACTH), antidiuretic hormone (ADH), aldosterone, cortisol, thyroid hormone and HCG.

Studies have shown:

■ a 45% increase in creatinine clearance by 9 weeks' gestation
■ a peak at about 32 weeks' gestation of about 50% above non-pregnant levels
■ a significant decrease towards non-pregnant levels prior to birth.

Plasma levels of urea and creatinine decrease in proportion with the increase in GFR during normal pregnancy. Many women with proteinuria before pregnancy experience a progressive increase in the amount of protein spilled during pregnancy; however, the upper limit of normal is considered to be 300 mg over 24 hours. The increased GFR coupled with impaired tubular reabsorption capacity for filtered glucose results in excretion of glucose (*glycosuria*) at some time during pregnancy in 50% of women.

The urine is more alkaline owing to the presence of glucose and to the increased renal loss of bicarbonate caused by the alkalaemia of pregnancy. Renin rises early in pregnancy and continues to increase until term. It acts on angiotensinogen to form increased amounts of angiotensin I and subsequently II (Fig. 7.1). Increased production of angiotensin II stimulates the release of increased levels of aldosterone.

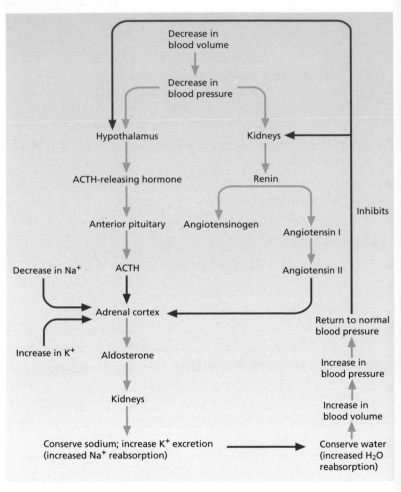

Fig. 7.1 The renin–angiotensin system.
(From Hinchcliff et al. 1996, p. 226, with permission of Baillière Tindall, London.)

Aldosterone prevents the increased loss of sodium that could occur as a result of the increased GFR and the natriuretic effects of progesterone. Despite elevated aldosterone levels, potassium excretion is decreased, possibly because of the effects of progesterone.

Changes in the Gastrointestinal System

- The gums become oedematous, soft and spongy during pregnancy, probably owing to the effect of oestrogen, which can lead to bleeding when the gums are mildly traumatised, as with a toothbrush. Occasionally a focal, highly vascular swelling known as *epulis* (or gingivitis) develops; it is caused by growth of the gum capillaries. It usually regresses spontaneously after delivery.

- Profuse salivation, or ptyalism, is an occasional complaint in pregnancy.

- Dietary changes in pregnancy, such as aversion to coffee, alcohol and fried foods, are very common, as are cravings for salted and spiced foods. Pica, the term given to the bizarre craving for and compulsive, secret chewing of food or ingestion of non-food substances (e.g. ice, coal, disinfectants), is also reasonably common.

- Although in early pregnancy many women experience nausea, an increase in appetite may also be noticed, with the daily food intake increasing by up to 200 kcal.

- Many women notice an increase in thirst in pregnancy because of the resetting of osmotic thresholds for thirst and vasopressin.

- As pregnancy progresses, the enlarging uterus displaces the stomach and intestines. At term the stomach attains a vertical position rather than its normal horizontal one. These mechanical forces lead to increased intragastric pressure and a change in the angle of the gastro-oesophageal junction, leading to greater oesophageal reflux.

- Marked reduction of gastric and intestinal tone and motility plus relaxation of the lower oesophageal sphincter predispose to heartburn, constipation and haemorrhoids.

Changes in Metabolism

In order to provide for increased basal metabolic rate and oxygen consumption, as well as the needs of the rapidly growing uterus, fetus and placenta, the pregnant woman undergoes many metabolic changes.

- Protein metabolism is enhanced to supply substrate for maternal and fetal growth.
- Fat metabolism increases, as evidenced by elevation of all lipid fractions in the blood.
- Carbohydrate metabolism, however, demonstrates the most dramatic changes.

The continuous supply of glucose required by the growing fetus is met by:

- the intake of glucose when the mother eats
- the enhanced secretion of insulin in response to glucose.

There is evidence that HPL or other growth-related hormones may contribute to the process by reducing peripheral insulin sensitivity. It has also been suggested that there may be alterations in the characteristics of insulin binding to its receptor.

Optimal blood glucose levels in the pregnant woman range between 4.4 and 5.5 mmol/L. In the pregnant woman hypoglycaemia is defined as a concentration below 3.3 mmol/L.

It is recommended that pregnant women do not:

- fast
- skip meals
- restrict carbohydrate intake.

Maternal blood glucose levels are of critical importance for fetal well-being and prolonged fasting in pregnancy produces a more intense ketonaemia, which is dangerous to fetal health.

Although Muslim women are exempt from fasting while pregnant, those who wish to fast during Ramadan may do so under medical supervision if it occurs during the second trimester. Fasting during the first and third trimesters, however, is not recommended, the main danger to the fetus possibly being from dehydration rather than from malnutrition.

Material Weight

Weight gain during pregnancy comprises:

- the products of conception (fetus, placenta and amniotic fluid)
- hypertrophy of several maternal tissues (uterus, breasts, blood, fat stores, and extracellular and extravascular fluid) (Table 7.4).

An optimal weight gain for an average pregnancy is 12.5 kg, 9 kg of which is gained in the last 20 weeks. Appropriate weight gain for each individual woman is now based on the pre-pregnancy BMI, which reflects the mother's weight-to-height ratio.

Table 7.4 Distribution of average increase in weight in pregnancy showing relative proportions of protein and fat

Site	Weight (kg)	Protein (%)	Fat (%)
Fetus	3.2	44	15
Placenta	0.6	10	
Amniotic fluid	0.8		
Uterus	0.9	17	
Breasts	0.4	8	
Blood	1.5	14	
Water	2.6		
Adipose tissue	2.5		85
Total	12.5		

Skeletal Changes

- During pregnancy, relaxation of the pelvic joints results from hormonal changes. Oestrogen, progesterone and relaxin all appear to be implicated.

- This allows some expansion of the pelvic cavity during descent of the fetal head in labour. The increase in width of the symphysis pubis, which has been associated with severe pelvic pain, occurs more in multiparous than in primigravid women, and returns to normal soon after birth.

- Posture usually alters to compensate for the enlarging uterus, particularly if abdominal muscle tone is poor. A progressive lordosis shifts the woman's centre of gravity back over her legs.

- There is also increased mobility of the sacroiliac and sacrococcygeal joints, which may contribute to the alteration in maternal posture, leading to low back pain in late pregnancy, particularly in the multiparous woman.

Skin Changes

Pigmentation

From the 3rd month until term, some degree of skin darkening is observed in 90% of all pregnant women:

- The pigmented linea alba, now called the *linea nigra*, runs from the os pubis to above the umbilicus.

- Pigmentation of the face, which affects at least half of all pregnant women, is called *chloasma* or *melasma*, or 'mask of pregnancy'.

Melasma is caused by melanin deposition into epidermal or dermal macrophages. Epidermal melanosis usually regresses postpartum but dermal melanosis may persist for up to 10 years in one-third of women. Chloasma can be minimised or prevented by avoiding sun exposure and using high-protection factor sun creams.

Stretch marks

As maternal size increases, stretching occurs in the collagen layer of the skin, particularly over the breasts, abdomen and thighs. In some women the areas of maximum stretch become thin and stretch marks, *striae gravidarum*, appear as red stripes changing to glistening, silvery white lines approximately 6 months after the birth.

Itching

Although not common, itching of the skin in pregnancy (not due to liver disease) can be distressing. Obstetric cholestasis (see ch. 12) must be excluded before assuming itching is a problem in pregnancy.

Hair

The proportion of growing hairs to resting hairs is increased in pregnancy so the woman reaches the end of pregnancy with many overaged hairs. This ratio is reversed after delivery so that sometimes alarming amounts of hair are shed during brushing or washing. Normal hair growth is usually restored by 6–12 months. Mild hirsutism is common during pregnancy, particularly on the face.

Other skin changes

A rise in temperature by 0.2–0.4°C occurs as a result of the effects of progesterone and the increased basal metabolic rate (BMR). Angiomas or *vascular spiders* (minute red elevations on the skin of the face, neck, arms and chest) and *palmar erythema* (reddening of the palms) frequently occur, possibly as a result of the high levels of oestrogen. They are of no clinical significance and disappear after pregnancy.

Changes in the Breasts

Major changes take place in the breasts during pregnancy owing to the increased blood supply; these changes are stimulated by secretion of oestrogen and progesterone from both corpus luteum and placenta. Among these changes is the formation of new ducts and acini cells (Box 7.2).

Box 7.2 Breast changes in chronological order

3–4 weeks

- There may be a prickling, tingling sensation due to increased blood supply, particularly around the nipple

6–8 weeks

- Breasts increase in size, becoming painful, tense and nodular due to hypertrophy of the alveoli
- Delicate bluish surface veins become visible just beneath the skin

8–12 weeks

- Montgomery's tubercles become more prominent on the areola; these hypertrophic sebaceous glands secrete sebum, which keeps the nipple soft and supple
- Pigmented areas around the nipple (the primary areola) darken, and may enlarge and become more erectile

16 weeks

- Colostrum can be expressed
- The secondary areola develops, with further extension of the pigmented areas that is often mottled in appearance

Late pregnancy

- Colostrum may leak from the breasts
- Progesterone causes the nipple to become more prominent and mobile

---

Changes in the Endocrine System

Endocrine changes in pregnancy are complex and understanding of them is incomplete. It is now clear, however, that during pregnancy the intrauterine tissues can also produce many of the peptide and steroid hormones that are produced by the endocrine glands in the non-pregnant state. Many hormones exert their actions indirectly by interacting with cytokines and chemokines. During pregnancy these substances are substantially altered. Early effects of placental hormones are described in chapter 3. Later physiological effects caused by hormones have been highlighted throughout this chapter as they impact on the various systems, and are now summarised.

Placental hormones

These are listed in Box 7.3.

Pituitary gland and its hormones

- The pituitary gland enlarges during pregnancy owing to hypertrophy of the anterior lobe. Secretion of FSH and LH is greatly inhibited during pregnancy by the negative feedback of progesterone and oestrogen.
- In contrast there is increased secretion of hormones by the pituitary gland.

The anterior lobe secretes:

- thyroid-stimulating hormone (TSH),
- ACTH
- prolactin
- melanocyte-stimulating hormone (MSH).

The posterior lobe of the pituitary gland secretes:

- oxytocin
- antidiuretic hormone (ADH, vasopressin).

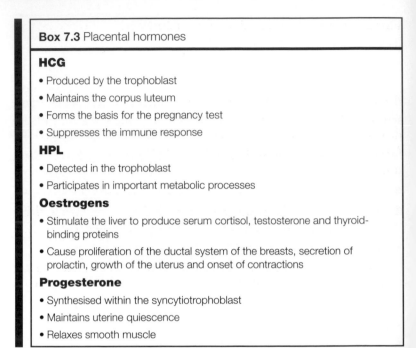

Box 7.3 Placental hormones

HCG

- Produced by the trophoblast
- Maintains the corpus luteum
- Forms the basis for the pregnancy test
- Suppresses the immune response

HPL

- Detected in the trophoblast
- Participates in important metabolic processes

Oestrogens

- Stimulate the liver to produce serum cortisol, testosterone and thyroid-binding proteins
- Cause proliferation of the ductal system of the breasts, secretion of prolactin, growth of the uterus and onset of contractions

Progesterone

- Synthesised within the syncytiotrophoblast
- Maintains uterine quiescence
- Relaxes smooth muscle

Prolactin is essential for lactation and levels rise up to 20-fold during pregnancy and lactation. Its effect of producing milk is suppressed during pregnancy by high levels of oestrogen and progesterone. There is also intrauterine production of prolactin from cells within the decidua.

The posterior pituitary gland releases oxytocin throughout pregnancy. Concentrations of oxytocin in the maternal circulation do not change significantly during pregnancy or prior to the onset of labour, but do rise late in the second stage of labour. There is, however, an increased uterine sensitivity to oxytocin during labour that is influenced by the ratio of oestrogen to progesterone. The pulsatile release produces more effective uterine contractions. Oxytocin is also important for successful lactation.

Thyroid function

Alterations in the structure and function of the thyroid gland cause many thyroid symptoms to be mimicked in pregnancy, resulting in diagnostic confusion in the interpretation of thyroid function tests. Overall control of the thyroid gland, however, is unaltered during normal pregnancy.

- There is a moderate increase in size early in pregnancy.
- There is a marked increase in thyroid-binding globulin, and the bound forms of thyroxine (T_4) and tri-iodothyronine (T_3) peak at about 12 weeks' gestation,

Circulating concentrations of unbound (inactive) T_3 and T_4 are essentially unaltered. Similarly, TSH shows no change in pregnancy.

Adrenal glands

- In early pregnancy the levels of ACTH are reduced, but from 3 months until term there is a significant rise, along with an increase in serum concentrations of circulating free cortisol.
- The placenta and the trophoblast cells also produce corticotrophin-releasing factor and ACTH. These hormones are important in relation to the priming of myometrial activity and may also influence the fetal adrenals.
- The raised levels of unbound cortisol are reflected in the excretion of double the amount of urinary cortisol.
- From 15 weeks' gestation until the third trimester there is a 10-fold increase in the secretion of aldosterone and deoxycorticosterone by the maternal adrenal glands and also by fetal intrauterine tissues, which is stimulated to a certain extent by the acute rise in ACTH. This rise was formerly attributed

entirely to progesterone; however, it is now clear that its main means of control is via the renin–angiotensin system (Fig. 7.1) with involvement of factors such as atrial natriuretic peptide and angiotensins.

Diagnosis of Pregnancy

- Amenorrhoea, breast changes, nausea, changes in food and drink preference, overwhelming tiredness, frequency of micturition and backache often convince women that they are pregnant (Table 7.5).

- The fluttering movements of the fetus felt by the mother, known as *quickening,* can be used to check the date of expected birth; a primigravid woman feels them at 18–20 weeks, and a multigravid woman at 16–18 weeks.

- Using transvaginal ultrasound, the gestational sac can be visualised at 4.5 weeks and heart pulsation can be seen at 5 weeks.

- Using transabdominal ultrasound, visualisation of gestational sac and heart pulsation is possible 1 week later.

- Doppler can detect the fetal heart at 11–12 weeks' gestation.

- The palpation of fetal parts and fetal movements from about 22 weeks are good positive signs of pregnancy.

- Biochemical pregnancy tests depend on the detection of HCG, produced by the trophoblast. HCG can be detected in blood as early as 6 days after conception, and in urine 26 days after conception. Many different pregnancy tests are available, but the most popular over-the-counter home pregnancy test is the *enzyme-linked immunosorbent assay* (ELISA).

Table 7.5 Signs of pregnancy

Sign	Time of occurrence (gestational age)	Differential diagnosis
Possible (presumptive) signs		
Early breast changes (unreliable in multigravida)	3–4 weeks +	Contraceptive pill
Amenorrhoea	4 weeks +	Hormonal imbalance
		Emotional stress
		Illness
Morning sickness	4–14 weeks	Gastrointestinal disorders
		Pyrexial illness
		Cerebral irritation, etc.
Bladder irritability	6–12 weeks	Urinary tract infections
		Pelvic tumour
Quickening	16–20 weeks +	Intestinal movement, 'wind'
Probable signs		
Presence of HCG in:		
Blood	9–10 days	Hydatidiform mole
Urine	14 days	Choriocarcinoma
Softened isthmus (Hegar's sign)	6–12 weeks	
Blueing of vagina (Chadwick's sign)	8 weeks +	
Pulsation of fornices (Osiander's sign)	8 weeks +	Pelvic congestion
Uterine growth	8 weeks +	Tumours
Changes in skin pigmentations	8 weeks +	

(Continued)

Table 7.5 (Continued)

Sign	Time of occurrence (gestational age)	Differential diagnosis
Uterine soufflé	12–16 weeks	Increased blood flow to uterus, as in large uterine myomas or ovarian tumours
Braxton Hicks contractions	16 weeks	
Ballottement of fetus	16–28 weeks	
Positive signs		
Visualisation of gestational sac by:		
Transvaginal ultrasound	4.5 weeks	
Transabdominal ultrasound	5.5 weeks	
Visualisation of heart pulsation by:		
Transvaginal ultrasound	5 weeks	
Transabdominal ultrasound	6 weeks	
Fetal heart sounds by:		
Doppler	11–12 weeks	
Fetal stethoscope	20 weeks +	
Fetal movements:		
Palpable	22 weeks +	
Visible	Late pregnancy	
Fetal parts palpated	24 weeks +	
Visualisation of fetus by:		
X-ray	16 weeks +	

Chapter 8

Common Disorders of and Exercises for Pregnancy

Common disorders experienced by some women as a consequence of the physiological changes occurring in their body are listed in Box 8.1.

Relief of Aches and Pains

Back and pelvic pain

- Backache can be eased by good posture and practice of the transversus and pelvic-tilting exercises in standing, sitting and lying positions.
- Women complaining of severe pain involving more than one area of the pelvis (*pelvic arthropathy*) should be referred to a women's health physiotherapist for assessment, advice and possible manipulation.
- Sciatica-like pain may be relieved by lying on the side away from the discomfort so that the affected leg is uppermost. Pillows should be placed strategically to support the whole limb.

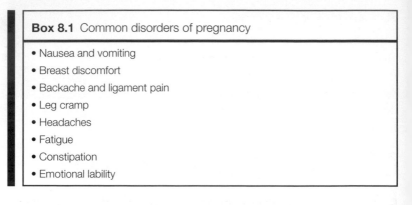

> **Box 8.1** Common disorders of pregnancy
>
> - Nausea and vomiting
> - Breast discomfort
> - Backache and ligament pain
> - Leg cramp
> - Headaches
> - Fatigue
> - Constipation
> - Emotional lability

- Symphysis pubis dysfunction (SPD), formerly known as diastasis of the symphysis pubis, is covered in chapter 11.

Midwives should be aware of necessary precautions and correct positions in relation to labour.

Cramp

Women can help prevent cramp in pregnancy by practising foot and leg exercises.

- To relieve sudden cramp in the calf muscles whilst in the sitting position, the woman should hold the knee straight and stretch the calf muscles by pulling the foot upwards (dorsiflexing) at the same time.

- Alternatively, standing firmly on the affected leg and striding forwards with the other leg will stretch the calf muscles and solve the problem.

Rib stitch or discomfort

Discomfort around the rib cage can often be relieved by:

- adopting a good posture
- specifically stretching one or both arms upwards, depending on which side the pain affects.

Antenatal Exercises

Before teaching exercises it is essential to understand the simple anatomy and functions of the muscles involved, in order to be able to select and/or adapt appropriate exercises in different circumstances. The positions that pregnant women adopt for exercises should be carefully considered:

■ Women should not be asked to lie flat in the later second and third trimesters because of the danger of supine hypotension.

■ Instead, a half-lying position with the back raised to an angle of approximately 35° can be used.

■ Foot and leg exercises and pelvic tilting can be performed in sitting or half-lying positions, whereas transversus and pelvic floor exercises can be carried out in any position.

Muscles of good tone are more elastic and will regain their former length more efficiently and more quickly after being stretched than muscles of poor tone. Exercising the abdominal muscles antenatally will ensure a speedy postnatal return to normal, effective pushing in labour and the lessening of backache in pregnancy. An important function of the abdominal muscles is the control of pelvic tilt. As the ligaments around the pelvis stretch and no longer give such firm support to the joints, the muscles become the second line of defence, helping to prevent an exaggerated pelvic tilt and unnecessary strain on the pelvic ligaments. Overstretched ligaments and weakened abdominal muscles during pregnancy can lead to chronic skeletal problems postnatally as well as backache antenatally. Exercises for the transversus muscles (transversus exercise) and rectus muscles (pelvic tilting) help to prevent this and maintain good abdominal tone.

Exercises that involve the oblique abdominal muscles should be avoided in later pregnancy as they may cause diastasis recti.

Transversus exercise

To tone the deep transverse abdominal muscles and to help prevent backache:

- Sit comfortably or kneel on all fours with a level spine.
- Breathe in and out, then gently pull in the lower part of the abdomen below the umbilicus, keeping the spine still and breathing normally.
- Hold for up to 10 seconds then relax gently.
- Repeat up to 10 times.

Pelvic tilting or rocking

To encourage good posture and ease backache:

- Adopt a half-lying position, well supported with pillows, and the knees bent and feet flat.
- One hand should be placed under the small of the back and the other on top of the abdomen.
- Tighten the abdominals and buttocks, and press the small of the back down on to the hand underneath.
- Breathe normally; hold for up to 10 seconds then relax.
- Repeat up to 10 times.

Pelvic tilting can also be performed sitting, standing or kneeling.

Pelvic floor exercise

To maintain the tone of the muscles so they retain their functions and to help the muscles to relax during parturition and regain their former strength quickly during the puerperium:

- Sit, stand or half-lie with legs slightly apart.
- Close and draw up around the back passage as though preventing a bowel action then repeat around the front two passages as though preventing the flow of urine.

- Draw up inside and hold for as long as possible, up to 10 seconds, breathing normally, then relax.
- Repeat up to 10 times.

All women should be able to perform this simple exercise, which can be practised anywhere and at any time. It will build up the endurance of the postural slow-twitch fibres in the pelvic floor but can also be performed quickly up to 10 times without holding the contraction. This works the fast-twitch fibres, which need to work quickly to prevent leakage (e.g. when coughing). All women should practise this exercise very regularly antenatally, particularly after emptying the bladder. For those with diminished pelvic floor awareness, attempting to 'stop midstream' occasionally or 'gripping' on to an imaginary tampon that is slipping out may assist the ability to contract the correct muscles.

Foot and leg exercises

To improve the circulation and prevent or alleviate cramp, oedema and varicose veins, each of the following should be repeated several times per day:

- Bend and stretch the ankles.
- Circle feet at the ankles.
- Brace the knees and let go.

Additional information

- Advise pregnant women to avoid long periods of standing, which may increase oedema, but encourage walking.
- Discourage sitting or lying with legs crossed, which can impede the circulation.
- Describe how to relieve cramp.
- Advise on correct use of support tights.
- Stress the importance of supporting footwear of sensible height.

■ Advise sitting with feet elevated whenever possible and with heels higher than hips if oedema is present.

Stress, Relaxation and Respiration

Tension manifests itself with muscle tightening and shows in the ways listed in Box 8.2.

When tension increases, breathing often becomes shallow and rapid; when severe, breath holding may feature. The higher the stress level, the greater is the degree of postural change that will be evident. Mental tension often leads to physical tension and a vicious circle is established. Muscles can work singly but usually they work in groups and when any group of muscles is working, the opposite group relaxes. This is a physiological fact and is known as *reciprocal inhibition* or *reciprocal relaxation*.

Reciprocal relaxation ensures that, when following a series of instructions for the whole body, one will be able to bring release of tension and relaxation to all areas.

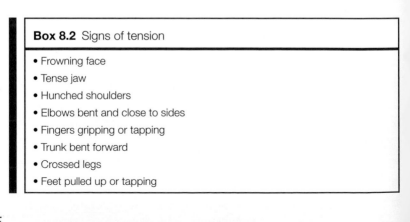

Box 8.2 Signs of tension

- Frowning face
- Tense jaw
- Hunched shoulders
- Elbows bent and close to sides
- Fingers gripping or tapping
- Trunk bent forward
- Crossed legs
- Feet pulled up or tapping

Respiration

Respiration is affected by stress and adapted breathing is one of the easiest ways of assisting relaxation. Breathing can be used to increase the depth of relaxation by varying its speed; slower breathing leads to deeper relaxation. Natural rhythmic breathing must not be confused with specific unnatural levels or rates of breathing. Women in labour frequently breathe very rapidly at the peak of a contraction but should be encouraged not to do so. Persistent rapid breathing or breath holding is usually a sign of panic.

Very slow deep breathing can cause hyperventilation, which produces tingling in the fingers and may proceed to carpopedal spasm and even tetany. Rapid shallow breathing or panting is only tracheal and can lead to hypoventilation with subsequent oxygen deprivation. During pregnancy, labour and birth, emphasis should be placed on easy, rhythmic breathing and on avoiding very deep breathing, shallow panting or long periods of breath holding.

Chapter 9

Antenatal Care

Aim of Antenatal Care

The aim is to monitor the progress of pregnancy in order to support maternal health and normal fetal development. It is essential that the midwife critically evaluates the physical, psychological and sociological effects of pregnancy on the woman and her family. The midwife achieves this by:

- developing a partnership with the woman
- providing a holistic approach to the woman's care that meets her individual needs
- promoting an awareness of the public health issues for the woman and her family
- exchanging information with the woman and her family and enabling them to make informed choices about pregnancy and birth
- being an advocate for the woman and her family during her pregnancy, supporting her right to choose care that is appropriate for her own needs and those of her family
- recognising complications of pregnancy and appropriately referring women within the multidisciplinary team

- assisting the woman and her family in their preparations to meet the demands of birth, and making a birth plan
- assisting the woman in making an informed choice about methods of infant feeding and giving appropriate and sensitive advice to support her decision
- offering education for parenthood within a planned programme or on an individual basis
- working in partnership with other pertinent organisations.

The Initial Assessment (Booking Visit)

The purpose of this visit is to:

- introduce the woman to the maternity service
- share information in order to discuss, plan and implement care for the duration of the pregnancy, the birth and postnatally.

The earlier the first contact is made with the midwife, the more appropriate and valuable the advice given relating to nutrition and care of the developing fetal organs, which are almost completely formed by 12 weeks' gestation. Medical conditions, infections, smoking, alcohol and drug taking may all have a profound and detrimental effect on the fetus during this time.

Models of midwifery care

Options for place of birth include:

- the home
- a birth centre
- a peripheral unit
- a tertiary hospital.

The majority of women receive antenatal care in the community, either in their own home or at a local clinic. Hospital-based clinics are available for women who receive care from an obstetrician or physician in addition to their midwife. Women who have risk factors identified or who develop complications during pregnancy will usually plan for a hospital birth.

Introduction to the midwifery service

The woman's introduction to midwifery care is crucial in forming her initial impressions of the maternity service. A friendly, professional approach will enable the development of a partnership between the woman and the midwife. The initial visit focuses on the exchange of information (Box 9.1). This helps the midwife and the woman to get to know each other, ideally within the woman's own environment. The midwife may meet other members of the family and in this way gain a more holistic view of the woman's needs. Nevertheless, the midwife will also recognise that there are occasions when the woman may need to spend time alone with her to facilitate discussion, which

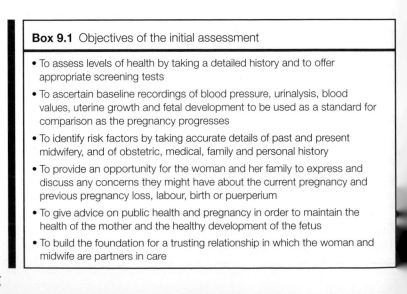

Box 9.1 Objectives of the initial assessment

- To assess levels of health by taking a detailed history and to offer appropriate screening tests
- To ascertain baseline recordings of blood pressure, urinalysis, blood values, uterine growth and fetal development to be used as a standard for comparison as the pregnancy progresses
- To identify risk factors by taking accurate details of past and present midwifery, and of obstetric, medical, family and personal history
- To provide an opportunity for the woman and her family to express and discuss any concerns they might have about the current pregnancy and previous pregnancy loss, labour, birth or puerperium
- To give advice on public health and pregnancy in order to maintain the health of the mother and the healthy development of the fetus
- To build the foundation for a trusting relationship in which the woman and midwife are partners in care

she may not feel able to do in the presence of family members — for example, in situations involving domestic abuse.

Communication

The midwife requires many skills in order to provide optimal antenatal care; one of the most fundamental of these is the ability to communicate effectively. Listening skills involve attending to or focusing on what the woman is saying, and considering the words, phrases and general content of what is said. In addition, non-verbal responses, including facial expression, body position, eye contact, proximity to the midwife and touch, will affect the flow of information between woman and midwife.

The midwife can promote communication with the woman by:

- using gentle questioning
- making open-ended statements
- reflecting back key words used during the discussion to encourage and facilitate exploration of what is being said.

Communication encompasses the writing of accurate, comprehensive and contemporaneous records of information given and received and the plan of care that has been agreed. This is essential when there is shared care within the multidisciplinary team, as well as to ensure that the woman understands the records she holds.

First impressions

A midwife can gain much from the initial observation and assessment of a woman at the start of their first meeting. The assessment should be carried out sensitively, enabling the woman to express her concerns about this or previous experiences of pregnancy or birth.

Observation of physical characteristics is also important. Posture and gait can indicate back problems or previous trauma to the pelvis. The woman may be lethargic, which could be an indication of extreme tiredness, anaemia, malnutrition or depression.

Social history

It is important to assess the response of the whole family to the pregnancy and to aim to improve health and reduce health inequalities in pregnant women and their young children. The midwife may, in partnership with the woman, advocate referral to a social worker, who has a role in alleviating some of these difficulties, or to other multi-professional agencies where assistance can be obtained.

General health

General health should be discussed and good habits reinforced, with further advice given when required. The midwife has a duty to help women set goals throughout their pregnancy and help them to cut down on their smoking, ideally giving up. The woman, her partner and other family members should be informed about the direct and passive effects of smoking on the baby. Alcohol abuse is less common but can affect the baby. It is recommended that women limit alcohol consumption to one standard unit per day.

Menstrual history

An accurate menstrual history is taken to determine the expected date of delivery (EDD). This will enable the midwife to predict a birth date and subsequently calculate gestational age at any point in the pregnancy. Abdominal assessment of uterine size can be made in conjunction with gestational age during the antenatal consultation. The midwife has a role in helping the woman to understand that an EDD is one day within a 5-week time frame during which her baby reaches term and may be born.

The EDD is calculated by adding 9 calendar months and 7 days to the date of the first day of the woman's last menstrual period. This method assumes that:

- The woman takes regular note of regularity and length of time between periods.
- Conception occurred 14 days after the first day of the last period; this is true only if the woman has a regular 28-day cycle.

- The last period of bleeding was true menstruation; implantation of the ovum may cause slight bleeding.

Naegele's rule suggests that the duration of a pregnancy is 280 days. However, controversy exists over the suitability of applying Naegele's rule to determine EDD; therefore ultrasound scanning has become the more accurate and commonly used method for predicting the EDD. This depends on an experienced ultrasonographer being both available and accessible, and also requires the woman's consent. Ultrasound before 16 weeks confirms the EDD; the 18–20 week scan identifies abnormalities.

If the woman has taken oral contraceptives within the previous 3 months, this may also confuse estimation of dates because breakthrough bleeding and anovular cycles lead to inaccuracies. Some women become pregnant with an intrauterine contraceptive device (IUCD) still in place. Although the pregnancy is likely to continue normally, the position of the IUCD may be determined using ultrasound techniques.

Obstetric history

In order to give a summary of a woman's childbearing history, the descriptive terms -*gravida* and -*para* are used:

- 'Gravid' means 'pregnant', 'gravida' means 'a pregnant woman', and a subsequent number indicates the number of times she has been pregnant regardless of outcome.
- 'Para' means 'having given birth'; a woman's parity refers to the number of times that she has given birth to a child, live or stillborn, excluding miscarriages and abortions.

A *grande multigravida* is a woman who has been pregnant five times or more irrespective of outcome. A *grande multipara* is a woman who has given birth five times or more.

Previous termination of pregnancy is usually discussed, although it may cause embarrassment or distress. Sometimes feelings are not expressed or resolved at the time of the miscarriage or termination, and this could interfere with emotional adjustment to the present pregnancy. Any form of abortion occurring in a Rhesus negative woman requires prophylactic administration of anti-D immunoglobulin to reduce the risk of Rhesus incompatibility in a subsequent pregnancy (see ch. 35).

Confidential information may be recorded in a clinic-held summary of the pregnancy and not in the woman's handheld record if she requests this.

Repeated spontaneous abortion (miscarriage) may indicate conditions such as genetic abnormality, hormonal imbalance or incompetent cervix. Screening or treatment may be necessary in the present pregnancy. The woman may be more anxious about this pregnancy, minor disturbances in pregnancy may be exacerbated and preoccupation with the pregnancy may lead to other psychological, social or physical problems. She is likely to feel reassured if she hears the fetal heart or sees the image on an ultrasound scan.

A risk assessment should be carried out based on the woman's obstetric and medical history and current pregnancy. This will enable the midwife and woman to:

- discuss the progress of the pregnancy
- determine the frequency of antenatal visits and the location of antenatal care
- identify appropriate screening techniques and other health professionals who may need to be involved.

Place of birth will also be influenced by the risk assessment but in all cases the ultimate decision is taken by the mother, who should make an informed choice (Box 9.2).

Medical history

During pregnancy both the mother and the fetus may be affected by a medical condition, or a medical condition may be altered by the pregnancy; if untreated, there may be serious consequences for the woman's health.

Box 9.2 Factors that may require additional antenatal surveillance or advice

Initial assessment

- Age less than 18 years or over 35 years
- Grande multiparity (more than five previous births)
- Vaginal bleeding at any time during pregnancy
- Unknown or uncertain EDD

Past obstetric history

- Stillbirth or neonatal death
- Baby small or large for gestational age
- Congenital abnormality
- Rhesus isoimmunisation
- Pregnancy-induced hypertension
- Two or more terminations of pregnancy
- Two or more spontaneous abortions
- Previous preterm labour
- Cervical cerclage in past or present pregnancy
- Previous caesarean section or uterine surgery
- Ante- or postpartum haemorrhage
- Precipitate labour
- Multiple pregnancy

Maternal health

- Previous history of deep vein thrombosis or pulmonary embolism
- Chronic illness
- Hypertension
- History of infertility
- Uterine anomaly, including fibroids
- Smoking
- Family history of diabetes
- Alcohol or drug-taking
- Psychological or psychiatric disorders

(Continued)

> **Box 9.2** (Continued)
>
> **Examination at the initial assessment**
> - Blood pressure 140/90 mmHg or above
> - Maternal obesity or underweight according to BMI
> - Maternal height less than 5 feet (150 cm or less)
> - Cardiac murmur detected
> - Other pelvic mass detected
> - Rhesus negative blood group
> - Blood disorders

Family history

Certain conditions are genetic in origin, others are familial or related to ethnicity, and some are associated with the physical or social environment in which the family lives.

Physical Examination

Prior to the physical examination of a pregnant woman, her consent and comfort are primary considerations. Sophisticated biochemical assessments and ultrasound investigations can enhance clinical observations.

Weight

- All women should be weighed or asked for a pre-pregnant weight at booking; if it is within the normal BMI range, repeated weighing is not recommended.
- Women with a BMI of 35 or above or 18 or under should be carefully monitored and offered nutritional counselling.

Blood pressure

Blood pressure is taken in order to ascertain normality and provide a baseline reading for comparison throughout pregnancy.

- The systolic recording may be falsely elevated if a woman is nervous or anxious; long waiting times can cause additional stress. A full bladder can also cause an increase in blood pressure.

- The woman should be comfortably seated or resting in a lateral position on the couch when the blood pressure is taken. Brachial artery pressure is highest when sitting and lower when in the recumbent position.

- A systolic blood pressure of 140 mmHg or diastolic pressure of 90 mmHg at booking is indicative of hypertension and will need careful monitoring during pregnancy with both midwife and obstetrician support.

Urinalysis

- At the first visit a midstream specimen should be sent to the laboratory for culture to exclude asymptomatic bacteriuria.

- Urinalysis for proteinuria is performed at every visit.

Blood tests in pregnancy

The midwife should explain why blood tests are carried out at the booking visit. Women should be assisted by the midwife to make an informed choice about the tests that are available. The midwife should be fully aware of the difference between screening and diagnostic tests, and of their accuracy, and should discuss these options with the women. Blood tests taken at the initial assessment include the ones listed in Box 9.3.

Rhesus negative women who have threatened miscarriage, amniocentesis or any other uterine trauma should be given anti-D gammaglobulin within a few days of the event. If the titration demonstrates

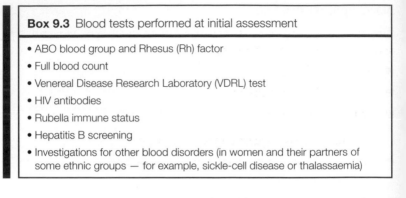

Box 9.3 Blood tests performed at initial assessment

- ABO blood group and Rhesus (Rh) factor
- Full blood count
- Venereal Disease Research Laboratory (VDRL) test
- HIV antibodies
- Rubella immune status
- Hepatitis B screening
- Investigations for other blood disorders (in women and their partners of some ethnic groups — for example, sickle-cell disease or thalassaemia)

a rising antibody response, then more frequent assessment will be made in order to plan management by a specialist in Rhesus disease.

The midwife's examination and advice

The midwife's general examination of the woman is holistic and should encompass her physical, social and psychological well-being. It is important for the midwife to have a knowledge and understanding of the common disorders of pregnancy in order to advise the woman on strategies that will help her to cope with the condition and to minimise the effects she experiences. If at any time the midwife notices any sign of ill health she should discuss this with the woman, and advocate referral to the most appropriate health professional.

The midwife should facilitate discussion about infant feeding. Breastfeeding should be promoted in a sensitive manner and information given about the benefits to both mother and baby. Some women will appreciate information about the body changes taking place during pregnancy. Partners may also be affected by the changes. A good relationship, in which the couple feels able to share anxieties and fears, may minimise some of the difficulties in making the transition to parenthood.

Nausea and vomiting

These are said to affect over 50% of pregnancies. The cause is thought to be a combination of:

- hormonal changes
- psychological adjustments
- neurological factors.

The midwife may suggest remedies such as:

- eating a dry biscuit or cracker with a drink before rising in the morning
- avoiding spicy or pungent odours
- eating little and often (helps to maintain the body's blood sugar levels; drinking small amounts of fluid between meals will help to maintain hydration).

Other suggested remedies have included:

- the use of neurological devices, which transmit electrical stimulation via the wrist, and are thought to trigger sensory and neurological impulses that control vomiting
- complementary therapies, such as acupuncture and homeopathic and herbal remedies, which may be of benefit in minimising discomfort.

Nausea and vomiting generally improve around the 16th week of pregnancy. A small proportion of affected women will develop a more serious condition known as hyperemesis gravidarum, which requires urgent referral to a doctor.

Bladder and bowel function

Bladder and bowel function may be discussed. Dietary advice may be necessary at this visit or later in the pregnancy, with reference to how hormonal changes may alter normal bowel and kidney function. The midwife should be able to advise women on how to avoid constipation: for example, by taking a high-fibre diet and maintaining an adequate fluid intake. If constipation persists, then haemorrhoids may develop, caused by straining at defecation.

Vaginal discharge

Vaginal discharge increases in pregnancy; the woman may discuss any increase or changes with the midwife. Once the woman has identified what is normal she will then be able to report any changes to the midwife during subsequent visits.

- If the discharge is itchy, causes soreness, is any colour other than creamy-white or has an offensive odour, then infection is likely and should be investigated further.

- Later in pregnancy the woman may report a change from leucorrhoea to a heavier mucous discharge. Mucoid loss is evidence of cervical changes, and if it occurs before the 37th week, may be an early sign of preterm labour.

- The obstetrician will investigate vaginal bleeding during pregnancy; however, in early pregnancy spotting may occur at the time when menstruation would have been due.

- Early bleeding is not uncommon; the midwife should advise the woman to rest at this time and to avoid sexual intercourse until the pregnancy is more stable.

Abdominal examination

This should be performed at each antenatal visit (see below). At the initial assessment the midwife will observe for signs of pregnancy. It is unlikely that the uterus will be palpable abdominally before the 12th week of gestation. If it has previously been retroverted, it may not be palpable until the 16th week.

Oedema

This is not likely to be in evidence during the initial assessment but may occur as the pregnancy progresses. Physiological oedema occurs after rising in the morning and worsens during the day; it is often associated with daily activities or hot weather. At visits later in pregnancy the midwife should observe for oedema and ask the woman about symptoms.

Varicosities

These are more likely to occur during pregnancy and are a predisposing cause of deep vein thrombosis. The woman should be asked to report any tenderness that she feels either during the examination or at any time during the pregnancy. Advice about support tights can be offered.

Abdominal Examination

The abdominal examination is carried out to establish and affirm that fetal growth is consistent with gestational age during the progression of pregnancy. Specific aims are listed in Box 9.4.

Preparation

It is important for the midwife to expose only that area of the abdomen she needs to palpate; the remainder of the woman's body should be covered to enhance privacy. The bladder should be emptied. The woman should be lying comfortably with her arms by her sides to relax the abdominal muscles. She should then sit up to discuss the findings with the midwife.

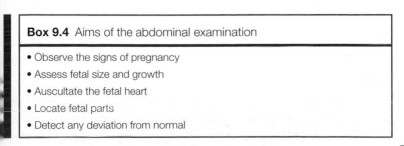

Box 9.4 Aims of the abdominal examination

- Observe the signs of pregnancy
- Assess fetal size and growth
- Auscultate the fetal heart
- Locate fetal parts
- Detect any deviation from normal

Method

Inspection

- The size of the uterus is assessed approximately by observation.

- The shape of the uterus is longer than it is broad when the lie of the fetus is longitudinal. If the lie is transverse, the uterus is low and broad.

- The multiparous uterus may lack the snug ovoid shape of the primigravid uterus. Often it is possible to see the shape of the fetal back or limbs.

- If the fetus is in an occipitoposterior position, a saucer-like depression may be seen at or below the umbilicus.

- The midwife may observe fetal movements or they may be felt by the mother; this can help the midwife determine the position of the fetus.

- Lax abdominal muscles in the multiparous woman may allow the uterus to sag forwards; this is known as *pendulous abdomen* or anterior obliquity of the uterus. In the primigravida it is a serious sign, as it may be due to pelvic contraction.

Skin changes

- Stretch marks known as *striae gravidarum* from previous pregnancies appear silvery and recent ones appear pink.

- A *linea nigra* may be seen; this is a normal dark line of pigmentation running longitudinally in the centre of the abdomen below and sometimes above the umbilicus.

- Scars may indicate previous obstetric or abdominal surgery.

Palpation

- To determine the height of the fundus the midwife places her hand just below the xiphisternum.

- Pressing gently, she moves her hand down the abdomen until she feels the curved upper border of the fundus, noting the number of fingerbreadths that can be accommodated between the two.

- Alternatively, the distance between the fundus and the symphysis pubis can be determined with a tape measure.

   The height of the fundus correlates well with gestational age, especially during the earlier weeks of pregnancy (Fig. 9.1).

- If the uterus is unduly big, the fetus may be large, but multiple pregnancy or polyhydramnios may be suspected.

- When the uterus is smaller than expected, the LMP date may be incorrect, or the fetus may be small for gestational age.

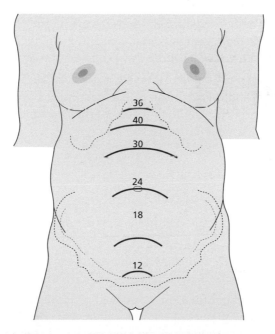

Fig. 9.1 Growth of the uterus, showing the fundal heights at various weeks of pregnancy.

Fundal palpation

This determines the presence of the breech or the head. This information will help to diagnose the lie and presentation of the fetus.

- Watching the woman's reaction to the procedure, the midwife lays both hands on the sides of the fundus, fingers held close together and curving round the upper border of the uterus.

- Gentle yet deliberate pressure is applied using the palmar surfaces of the fingers to determine the soft consistency and indefinite outline that denotes the breech. Sometimes the buttocks feel rather firm but they are not as hard, smooth or well defined as the head.

- With a gliding movement the fingertips are separated slightly in order to grasp the fetal mass, which may be in the centre or deflected to one side, to assess its size and mobility. The breech cannot be moved independently of the body, as the head can.

- The head is much more distinctive in outline than the breech, being hard and round; it can be balloted (moved from one hand to the other) between the fingertips of the two hands because of the free movement of the neck.

Lateral palpation

This is used to locate the fetal back in order to determine position.

- The hands are placed on either side of the uterus at the level of the umbilicus.

- Gentle pressure is applied with alternate hands in order to detect which side of the uterus offers the greater resistance.

- More detailed information is obtained by feeling along the length of each side with the fingers. This can be done by sliding the hands down the abdomen while feeling the sides of the uterus alternately.

- Some midwives prefer to steady the uterus with one hand and, using a rotary movement of the opposite hand, to map out the back as a continuous smooth resistant mass from the breech down to the neck; on the other side the same movement reveals the limbs as small parts that slip about under the examining fingers.

- 'Walking' the fingertips of both hands over the abdomen from one side to the other is an excellent method of locating the back. The fingers should be dipped deeply into the abdominal wall. The firm back can be distinguished from the fluctuating amniotic fluid and the receding knobbly small parts. To make the back more prominent, fundal pressure can be applied with one hand and the other used to 'walk' over the abdomen. Palpating from the neck upwards and inwards can locate the anterior shoulder.

Pelvic palpation

Pelvic palpation will identify the fetal presentation; however, as this can cause discomfort to the woman it is not recommended before 36 weeks.

- Ask the woman to bend her knees slightly in order to relax the abdominal muscles.

- Suggest that she breathe steadily; relaxation may be helped if she sighs out slowly.

- The sides of the uterus just below umbilical level are grasped snugly between the palms of the hands with the fingers held close together, and pointing downwards and inwards.

If the head is presenting, a hard mass with a distinctive round, smooth surface will be felt. The midwife should also estimate how much of the fetal head is palpable above the pelvic brim to determine engagement. The two-handed technique appears to be the more comfortable for the woman and gives the most information.

Pawlik's manœuvre is sometimes used to judge the size, flexion and mobility of the head but the midwife must be careful not to apply undue pressure. It should be used only if absolutely necessary. The midwife grasps the lower pole of the uterus between her fingers and thumb, which should be spread wide enough apart to accommodate the fetal head.

Auscultation

Routine auscultation of the fetal heart is not recommended; however, when requested by the mother it may provide some reassurance.

- A Pinard's stethoscope is placed on the mother's abdomen, at right angles to it over the fetal back (Fig. 9.2).

- The ear must be in close, firm contact with the stethoscope but the hand should not touch it while listening.

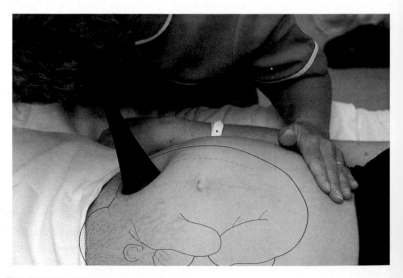

Fig. 9.2 Auscultation of the fetal heart.

- The stethoscope should be moved about until the point of maximum intensity is located where the fetal heart is heard most clearly.

- The midwife should count the beats per minute, which should be in the range of 110–160.

- The midwife should take the woman's pulse at the same time as listening to the fetal heart to enable her to distinguish between the two.

In addition, ultrasound equipment (e.g. a Sonicaid or Doppler) can be used for this purpose, so that the woman may also hear the fetal heartbeat.

Findings

The findings from the abdominal examination should be considered as part of the holistic picture of the pregnant woman. The midwife assesses all the information which she has gathered and critically evaluates the well-being of the mother and the fetus. Deviation from the expected growth and development should be referred to the obstetrician.

Gestational age

During pregnancy the uterus is expected to grow at a predicted rate and in early pregnancy uterine size will usually equate with the gestation estimated by dates. Later in pregnancy, increasing uterine size gives evidence of continuing fetal growth but is less reliable as an indicator of gestational age.

Multiple pregnancy increases the overall uterine size and should be diagnosed by 24 weeks' gestation. In a singleton pregnancy the fundus reaches the umbilicus at 22–24 weeks and the xiphisternum at 36 weeks. In the last month of pregnancy lightening occurs as the fetus sinks down into the lower pole of the uterus. The uterus becomes broader and the fundus lower. In the primigravida strong, supportive abdominal muscles encourage the fetal head to enter the brim of the pelvis.

Lie

The lie of the fetus is the relationship between the long axis of the fetus and the long axis of the uterus. In the majority of cases the lie is *longitudinal* owing to the ovoid shape of the uterus; the remainder are oblique or transverse.

Attitude

Attitude is the relationship of the fetal head and limbs to its trunk. The attitude should be one of flexion.

Presentation

Presentation refers to the part of the fetus that lies at the pelvic brim or in the lower pole of the uterus. Presentations can be:

- vertex
- breech
- shoulder
- face
- brow.

Vertex, face and brow are all head or cephalic presentations.

Denominator

The denominator is the name of the part of the presentation, which is used when referring to fetal position. Each presentation has a different denominator and these are as follows:

- In the vertex presentation it is the occiput.
- In the breech presentation it is the sacrum.
- In the face presentation it is the mentum.

Although the shoulder presentation is said to have the acromion process as its denominator, in practice the dorsum is used to describe the position. In the brow presentation no denominator is used.

Position

The position is the relationship between the denominator of the presentation and six points on the pelvic brim. In addition, the denominator may be found in the midline either anteriorly or posteriorly, especially late in labour. This position is often transient and is described as *direct anterior* or *direct posterior*.

Anterior positions are more favourable than posterior positions because, when the fetal back is in front, it conforms to the concavity of the mother's abdominal wall and can therefore flex more easily. When the back is flexed, the head also tends to flex and a smaller diameter presents to the pelvic brim. There is also more room in the anterior part of the pelvic brim for the broad biparietal diameter of the head.

The positions in a vertex presentation are summarised in Box 9.5 and Figures 9.3–9.8.

Box 9.5 Positions in a vertex presentation

Left occipitoanterior (LOA)

- The occiput points to the left iliopectineal eminence
- The sagittal suture is in the right oblique diameter of the pelvis (Fig. 9.3)

Right occipitoanterior (ROA)

- The occiput points to the right iliopectineal eminence
- The sagittal suture is in the left oblique diameter of the pelvis (Fig. 9.4)

Left occipitolateral (LOL)

- The occiput points to the left iliopectineal line midway between the iliopectineal eminence and the sacroiliac joint
- The sagittal suture is in the transverse diameter of the pelvis (Fig. 9.5)

Right occipitolateral (ROL)

- The occiput points to the right iliopectineal line midway between the iliopectineal eminence and the sacroiliac joint
- The sagittal suture is in the transverse diameter of the pelvis (Fig. 9.6)

(Continued)

Box 9.5 (Continued)

Left occipitoposterior (LOP)

- The occiput points to the left sacroiliac joint; the sagittal suture is in the left oblique diameter of the pelvis (Fig. 9.7)

Right occipitoposterior (ROP)

- The occiput points to the right sacroiliac joint; the sagittal suture is in the right oblique diameter of the pelvis (Fig. 9.8)

Direct occipitoanterior (DOA)

- The occiput points to the symphysis pubis; the sagittal suture is in the anteroposterior diameter of the pelvis

Direct occipitoposterior (DOP)

- The occiput points to the sacrum; the sagittal suture is in the anteroposterior diameter of the pelvis

In breech and face presentations the positions are described in a similar way using the appropriate denominator.

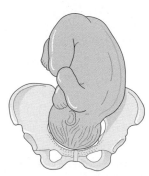 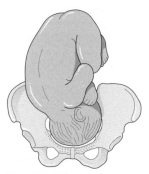

Fig. 9.3 Left occipitoanterior.　　**Fig. 9.4** Right occipitoanterior.

Engagement

Engagement is said to have occurred when the widest presenting transverse diameter has passed through the brim of the pelvis. In cephalic presentations this is the biparietal diameter, and in breech

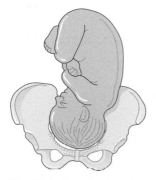

Fig. 9.5 Left occipitolateral.

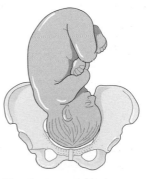

Fig. 9.6 Right occipitolateral.

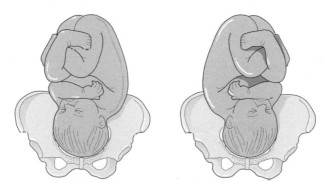

Fig. 9.7 Left occipitoposterior.   **Fig. 9.8** Right occipitoposterior.

presentations the bitrochanteric diameter. Engagement in a cephalic presentation demonstrates that the maternal pelvis is likely to be adequate for the size of the fetus and that the baby will birth vaginally.

In a primigravid woman the head normally engages at any time from about 36 weeks of pregnancy, but in a multipara this may not occur until after the onset of labour. When the vertex presents and the head is engaged the following will be evident on clinical examination:

■ Only two-fifths to three-fifths of the fetal head is palpable above the pelvic brim (Fig. 9.9).

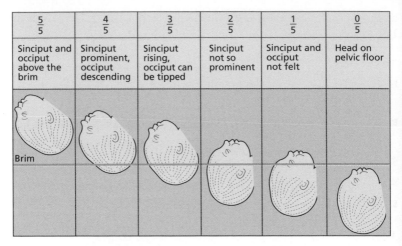

$\frac{5}{5}$	$\frac{4}{5}$	$\frac{3}{5}$	$\frac{2}{5}$	$\frac{1}{5}$	$\frac{0}{5}$
Sinciput and occiput above the brim	Sinciput prominent, occiput descending	Sinciput rising, occiput can be tipped	Sinciput not so prominent	Sinciput and occiput not felt	Head on pelvic floor

Fig. 9.9 Descent of the fetal head estimated in fifths palpable above the pelvic brim.

- The head is not mobile.

On rare occasions the head is not palpable abdominally because it has descended deeply into the pelvis. If the head is not engaged, the findings are as follows:

- More than half of the head is palpable above the brim.
- The head may be high and freely movable (ballotable) or partly settled in the pelvic brim and consequently immobile.

If the head does not engage in a primigravid woman at term, there is a possibility of a malposition or cephalopelvic disproportion. Referral to an obstetrician should be made.

Ongoing Antenatal Care

The information gathered during the antenatal visits will enable the midwife and pregnant woman to determine the appropriate pattern of antenatal care. The following schedule is based on guidelines from the UK's National Institute for Health and Clinical Excellence (NICE).

16 weeks

- Review, discuss and document results of screening tests undertaken at initial assessment.
- Investigate a haemoglobin level below 11 g/dl and consider iron supplementation.
- Measure blood pressure.
- Urinalysis for proteinuria.
- Information exchange and review of care plan.

18–20 weeks

- Ultrasound scan to detect fetal anomalies.

25 weeks

- Measure fundal height.
- Measure blood pressure.
- Urinalysis for proteinuria.
- Information exchange and review of care plan.

28 weeks

- Offer repeat screening for anaemia and atypical red-cell alloantibodies.
- Investigate a haemoglobin level below 10.5 g/dl and consider iron supplementation.
- Offer anti-D to Rh negative women.
- Measure fundal height.
- Measure blood pressure.
- Urinalysis for proteinuria.
- Information exchange and review of care plan.

31 weeks (nulliparous women)

- Measure fundal height.
- Measure blood pressure.
- Urinalysis for proteinuria.
- Review, discuss and document results of screening tests undertaken at 28-week assessment.
- Information exchange and review of care plan.

34 weeks

- Offer a second dose of anti-D to Rhesus negative women.
- Measure fundal height.
- Measure blood pressure.
- Urinalysis for proteinuria.
- *Multiparous women* — review, discuss and document results of screening tests undertaken at 28-week assessment.
- Information exchange and review of care plan.

36 weeks

- Measure blood pressure.
- Urinalysis for proteinuria.
- Measure fundal height.
- Check presentation of fetus; refer to obstetrician if breech.
- Information exchange and review of care plan.

38 weeks

- Measure blood pressure.
- Urinalysis for proteinuria.
- Measure fundal height.
- Information exchange and review of care plan.

40 weeks (nulliparous women)

- Measure blood pressure.
- Urinalysis for proteinuria.
- Measure fundal height.
- Information exchange and review of care plan.

41 weeks

- Measure blood pressure.
- Urinalysis for proteinuria.
- Measure fundal height.
- Information exchange and review of care plan.
- Offer a membrane sweep.
- Offer induction of labour.

Chapter 10

Specialised Fetal Investigations

Advances in technology mean that assessment of the fetus during pregnancy has become increasingly sophisticated and more widespread. Biochemical tests on maternal serum are commonly performed in order to identify which pregnancies carry a high risk of Down syndrome (trisomy 21) and ultrasound scanning is continually being refined. Therefore more potential abnormalities are identified in the antenatal period, which increases the number of mothers who may be defined as being at 'high risk' of having a fetal abnormality.

Psychological Aspects of Prenatal Testing

Prenatal testing is a two-edged sword. It enables midwives and doctors to give people choices that were unheard of in previous generations and that may prevent much suffering. However, in some circumstances they actually increase the amount of anxiety and psychological trauma experienced in pregnancy.

Anxiety caused by consideration of possible fetal abnormality may be accompanied by moral or religious dilemmas. This is because parents may be faced with several difficult decisions. For instance tests that can diagnose chromosomal or genetic abnormalities also

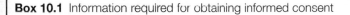

Box 10.1 Information required for obtaining informed consent

- Purpose of the procedure
- All risks and benefits to be reasonably expected
- Details of all possible future treatments that could arise as a consequence of testing
- Disclosure of all appropriate techniques that may be advantageous
- The option of refusing any tests
- The offer to answer any queries

---

carry a risk of procedure-induced miscarriage. Many parents agonise about whether to subject a potentially normal fetus to this risk in order to obtain this information. Parents may then need to consider whether they wish to terminate or continue with an affected pregnancy. Such dilemmas are an unfortunate but inevitable cost of the choices associated with the availability of some fetal investigations.

The Role of the Midwife

It will often be necessary for the midwife to present and discuss options with women, so that they can make a choice that best suits their circumstances and preferences (Box 10.1). The midwife must strive to obtain informed consent *before* any tests are undertaken.

Tests for Fetal Abnormality

Broadly speaking, there are two types of test for fetal anomaly. They are classified as:

- screening tests
- diagnostic tests.

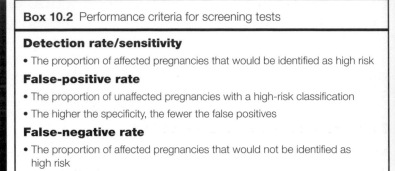

Box 10.2 Performance criteria for screening tests

Detection rate/sensitivity
• The proportion of affected pregnancies that would be identified as high risk

False-positive rate
• The proportion of unaffected pregnancies with a high-risk classification
• The higher the specificity, the fewer the false positives

False-negative rate
• The proportion of affected pregnancies that would not be identified as high risk
• The higher the sensitivity, the fewer the false negatives

Screening for fetal abnormality

Screening tests aim to identify a proportion of individuals (often around 5% of a population) who have the highest chances of a named disorder. This makes it possible to target further investigations towards those with the best indication. Mothers who undergo screening tests will be classified as above or below an action limit, whereby they are recalled and offered follow-up procedures.

The performance of a screening test is defined in a number of ways (Box 10.2).

Diagnosis of fetal abnormality

Diagnostic tests are performed in order to confirm or disprove the presence of a particular abnormality.

The Use of Ultrasound in Obstetrics

Most mothers undergo at least one ultrasound scan during pregnancy. This procedure can enable assessment and monitoring of many aspects of the pregnancy and is often presented as 'routine'. It can be used in order to screen for and to diagnose fetal abnormalities

Ultrasound works by transmitting sound at a very high pitch, via a probe, in a narrow beam. When the sound waves enter the body and encounter a structure, some of that sound is reflected back. The amount of sound reflected varies according to the type of tissue encountered. Generally, pictures are transmitted in 'real time', which enables fetal movements to be seen.

First trimester pregnancy scans

Many areas offer mothers a scan in early pregnancy, often around 12–14 weeks' gestation. The purpose of this is to establish:

- that the pregnancy is viable and intrauterine
- gestational age
- fetal number (and chorionicity or amnionicity in multiple pregnancies)
- detection of gross fetal abnormalities, such as anencephaly.

There is evidence to suggest that at least one scan is beneficial, mainly in reducing the need to induce labour for postmaturity. A gestation sac can usually be visualised from 5 weeks' gestation and a small embryo from 6 weeks. Until 13 weeks, gestational age can be accurately assessed by crown–rump length (CRL) measurement. Mothers are asked to attend with a full bladder, since this aids visualisation of the uterus at an early gestation.

Measurement of nuchal translucency at 10–14 weeks as a screen for Down syndrome

Information about the fetus can be gained by observation of the nuchal translucency (NT) at 10–14 weeks' gestation. This involves measuring the thickness of the subcutaneous collection of fluid at the back of the neck. Increased NT is used as a basis upon which to screen for Down syndrome. The main advantage of this test is that it offers an early way of assessing the mother's risk for Down syndrome. Increased NT is also associated with other structural (mainly cardiac) and genetic syndromes, and this enables increased pregnancy surveillance to be arranged. However, a disadvantage of this knowledge is that parents may suffer considerable anxiety until later scans offer some degree of reassurance.

Second trimester ultrasound scans

After 13 weeks of pregnancy, gestational age is primarily assessed using the biparietal diameter (BPD). It is a very useful measurement during the second trimester, but becomes less accurate towards the end of pregnancy because the shape of the head may alter. Limbs are also measured, most notably the femur.

The detailed fetal anomaly scan

This scan is usually performed at 18–22 weeks of pregnancy. Visualisation of fetal anatomy is more difficult before that time, although some ultrasound departments have very sophisticated equipment which can identify anomalies much earlier. The purpose of this scan is to reassure the mother that the fetus has no obvious structural abnormalities. Detection rates vary considerably, but it is thought that around 50% of significant abnormalities are identified at this time.

Some structural problems do not have associated sonographic signs and some fetal abnormalities may not appear until later in pregnancy. Diagnosis may therefore be missed.

Markers for chromosomal abnormality

Markers are minor sonographic clue signs that increase the chance that the fetus has a chromosomal abnormality. (Most are associated with Down syndrome.) The strength of association between each individual marker and Down syndrome varies considerably. When markers are identified, it is important to consider whether there are other risk factors, such as advancing maternal age or increased NT measurement at 10–14 weeks. The mother's aggregate risk for Down syndrome can then be calculated, taking all these factors into account.

Third trimester pregnancy scans

In general, late pregnancy scans are performed in response to a specific clinical need and not as a screen of the low-risk pregnant population. However, fetal abnormalities may come to light or be reassessed at this time. Many late scans are performed as a means of monitoring fetal well-being, growth and development.

Fetal growth

Many scans are performed in order to detect instances when growth deviates from normal.

- Fetuses with excessive growth (*macrosomia*) have increased perinatal mortality and morbidity.
- Fetuses may be small because they are preterm or because they are small for dates.

Sometimes, these two problems overlap.

In general, growth-restricted babies can be divided into two groups:

- those with symmetrical growth restriction
- those with asymmetrical growth restriction.

Symmetrical growth restriction

Most symmetrically small fetuses are entirely normal and may be genetically predetermined to be small. However, in some instances this may be caused by chromosomal abnormalities, infection or environmental factors such as maternal substance misuse.

Asymmetrical growth restriction

These fetuses have a head size appropriate for gestational age, but thin bodies. This is generally caused by placental insufficiency. Glycogen stores in the liver are reduced, so there are fewer energy reserves for the fetus during labour. Asymmetrically growth-restricted fetuses are therefore more likely to suffer antenatal or perinatal asphyxia, or both. Other potential problems include hypoglycaemia, hypothermia and premature birth.

In order to assess fetal growth, the gestational age must be accurately assessed on scan before 24 weeks. Women at high risk of having an abnormally grown fetus should have serial scans — often at 28, 32 and 36 weeks. Where there is a particular concern, growth may be measured every 2 weeks. The most important measurements are head circumference and abdominal circumference. In this way, trends in fetal growth can be assessed.

Doppler ultrasonography

In recent years, there have been major developments in the use of Doppler ultrasound techniques for the study of maternal and fetal circulation. Abnormalities in Doppler measurements may be detected before growth becomes impaired and can be used as a prognostic indicator.

Biophysical profiling

Another ultrasound measure of fetal well-being is the fetal biophysical profile. This is used to determine whether there are signs of fetal hypoxia or compromised placental function, or both. A score is calculated on the basis of five criteria (Box 10.3).

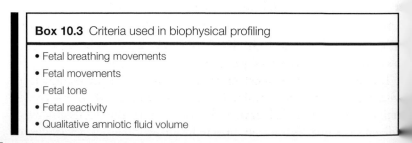

Box 10.3 Criteria used in biophysical profiling

- Fetal breathing movements
- Fetal movements
- Fetal tone
- Fetal reactivity
- Qualitative amniotic fluid volume

Findings from growth scans, biophysical profile scores and cardiotocography (CTG) recordings should be considered collectively, taking into account the full clinical picture and obstetric history.

Screening for Fetal Abnormality from Maternal Serum

Neural tube defect screening

Alpha fetoprotein (AFP) is present in fetal serum and amniotic fluid by 6 weeks' gestation. Thereafter, the levels alter according to gestation. When the fetus has an open neural tube defect, AFP can escape in increased amounts, causing levels to be raised in maternal serum. A blood sample from the mother at 15–18 weeks' gestation has a detection rate of 98%. Since the AFP level varies according to gestational age, it is important to assess the gestation accurately before results can be reliably interpreted.

Down syndrome screening from maternal serum

A variety of biochemical markers in maternal serum have been used, in order to assess the risk of Down syndrome. The most common ones are:

- AFP (reduced in many affected pregnancies)
- HCG (which is usually raised)
- unconjugated oestriol (uE_3, which is usually low).

If all three markers are used, this is called the *triple test*. If only AFP and HCG are used, this is called the *double test*. Maternal blood is sampled at 15–18 weeks' gestation.

The levels of biochemical markers are considered in conjunction with maternal age. A combined risk is then calculated. If this risk is greater than a specified limit (often 1 in 250), the mother is considered to be in a high-risk group and is offered further diagnostic tests.

Invasive Diagnostic Tests

If mothers are found to have an increased risk of chromosomal or genetic problems, they may wish to undergo a diagnostic procedure. The two most frequently used tests are:

- chorionic villus sampling (CVS)
- amniocentesis.

These tests provide the opportunity to examine the fetal karyotype (the number and structure of chromosomes, visible through a microscope during mitotic metaphase) or for DNA analysis for particular gene mutations, or both.

Chorionic villus sampling

CVS is the acquisition of chorionic villi (placental tissue) under continuous ultrasound guidance. This may be performed at any stage after 10 weeks of pregnancy.

Access may be achieved transcervically (until 13 weeks' gestation) or via the transabdominal route.

The main advantage of CVS is that this is the earliest way mothers can obtain definitive information about the chromosomal/genetic status of the fetus. The main disadvantage with CVS is the procedure-induced risk of miscarriage, which is 0.5–2%.

Amniocentesis

This is usually performed after 15 weeks' gestation, as early amniocentesis has a higher loss rate than early CVS. The procedure involves transabdominal insertion of a fine needle into the amniotic fluid cavity, under continuous ultrasound guidance; 15 ml of amniotic fluid are aspirated. Cytogenetic, molecular (DNA) and biochemical analyses are possible. Amniocytes are often examined. These comprise cells that have been shed from several fetal sites, including skin, lungs and renal tract. The risk of procedure-induced miscarriage is 1%.

Recent advances in cytogenetic techniques mean that mothers can obtain an initial set of results (usually for Down syndrome) and then a full culture result after 2–3 weeks. This involves the use of fluorescent in-situ hybridisation (FISH), whereby a specific probe 'paints' the chromosomes to be examined. Cells are examined to determine whether there are two or three signals for this chromosome. Two is the normal count, whereas three indicates Down syndrome.

Fetal blood sampling

The use of this technique has declined in recent years because improved molecular and cytogenetic techniques allow more diagnoses to be made from chorionic villi or amniotic fluid. However, fetal blood may be advantageous when there are ambiguous findings from placental tissue. Also, when there is Rhesus isoimmunisation, it may be necessary to determine the fetal haemoglobin. When this is low, an intrauterine transfusion may be performed. Blood can be sampled from the umbilical cord or intrahepatic umbilical vein; the latter is less risky. The loss rate also depends upon the gestation and condition of the fetus. In uncomplicated procedures after 20 weeks, the loss rate is around 1%.

Chapter 11

Abnormalities of Early Pregnancy

Bleeding in Pregnancy

Vaginal bleeding during pregnancy is abnormal. It is a cause of concern to mothers, particularly those who have had a previous experience of fetal loss. If the woman presents with a history of bleeding in the current pregnancy, it is important to establish when it occurred. How much blood was lost, the colour of the loss and whether it was associated with any pain should be noted. If the symptoms have subsided, it is important to advise the mother to report any recurrence.

Assessment of fetal condition will depend on gestation. Ultrasound scanning can confirm viability of the pregnancy before heart sounds are audible or movements felt. In the second trimester the use of ultrasound equipment can elicit the heart sounds, and note of fetal movements may also be made.

Implantation bleeding

As the trophoblast erodes the endometrial epithelium and the blastocyst implants, a small vaginal blood loss may be apparent to the woman. It occurs around the time of expected menstruation and may be mistaken for a period, although lighter. It is of significance if the estimated date of delivery is to be calculated from menstrual history.

Cervical ectropion

This condition is commonly and erroneously known as a cervical erosion. High levels of oestrogen cause proliferation of columnar epithelial cells, found in the cervical canal. These occupy a wider area, including the vaginal aspect of the cervix, encroaching on the squamous epithelial cells (metaplasia). The junction between is everted into the vagina. This ectropion is a physiological response to the hormonal changes in pregnancy. As the cells are vascular it may cause intermittent blood-stained loss, or spontaneous bleeding particularly following sexual intercourse. Normally, treatment is not required in pregnancy and the ectropion will usually disappear during the puerperium.

Cervical polyps

Small, vascular pedunculated growths attached to the cervix may bleed during pregnancy. They can be visualised on speculum examination and no treatment is required during pregnancy, unless bleeding is profuse or a cervical smear suggests malignancy.

Carcinoma of the cervix

Carcinoma of the cervix is the most frequently diagnosed cancer in pregnancy. It is a treatable condition if detected early.

Cervical intraepithelial neoplasia (CIN) is the precursor to invasive cancer of the cervix. If the condition is detected at this stage, treatment can be given and the cytology reverts to normal. The principal screening test used is the Papanicolaou smear (Pap smear).

Types

There are two main types of cervical cancer:

- squamous cell carcinoma
- adenocarcinoma.

The latter is less common.

Clinical presentation

- Bleeding is the most common symptom.
- Vaginal discharge is the next most common.

As symptoms may be mistakenly diagnosed as symptoms of pregnancy, there may be delay in diagnosis.

Investigation

- A Papanicolaou smear test will detect atypical cells on the surface of the cervix, or within the endocervix.
- When changes are detected, a repeat smear test, followed by colposcopy, is indicated.
- Biopsies can be taken to reveal the extent of the lesion.

As with any investigation, the mother and her partner should be fully informed about any tests and treatments that are offered. She should be aware of when and from whom results will be available. Adequate time should be made to ensure that the results are discussed in a non-hurried manner. A positive test result following a smear test will cause anxiety to the mother and her family and it is important that accurate information is available, along with supportive counselling.

Treatment

Treatment depends on the stage of the disease and gestation. Laser treatment or cryotherapy following colposcopy can be carried out on an outpatient basis and will result in the destruction of the abnormal area of cells.

Cone biopsy under general anaesthesia involves excision of cervical tissue and is both a diagnostic tool and a treatment, but it may increase the risk to the mother. The cervix is highly vascular in pregnancy and the risk of haemorrhage is high, as is the possibility of causing the mother to miscarry. Delaying treatment until the end of pregnancy is an option for women who are found to have early changes in cervical cytology.

If the changes to the cervix are advanced and diagnosis is made in the first or second trimester, the mother may have to make a choice as to whether to terminate the pregnancy in order to undergo treatment. If diagnosis is made later in pregnancy, a decision to deliver the fetus may be taken to allow the mother to commence treatment.

Spontaneous miscarriage

Spontaneous miscarriage is defined as the involuntary loss of the products of conception prior to 24 weeks' gestation.

Incidence

Fifteen per cent of all confirmed pregnancies are said to result in miscarriages, the majority of which happen in the first trimester. The different types of spontaneous miscarriage (abortion) have varying signs and symptoms (Fig. 11.1 and Table 11.1).

Sequelae to early pregnancy loss

- All staff should pay particular attention to avoiding the use medical jargon that cannot be understood by the client. Language should be appropriate, avoiding terms such as 'products' or 'scrape', recognising that most women will be grieving for the lost baby.
- Regardless of gestation, the parents may want to see and hold the baby. Some parents may want to see the loss when there is no body and should be given the opportunity to do so.

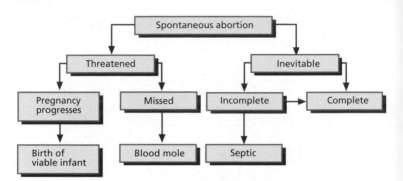

Fig. 11.1 Spontaneous miscarriage: summary of key practice points.

- Creation of memories is important for the grieving process, and midwives can assist by taking photographs of the baby for the parents, and by providing a letter or certificate to confirm the loss.

- Parents need information on how the remains will be disposed of. Under 24 weeks' gestation the baby is not registrable in the UK; it is therefore not a legal requirement for the baby to be buried or cremated but nevertheless respectful disposal is paramount. At no time should any fetal remains be included with hospital clinical waste. Parents may wish to take the remains home; burial in a garden is not precluded in this instance. If cremation is considered, then midwives should be aware that the size of the fetus may result in few ashes, if any.

- Full written consent must be given by the mother for postmortem or any other investigations involving fetal tissue. Follow-up after miscarriage is needed, with parents being given the opportunity to receive further information about their loss and be offered advice regarding future pregnancies.

Induced abortion

Termination of pregnancy before 24 weeks' gestation is legal in the UK within the terms of current legislation.

Table 11.1 Signs of miscarriage

Signs and symptoms	Threatened miscarriage	Inevitable miscarriage	Incomplete miscarriage	Complete miscarriage	Delayed miscarriage	Septic miscarriage
Pain	Variable	Severe/rhythmical	Severe	Diminishing/none	None	Severe/variable
Bleeding	Scanty	Heavy/clots	Heavy profuse	Minimal/none	Some spotting possible Brown loss	Variable May smell offensive
Cervical os	Closed	Open	Open	Closed	Closed	Open
Uterus (if palpable)	Soft, no tenderness	Tender, may be smaller than expected	Tender/painful	Firm, contracted	Smaller than expected	Bulky/tender/painful
Additional signs and symptoms			Tissue present in cervix Shock			

Methods

- Abortion can be carried out in the first trimester, using vacuum aspiration, dilatation and evacuation under general anaesthetic. Medical methods using mifepristone and prostaglandin are licensed for use up to the 63rd day from the first day of a woman's last menstrual period.

- In the second trimester, medical methods are used. Extrauterine prostaglandin, accompanied by large doses of oxytocin, produces uterine contractions. The mother experiences labour pains and the process may be protracted.

- Prophylactic antibiotics may be given following termination, and for non-sensitised Rhesus negative women, anti-D immunoglobulin is recommended.

Recurrent miscarriage

Recurrent miscarriage is defined as the loss of three or more consecutive pregnancies. The incidence of recurrent miscarriage suggests that there are significant underlying causes and the loss of the pregnancy is not chance. Factors associated with recurrent miscarriage are listed in Box 11.1. In many cases no causative factor is identified. Women should be referred to specialist clinics where a screening service is available.

Box 11.1 Some factors associated with recurrent miscarriage

- Genetic causes
- Immunological factors
- Hypersecretion of LH
- Infection
- Structural anomalies

Cervical incompetence

Cervical incompetence describes painless dilatation of the cervix in the second or early third trimester, allowing bulging membranes through the cervical os into the vagina. Miscarriage or preterm birth may occur if the membranes rupture. Cervical incompetence recurs in subsequent pregnancies.

Causes

- Trauma to the cervix during dilatation and curettage or induced abortion.
- Cone biopsy or congenital weakness of the cervix.

Treatment

Treatment for subsequent pregnancies by cervical cerclage remains controversial. If undertaken, it is carried out after the risk of early miscarriage is thought to be past. At 14 weeks' gestation a non-absorbable suture may be inserted at the level of the internal os. This remains in situ until 38 weeks or the onset of labour, when it is removed.

The use of the term 'cervical incompetence' is now questioned because of the negative context it engenders.

Ectopic Pregnancy

An ectopic pregnancy is one where implantation occurs at a site other than the uterine cavity. Sites can include:

- the uterine tube
- an ovary
- the cervix
- the abdomen.

Women require prompt, appropriate treatment for this life-threatening condition. Midwives need to consider the possibility of

---

Box 11.2 Risk factors for ectopic pregnancy

- Previous ectopic pregnancy
- Previous surgery on the uterine tube
- Exposure to diethylstilboestrol in utero
- Congenital abnormalities of the tube
- Previous infection including chlamydia, gonorrhoea and pelvic inflammatory disease
- Use of intrauterine contraceptive devices
- Assisted reproductive techniques

Box 11.3 Signs of ectopic pregnancy

Typical signs
- Localised/abdominal pain
- Amenorrhoea
- Vaginal bleeding or spotting

Atypical signs
- Shoulder pain
- Abdominal distension
- Nausea, vomiting
- Dizziness, fainting

---

ectopic pregnancy being responsible for unexplained abdominal pain and bleeding in early pregnancy.

Risk factors for ectopic pregnancy

Any of the alterations of the normal function of the uterine tube in transporting the gametes listed in Box 11.2 contributes to the risk of ectopic pregnancy.

Clinical presentation (Box 11.3)

Tubal pregnancy rarely remains asymptomatic beyond 8 weeks.

- Pelvic pain can be severe.
- Acute symptoms are the result of tubal rupture and relate to the degree of haemorrhage there has been.
- Ultrasound enables an accurate diagnosis of tubal pregnancy, making management more proactive.
- Vaginal ultrasound, combined with the use of sensitive blood and urine tests which detect the presence of HCG, helps to ensure diagnosis is made earlier.
- If the tube ruptures, shock may ensue; therefore resuscitation, followed by laparotomy, is needed.
- The mother should be offered follow-up support and information regarding subsequent pregnancies.

Gestational Trophoblastic Disease

Gestational trophoblastic disease is a general term covering:
- hydatidiform mole (benign)
- choriocarcinoma (malignant).

Hydatidiform mole

Hydatidiform mole applies to a gross malformation of the trophoblast in which the chorionic villi proliferate and become avascular. They are found in the cavity of the uterus and, very rarely, within uterine tube. As this condition can lead to the development of cancer, accurate diagnosis, treatment and follow-up are essential.

Two forms of mole have been identified:
- complete hydatidiform mole
- partial mole.

The complete form carries an increased risk of choriocarcinoma.

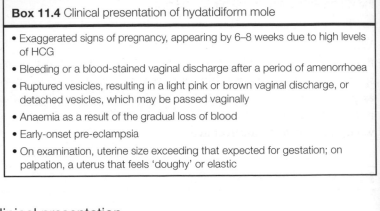

Box 11.4 Clinical presentation of hydatidiform mole

- Exaggerated signs of pregnancy, appearing by 6–8 weeks due to high levels of HCG
- Bleeding or a blood-stained vaginal discharge after a period of amenorrhoea
- Ruptured vesicles, resulting in a light pink or brown vaginal discharge, or detached vesicles, which may be passed vaginally
- Anaemia as a result of the gradual loss of blood
- Early-onset pre-eclampsia
- On examination, uterine size exceeding that expected for gestation; on palpation, a uterus that feels 'doughy' or elastic

Clinical presentation

See Box 11.4. Diagnosis is confirmed by ultrasound scan and serum HCG levels.

Treatment

The aim of treatment is to remove all trophoblast tissue. In some cases the hydatidiform mole aborts spontaneously. Where this does not occur, vacuum aspiration or dilatation and curettage is necessary. Spontaneous expulsion of the mole carries less risk of malignant change.

All women who have been treated for hydatidiform mole in the UK are recorded on a central register. Women confirmed as having a complete mole require follow-up over a 2-year period. Pregnancy should be avoided during the follow-up period. IUCDs are contra-indicated and hormonal methods of contraception should not be used until levels of HCG have returned to normal.

Administration of anti-D immunoglobulin in early pregnancy

Significant fetomaternal haemorrhage can occur following early pregnancy loss; therefore anti-D immunoglobulin should be administered to reduce the risk of isoimmunisation in Rhesus negative women.

Retroversion of the Uterus

When the long axis of the uterus is directed backwards during pregnancy, the uterus is said to be retroverted. In most cases it corrects spontaneously, the uterus rising out of the pelvis into the abdomen as pregnancy progresses, and there are no further problems. If the retroverted uterus fails to rise out of the pelvic cavity by the 14th week, it is said to be incarcerated.

Fibroids (Leiomyomas)

These are firm, benign tumours of muscular and fibrous tissue, ranging in size from very small to very large.

Effect of pregnancy on fibroids

Fibroids do not significantly increase in size during pregnancy; however, they may become more vascular and oedematous, making it softer and more difficult to detect on palpation.

Effect of fibroids on pregnancy

- Early pregnancy loss is associated with submucosal fibroids. Outcome of pregnancy is dependent on the position of the fibroid.

- Lesser effects include mild abdominal pain.

- Fibroids located in the lower segment or on the cervix can prevent descent of the fetal head, causing malpresentation and obstructed labour and resulting in the need for caesarean section.

- Severe postpartum haemorrhage may be caused if the fibroids prevent the complete separation of the placenta or contraction of the uterus. In anticipation of this, blood should be available for urgent cross-matching.

Removal of fibroids during caesarean section should be avoided because of the risk of profuse haemorrhage.

Red degeneration of fibroids

Degeneration of a fibroid occurs if a rapidly growing fibroid exceeds the available blood supply.

Hyperemesis Gravidarum

Excessive nausea and vomiting that start between 4 and 10 weeks' gestation, resolve before 20 weeks, and require intervention are known as hyperemesis gravidarum. The aetiology of hyperemesis is uncertain, with multifactorial causes such as endocrine, gastrointestinal and psychological factors proposed. Rising levels of oestrogen and HCG appear to be significant.

Diagnosis is made where there is a history of persistent, severe nausea and vomiting in early pregnancy; causes of vomiting not due to pregnancy need to be excluded. A mother suspected of suffering from hyperemesis presents as being unable to retain food or fluids. She may have lost weight, and be distressed and debilitated by her symptoms. The impact of nausea and vomiting on the woman and her daily life should not be underestimated. The woman requires admission to hospital for assessment and for management of symptoms.

Clinical presentation

- A history of the frequency and severity of the bouts of vomiting is taken.
- The mother's appearance is noted, including any dryness or inelasticity of the skin. In severe cases jaundice may be apparent.
- Additional signs of dehydration, such as rapid pulse, low blood pressure and dry furred tongue, may be seen.
- The mother's breath may smell of acetone, a sign of ketosis.

- Elevated haematocrit, alterations in electrolyte levels and ketonuria are associated with dehydration.

Management

- Hypovolaemia and electrolyte imbalance are corrected by intravenous infusion.

- Vitamin supplements can be given parenterally, particularly where hyperemesis has been prolonged.

- Initially nothing is given by mouth, to allow time for the vomiting to be controlled.

- Fluids and diet are gradually reintroduced as the woman's condition improves, but this is closely monitored.

- Antiemetics may be prescribed.

Chapter 12

Problems of Pregnancy

Abdominal Pain in Pregnancy

Abdominal pain is a common complaint in pregnancy. It is probably suffered by all women at some stage, and therefore presents a problem for the midwife of how to distinguish between:

- the physiologically normal (e.g. mild indigestion or muscle stretching)
- the pathological but not dangerous (e.g. degeneration of a fibroid)
- the dangerously pathological requiring immediate referral to the appropriate medical practitioner for urgent treatment (e.g. ectopic pregnancy or appendicitis).

The midwife should take a detailed history and perform a physical examination in order to reach a decision about whether to refer the woman. Treatment will depend on the cause (Box 12.1) and the maternal and fetal conditions.

Uterine fibroid degeneration

Uterine fibroid degeneration may cause recurrent acute pain during pregnancy and is due to a diminished blood supply that may cause central core necrosis of a fibroid or fibroids.

Box 12.1 Causes of abdominal pain in pregnancy

Pregnancy-specific causes

Physiological
- Heartburn, excessive vomiting, constipation
- Round ligament pain
- Severe uterine torsion
- Braxton Hicks contractions
- Miscellaneous discomfort in late pregnancy

Pathological
- Ectopic pregnancy
- Miscarriage
- Uterine fibroids
- Placental abruption
- Preterm labour
- Severe pre-eclampsia
- Uterine rupture

Incidental causes

Common pathology
- Appendicitis
- Intestinal obstruction
- Cholecystitis
- Inflammatory bowel disease
- Peptic ulcer
- Renal disease
- Ovarian pathology, e.g. torsion
- Acute pancreatitis
- Urinary tract infection
- Malaria
- Tuberculosis (may be associated with HIV infection)

Rare pathology
- Rectus haematoma
- Sickle-cell crisis
- Porphyria
- Arteriovenous haemorrhage
- Malignant disease

Management

- Rest and analgesia are required.
- Be aware that enlargement of the fibroid may occasionally impede the progress of labour and lead to rupture of the uterus.

Severe uterine torsion

Severe uterine torsion refers to rotation of the uterus by more than 90º, which may cause pain in the latter half of pregnancy.

Management

- Bed rest is necessary, altering the maternal position to correct the torsion spontaneously
- Analgesia is required.
- In severe cases a laparotomy will need to be performed in order for a clear diagnosis to be made.
- Delivery by caesarean section may be performed, either preceded or followed by manipulation of the uterus.

Symphysis pubis dysfunction (diastasis symphysis pubis)

This refers to abnormal relaxation of ligaments, causing increased mobility of the pubic joint. The woman may complain of pain at any time from the 28th week of pregnancy.

Management

- Reduce non-essential weight-bearing activities and avoid straddle movements that abduct the hips, e.g. squatting.
- A supportive panty girdle or 'tubigrip' and comfortable shoes may help when the woman is up and about.
- Refer to an obstetric physiotherapist for advice and treatment.

- In severe cases, bed rest on a firm mattress may be necessary.
- Postnatal physiotherapy will aid the strengthening and stabilisation of the joint.

Antepartum Haemorrhage (APH)

Antepartum haemorrhage is bleeding from the genital tract after the 24th week of gestation and before the onset of labour.

Effect on the fetus

Fetal mortality and morbidity are increased as a result of severe vaginal bleeding in pregnancy. Stillbirth or neonatal death may occur. Premature placental separation and consequent hypoxia may result in severe neurological damage in the baby.

Effect on the mother

If bleeding is severe, it may be accompanied by shock and disseminated intravascular coagulation (DIC). The mother may die or be left with permanent ill health.

Types of APH (Table 12.1)

- Bleeding from local lesions of the genital tract (*incidental causes*).
- Placental separation due to *placenta praevia* or *placental abruption*.

Initial appraisal of a woman with APH

APH is unpredictable and the woman's condition can deteriorate rapidly at any time. A rapid decision about the urgency of need for a medical or paramedic presence, or both, must be made, often at the same time as observing and talking to the woman and her partner.

Table 12.1 Causes of bleeding in late pregnancy

Cause	Incidence (%)
Placenta praevia	31.0
Abruption	22.0
'Unclassified bleeding', e.g.	47.0
Marginal	
Show	
Cervicitis	
Trauma	
Vulvovaginal varicosities	
Genital tumours	
Genital infections	
Haematuria	
Vasa praevia	
Other	

Assessment of physical condition

Maternal condition

- Take a history from the woman.
- Observe pulse rate, respiratory rate, blood pressure and temperature.
- Look for any pallor or breathlessness.
- Assess the amount of blood lost.
- Perform a gentle abdominal examination, observing for signs that the woman is going into labour.
- *On no account must any vaginal or rectal examination be done; nor may an enema or suppository be given to a woman suffering from an APH.*

Fetal condition

■ The mother should be asked if the baby has been moving as much as normal.

■ Attempt to auscultate the fetal heart; ultrasound apparatus made be used in order to obtain information.

Factors to aid differential diagnosis

The location of the placenta is perhaps the most critical piece of information that will be needed in order to make a correct diagnosis; initially, the midwife may not have this fact at her disposal. However, if she is able to elicit the information listed in Box 12.2 from her

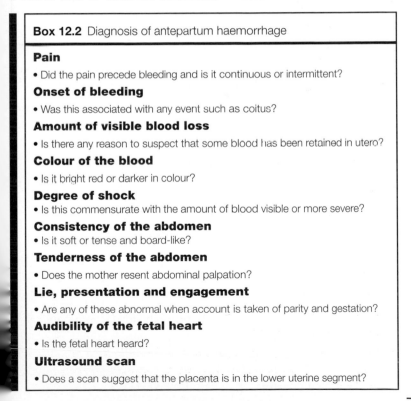

Box 12.2 Diagnosis of antepartum haemorrhage

Pain
• Did the pain precede bleeding and is it continuous or intermittent?

Onset of bleeding
• Was this associated with any event such as coitus?

Amount of visible blood loss
• Is there any reason to suspect that some blood has been retained in utero?

Colour of the blood
• Is it bright red or darker in colour?

Degree of shock
• Is this commensurate with the amount of blood visible or more severe?

Consistency of the abdomen
• Is it soft or tense and board-like?

Tenderness of the abdomen
• Does the mother resent abdominal palpation?

Lie, presentation and engagement
• Are any of these abnormal when account is taken of parity and gestation?

Audibility of the fetal heart
• Is the fetal heart heard?

Ultrasound scan
• Does a scan suggest that the placenta is in the lower uterine segment?

observations and from talking to the woman and her partner, then this will help her to arrive at a provisional diagnosis.

Supportive treatment

- Provide emotional reassurance.
- Give rapid fluid replacement (warmed) with a plasma expander, and later with whole blood if necessary.
- Give analgesia.
- If at home, arrange transfer to hospital.
- Subsequent management depends on the definite diagnosis.

Placenta praevia

In this condition the placenta is partially or wholly implanted in the lower uterine segment on either the anterior or posterior wall.

The lower uterine segment grows and stretches progressively after the 12th week of pregnancy. In later weeks this may cause the placenta to separate and severe bleeding can occur.

Degrees of placenta praevia

See Box 12.3.

Indications of placenta praevia

Bleeding from the vagina is the only sign and it is painless. The uterus is not tender or tense. The presence of placenta praevia should be considered when:

- the fetal head is not engaged in a primigravida (after 36 weeks)
- there is a malpresentation, especially breech
- the lie is oblique or transverse
- the lie is unstable, usually in a multigravida.

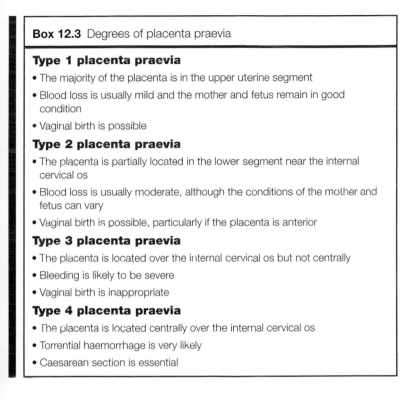

Box 12.3 Degrees of placenta praevia

Type 1 placenta praevia
- The majority of the placenta is in the upper uterine segment
- Blood loss is usually mild and the mother and fetus remain in good condition
- Vaginal birth is possible

Type 2 placenta praevia
- The placenta is partially located in the lower segment near the internal cervical os
- Blood loss is usually moderate, although the conditions of the mother and fetus can vary
- Vaginal birth is possible, particularly if the placenta is anterior

Type 3 placenta praevia
- The placenta is located over the internal cervical os but not centrally
- Bleeding is likely to be severe
- Vaginal birth is inappropriate

Type 4 placenta praevia
- The placenta is located centrally over the internal cervical os
- Torrential haemorrhage is very likely
- Caesarean section is essential

Localisation of the placenta using ultrasonic scanning will confirm the existence of placenta praevia and establish its degree.

Management of placenta praevia

The management of placenta praevia depends on:
- the amount of bleeding
- the condition of mother and fetus
- the location of the placenta
- the stage of the pregnancy.

> **Box 12.4** Predisposing factors in placental abruption
>
> - Pregnancy-induced hypertension
> - A sudden reduction in uterine size: e.g. when the membranes rupture or after the birth of a first twin
> - Direct trauma to the abdomen
> - High parity
> - Previous caesarean section
> - Cigarette smoking

Placental abruption

Premature separation of a normally situated placenta occurring after the 24th week of pregnancy is referred to as *placental abruption*.

The aetiology is not always clear; some predisposing factors are listed in Box 12.4.

Blood loss may be:

- revealed
- concealed
- mixed.

Management of different degrees of placental abruption

Mild separation of the placenta

In this case the placental separation and the haemorrhage are slight. Mother and fetus are in a stable condition. There is no indication of maternal shock and the fetus is alive with normal heart sounds. The consistency of the uterus is normal and there is no tenderness on abdominal palpation.

- An ultrasound scan can determine the placental location and identify any degree of concealed bleeding.
- Fetal condition should be assessed while bleeding persists by frequent or continuous monitoring of the fetal heart rate.

Subsequently, CTG should be carried out once or twice daily.

- If the woman is not in labour and the gestation is less than 37 weeks she may be cared for in an antenatal ward for a few days. She may then go home if there is no further bleeding and the placenta has been found to be in the upper uterine segment.

- Women who have passed the 37th week of pregnancy may be offered induction of labour, especially if there has been more than one episode of mild bleeding.

- Further heavy bleeding or evidence of fetal distress may indicate that a caesarean section is necessary.

Moderate separation of the placenta

This describes placental separation of about one-quarter. A considerable amount of blood may be lost, some of which will escape from the vagina and some of which will be retained as a retroplacental clot or an extravasation into the uterine muscle. The mother will be shocked, with a raised pulse rate and a lowered blood pressure. There will be a degree of uterine tenderness and abdominal guarding. The fetus may be alive, although hypoxic; intrauterine death is also a possibility.

The immediate aims of care are to reduce shock and to replace blood loss:

- Fluid replacement should be monitored with the aid of a central venous pressure line.

- The fetal condition should be assessed with continuous CTG if the fetus is alive, in which case immediate caesarean section may be indicated once the woman's condition is stabilised.

If the fetus is in good condition or has already died, vaginal birth may be contemplated. Such a birth is advantageous because it enables the uterus to contract and control the bleeding. The spontaneous onset of labour frequently accompanies moderately severe placental abruption, but if it does not, then amniotomy is usually sufficient to induce labour. Oxytocin may be used with great care, if necessary. Delivery is often quite sudden after a short labour. The use of drugs to attempt to stop labour is usually inappropriate.

Severe separation of the placenta

This is an acute obstetric emergency; at least two-thirds of the placenta has become detached and 2000 ml of blood or more are lost from the circulation. Most or all of the blood can be concealed behind the placenta. The woman will be severely shocked, perhaps to a degree far beyond what might be expected from the amount of visible blood loss. The blood pressure will be lowered; the reading may lie within the normal range owing to a preceding hypertension. The fetus will almost certainly be dead. The woman will have very severe abdominal pain with excruciating tenderness; the uterus has a board-like consistency.

Features associated with severe haemorrhage are:

- coagulation defects
- renal failure
- pituitary failure.

Treatment is the same as for moderate haemorrhage.

- Whole blood should be transfused rapidly and subsequent amounts calculated in accordance with the woman's central venous pressure.

- Labour may begin spontaneously in advance of amniotomy and the midwife should be alert for signs of uterine contraction causing periodic intensifying of the abdominal pain.

- However, if bleeding continues or a compromised fetal heart rate is present, caesarean section may be required as soon as the woman's condition has been adequately stabilised.

- The woman requires constant explanation and psychological support, despite the fact that, because of her shocked condition, she may not be fully conscious.

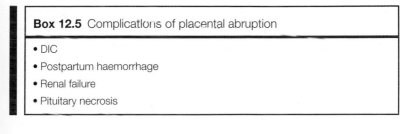

> **Box 12.5** Complications of placental abruption
>
> - DIC
> - Postpartum haemorrhage
> - Renal failure
> - Pituitary necrosis

- Pain relief must also be considered.
- The woman's partner will also be very concerned, and should not be forgotten in the rush to stabilise the woman's condition.

Complications

See Box 12.5.

Blood Coagulation Failure

Disseminated intravascular coagulation (DIC)

This is a situation of inappropriate coagulation within the blood vessels, which leads to the consumption of clotting factors. As a result clotting fails to occur at the bleeding site. DIC is rare when the fetus is alive and it usually starts to resolve when the baby is born. DIC is never a primary disease — it always occurs as a response to another disease process.

Events that trigger DIC include:

- placental abruption
- intrauterine fetal death, including delayed miscarriage
- amniotic fluid embolism
- intrauterine infection, including septic abortion
- pre-eclampsia and eclampsia.

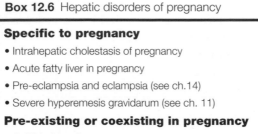

Box 12.6 Hepatic disorders of pregnancy

Specific to pregnancy
- Intrahepatic cholestasis of pregnancy
- Acute fatty liver in pregnancy
- Pre-eclampsia and eclampsia (see ch.14)
- Severe hyperemesis gravidarum (see ch. 11)

Pre-existing or coexisting in pregnancy
- Gall bladder disease
- Hepatitis

Management

The midwife should be alert for signs that clotting is abnormal, and the assessment of the nature of the clot should be part of her routine observation during the third stage of labour. Oozing from a venepuncture site or bleeding from the mucous membrane of the mother's mouth and nose must be noted and reported. Blood tests should include full blood count and blood grouping, clotting studies and the levels of platelets, fibrinogen and fibrin degradation products (FDPs).

Treatment involves the replacement of blood cells and clotting factors in order to restore equilibrium. This is usually done by the administration of fresh frozen plasma and platelet concentrates. Banked red cells will be transfused subsequently.

Hepatic Disorders and Jaundice in Pregnancy

Some liver disorders are specific to pregnant women, and some pre-existing or coexisting disorders may complicate the pregnancy (Box 12.6).

Intrahepatic cholestasis of pregnancy (ICP)

This is an idiopathic condition that begins in pregnancy, usually in the third trimester but occasionally as early as the first trimester. It resolves spontaneously following birth, but has a 60–80% recurrence rate in subsequent pregnancies. It is not a life-threatening condition for the mother, but she is at increased risk of preterm labour, fetal compromise and meconium staining and her stillbirth risk is increased by 15% unless there is active management of her pregnancy.

Clinical presentation

- There is pruritus at night.
- Fifty per cent of women affected will develop mild jaundice.
- Fever, abdominal discomfort and nausea and vomiting may occur.
- Urine may be darker and stools paler than usual.

Investigation

- Blood tests for an increase in bile acids, serum alkaline phosphatase, bilirubin and transaminases.
- Differential diagnosis: hepatic viral studies, an ultrasound scan of the hepatobiliary tract, an autoantibody screen.

Management

- Apply local antipruritic agents.
- Give vitamin K supplements for the mother.
- Monitor fetal well-being.
- Consider elective delivery when the fetus is mature, or earlier if the fetal condition appears to be compromised by the intrauterine environment.
- Give sensitive psychological care.
- Monitor the mother if she uses oral contraception in the future.

Gall bladder disease

Pregnancy appears to increase the likelihood of gallstone formation but not the risk of developing acute cholecystitis.

Diagnosis

- Previous history.
- An ultrasound scan of the hepatobiliary tract.

Treatment

- Provide symptomatic relief of biliary colic by analgesia, hydration, nasogastric suction and antibiotics.
- Surgery should be avoided, if possible.

Viral hepatitis (B)

Viral hepatitis is the most common cause of jaundice in pregnancy. Acute infection affects approximately 1 in 1000 pregnancies and has an incubation period of 1–6 months.

Clinical presentation

- Nausea, vomiting, anorexia.
- Pain over the liver.
- Mild diarrhoea.
- Jaundice lasting several weeks.
- Malaise.

The main means of spread is via blood, blood products and sexual activity. The virus can also be transmitted across the placenta. In healthy adults 90% of cases resolve completely within 6 months. In the remaining 10%, hepatitis B surface antigen (HBsAg) remains in the serum and the woman is considered to be a chronic carrier.

Diagnosis

- The woman's history of her symptoms and lifestyle.
- Serological studies.

Management

- Provide relief of symptoms
- Implement infection control measures if the woman is considered to be infectious.
- Provide information about the disease, nutrition and sexual health.
- Monitor liver function/fetal well-being.
- Assess fetal well-being.
- Offer immunisation to household contacts once their HBsAg seronegativity is established.
- Sexual partners should be traced and offered testing and vaccination.
- Postnatally, the mother should be encouraged to accept vaccination for the baby.
- Advice about breastfeeding remains controversial.

Skin Disorders

Many women suffer from physiological pruritus in pregnancy, especially over the abdomen.

Management

- Give reassurance and apply calamine lotion over the affected area.
- If pruritus is generalised, exclude other causes, e.g. intrahepatic cholestasis.

Disorders of the Amniotic Fluid

There are two chief abnormalities of amniotic fluid: polyhydramnios (or hydramnios) and oligohydramnios.

Polyhydramnios

The amount of liquor present in a pregnancy is estimated by measuring 'pools' of liquor around the fetus with ultrasound scanning. The single deepest pool is measured to calculate the amniotic fluid volume (AFV). However, where possible, a more accurate diagnosis may be gained by measuring the liquor in each of four quadrants around the fetus in order to establish an amniotic fluid index (AFI).

Polyhydramnios is said to be present when the AFV exceeds 8 cm, or the calculated AFI is more than 24 cm.

Causes

These include:

- oesophageal atresia
- open neural tube defect
- multiple pregnancy, especially in the case of monozygotic twins
- maternal diabetes mellitus
- rarely, an association with Rhesus isoimmunisation
- chorioangioma, a rare tumour of the placenta
- in many cases, an unknown cause.

Types

Chronic polyhydramnios

This is gradual in onset, usually starting from about the 30th week of pregnancy. It is the most common type.

Acute polyhydramnios

This is very rare. It usually occurs at about 20 weeks and comes on very suddenly. The uterus reaches the xiphisternum in about 3 or 4 days. It is frequently associated with monozygotic twins or severe fetal abnormality.

Diagnosis

The mother may complain of breathlessness and discomfort. If the polyhydramnios is acute in onset, she may have severe abdominal pain. The condition may cause exacerbation of symptoms associated with pregnancy, such as indigestion, heartburn and constipation. Oedema and varicosities of the vulva and lower limbs may be present.

Abdominal examination

- On inspection the uterus is larger than expected for the period of gestation and is globular in shape. The abdominal skin appears stretched and shiny with marked striae gravidarum and obvious superficial blood vessels.

- On palpation the uterus feels tense and it is difficult to feel the fetal parts, but the fetus may be balloted between the two hands. A fluid thrill may be elicited by placing a hand on one side of the abdomen and tapping the other side with the fingers.

- Ultrasonic scanning is used to confirm the diagnosis of polyhydramnios and may also reveal a multiple pregnancy or fetal abnormality.

Complications

These include:

- maternal ureteric obstruction
- increased fetal mobility leading to unstable lie and malpresentation
- cord presentation and prolapse

- prelabour (and often preterm) rupture of the membranes
- placental abruption when the membranes rupture
- preterm labour
- increased incidence of caesarean section
- postpartum haemorrhage
- raised perinatal mortality rate.

Management

Care will depend on the condition of the woman and fetus, the cause and degree of the polyhydramnios and the stage of pregnancy. The presence of fetal abnormality will be taken into consideration in choosing the mode and timing of delivery. If gross abnormality is present, labour may be induced; if the fetus is suffering from an operable condition such as oesophageal atresia, it may be appropriate to arrange transfer to a neonatal surgical unit.

Mild asymptomatic polyhydramnios is managed expectantly.

For a woman with symptomatic polyhydramnios:

- An upright position will help to relieve any dyspnoea and she may be given antacids to relieve heartburn and nausea.

- If the discomfort from the swollen abdomen is severe, then therapeutic amniocentesis, or amnioreduction, may be considered. However, this is not without risk, as infection may be introduced or the onset of labour provoked. No more than 500 ml should be withdrawn at any one time. It is at best a temporary relief as the fluid will rapidly accumulate again and the procedure may need to be repeated. Acute polyhydramnios managed by amnioreduction has a poor prognosis for the baby.

- Labour may need to be induced in late pregnancy if the woman's symptoms become worse.

- The lie must be corrected if it is not longitudinal and the membranes will be ruptured cautiously, allowing the amniotic fluid to drain out slowly in order to avoid altering the lie and to prevent cord prolapse.

- Placental abruption is also a hazard if the uterus suddenly diminishes in size.

Labour is usually normal but the midwife should be prepared for the possibility of postpartum haemorrhage. The baby should be carefully examined for abnormalities and the patency of the oesophagus ascertained by passing a nasogastric tube.

Oligohydramnios

Oligohydramnios is an abnormally small amount of amniotic fluid. At term it may be 300–500 ml but amounts vary and it can be even less. When diagnosed in the first half of pregnancy the condition is often found to be associated with renal agenesis (absence of kidneys) or Potter syndrome, in which the baby also has pulmonary hypoplasia. When diagnosed at any time in pregnancy before 37 weeks, it may be due to fetal abnormality or to preterm premature rupture of the membranes where the amniotic fluid fails to reaccumulate. The lack of amniotic fluid reduces the intrauterine space and over time will cause compression deformities. The baby has a squashed-looking face, flattening of the nose, micrognathia and talipes. The skin is dry and leathery in appearance.

Oligohydramnios sometimes occurs in the post-term pregnancy.

Diagnosis

- On inspection, the uterus may appear smaller than expected for the period of gestation.
- The mother who has had a previous normal pregnancy may have noticed a reduction in fetal movements.
- When the abdomen is palpated, the uterus is small and compact and fetal parts are easily felt.

- Ultrasonic scanning will enable differentiation of oligohydramnios from intrauterine growth restriction. Renal abnormality may be visible on the scan.

Management

If the ultrasound scan demonstrates renal agenesis, the baby will not survive. Liquor volume will also be estimated from the ultrasound scan, and if renal agenesis is not present, then further investigations will include careful questioning of the woman to check the possibility of preterm rupture of the membranes. Placental function tests will also be performed.

- Where fetal anomaly is not considered to be lethal, or the cause of the oligohydramnios is not known, prophylactic amnioinfusion with normal saline, Ringer's lactate or 5% glucose may be performed in order to prevent compression deformities and hypoplastic lung disease, and prolong the pregnancy.

- Labour may occur spontaneously or be induced because of the possibility of placental insufficiency.

- Epidural analgesia may be indicated because uterine contractions are often unusually painful.

- Continuous fetal heart rate monitoring is desirable.

Preterm Prelabour Rupture of the Membranes (PPROM)

This condition occurs before 37 completed weeks of gestation where rupture of the fetal membranes takes place without the onset of spontaneous uterine activity resulting in cervical dilatation.

Risks of PPROM

See Box 12.7.

> **Box 12.7** Some risks involved in preterm prelabour rupture of the membranes (PPROM)
>
> - Labour, which may result in a preterm birth
> - Chorioamnionitis, which may be followed by fetal and maternal systemic infection if not treated promptly
> - Oligohydramnios if prolonged PPROM occurs
> - Psychosocial problems resulting from uncertain fetal and neonatal outcome and long-term hospitalisation
> - Cord prolapse
> - Malpresentation associated with prematurity
> - Primary antepartum haemorrhage

Management

If PPROM is suspected, the woman will be admitted to the labour suite. A careful history is taken and rupture of the membranes confirmed by a sterile speculum examination of any pooling of liquor in the posterior fornix of the vagina. A fetal fibronectin immunoenzyme test may be used to confirm rupture of the membranes.

Digital vaginal examination should be avoided to reduce the risk of introducing infection. Observations must also be made of the fetal condition from the fetal heart rate (an infected fetus may have a tachycardia) and maternal infection screen, temperature and pulse, uterine tenderness and any purulent or offensively smelling vaginal discharge. A decision on future management will then be made.

If the woman has a gestation of less than 32 weeks, the fetus appears to be uncompromised, and APH and labour have been excluded, she will be managed expectantly:

- Admit to hospital.
- Offer frequent ultrasound scans to check the growth of the fetus and the extent and complications of any oligohydramnios.
- Administer corticosteroids.

- If labour intervenes, consider tocolytic drugs to prolong the pregnancy.
- Treat known vaginal infection with antibiotics. Prophylactic antibiotics may be offered to women without symptoms of infection.

If the woman is more than 32 weeks pregnant, the fetus appears to be compromised, and APH or intervening labour is suspected or confirmed, active management will ensue.

Malignant Disease in Pregnancy

If cancer is discovered before pregnancy is embarked upon, it should be treated and followed up before pregnancy is attempted. Once successfully treated, and as long as the reproductive organs are not damaged, pregnancy is rarely contraindicated for medical reasons. However, cancer discovered during pregnancy leads to a host of management dilemmas. The options involve balancing the effects of the treatment, the disease and delivery on both the mother and her fetus.

Obesity or Failure to Gain Weight in Pregnancy

Although evidence exists to refute strongly the value of routine weighing of pregnant women in predicting various perinatal outcomes, surprisingly little is known about optimal weight gain and the effects of large and low weight gain in pregnancy.

A woman who starts pregnancy while obese, or puts on an excessive amount of weight during pregnancy, appears to be:

- at greater risk of hypertensive disturbances, including pregnancy-induced hypertension, gestational diabetes, urinary tract infection, uncertain fetal position, postpartum haemorrhage and thrombophlebitis

- more likely to be delivered by caesarean section
- more likely to give birth to a baby who is either small or large for gestational age
- more prone to wound infection following operative delivery.

Obesity may also be associated with malnourishment from essential nutrient deficiency.

Ideally, all women should be given the opportunity to discuss diet, as well as other general lifestyle factors, from as early on in their pregnancy as possible, and at regular intervals thereafter. Referral to a dietitian may be helpful.

Blood pressure measurements should always be taken accurately with a correctly sized cuff, and screening carried out for gestational diabetes and urinary tract infection. Routine weighing is rarely of any practical benefit, and may only reduce a woman's self-esteem and make her dread her antenatal appointments. The midwife should also bear in mind that obesity can be a symptom of another disease.

Conversely, the midwife may observe that a woman appears to be thin during her pregnancy and not laying down healthy fat stores. Detailed discussion should attempt to elicit the quality and quantity of the woman's diet and her weight pattern over previous years.

Where a woman is suffering from nutritional deprivation she is at greater risk of:

- anaemia
- preterm birth
- intrauterine growth restriction and its sequelae, including birth asphyxia and perinatal death.

Chapter 13

Common Medical Disorders Associated with Pregnancy

Cardiac Disease

In most pregnancies, heart disease is diagnosed before pregnancy. There is, however, a small but significant group of women who will present at an antenatal clinic with an undiagnosed heart condition. Cardiac disease takes a variety of forms. Those more likely to be seen in pregnancy are:

- rheumatic heart disease
- congenital heart disease.

The most common congenital heart defects found in pregnancy are shown in Box 13.1.

Some congenital heart conditions are listed in Box 13.2.

Changes in cardiovascular dynamics during pregnancy

In normal pregnancy the haemodynamic profile alters in order to meet the increasing demands of the growing fetoplacental unit. Although this increases the workload of the heart quite significantly, normal

---

> **Box 13.1** Common congenital heart defects in pregnancy
>
> - Atrial septal defect (ASD)
> - Ventricular septal defect (VSD)
> - Patent ductus arteriosus (PDA)
> - Pulmonary stenosis
> - Aortic stenosis
> - Tetralogy of Fallot

> **Box 13.2** Some congenital heart conditions
>
> - Eisenmenger syndrome
> - Marfan syndrome
> - Ischaemic heart disease (IHD)
> - Endocarditis
> - Peripartum cardiomyopathy

---

healthy pregnant women are able to adjust to these physiological changes easily. In women with coexisting heart disease, however, the added workload can precipitate complications.

- The haemodynamic changes commence early in pregnancy and gradually reach their maximum effect between 28 and 32 weeks.
- During labour there is a significant increase in cardiac output as a result of uterine contractions.
- In the 12–24 hours following birth there is further alteration with the shift of blood (approximately 1 L) from the uterine to the systemic circulation.

Diagnosis

The recognition of heart disease in pregnancy may be difficult, as many of the symptoms of normal pregnancy resemble those of heart disease. The signs and symptoms of cardiac compromise are listed in Box 13.3.

> **Box 13.3** Common signs and symptoms of cardiac compromise in pregnancy
>
> - Fatigue
> - Shortness of breath (dyspnoea)
> - Difficulty in breathing unless upright (orthopnoea)
> - Palpitations
> - Bounding/collapsing pulse
> - Chest pain
> - Development of peripheral oedema
> - Distended jugular veins
> - Progressive limitation of physical activity

Laboratory tests can assist with the diagnosis of cardiac disease and determine the type of lesion, together with giving an assessment of current functional capacity. Tests include:

- full blood count (FBC)
- electrocardiography (ECG)
- chest radiograph to assess cardiac size and outline, pulmonary vasculature and lung fields
- clotting studies
- echocardiography.

Risks to mother and fetus

The majority of pregnancies complicated by maternal heart disease can be expected to have a favourable outcome for both mother and fetus. The risk for morbidity and mortality depends on:

- the nature of the cardiac lesion
- its effect on the functional capacity of the heart
- the development of pregnancy-related complications such as hypertensive disorders of pregnancy, infection, thrombosis and haemorrhage.

Preconception care

Women with known heart disease should seek advice from a cardiologist and an obstetrician before becoming pregnant, so that the risks of the condition can be discussed.

Antenatal care

The symptoms of normal pregnancy, together with the haemodynamic changes, can mimic the signs and symptoms of heart disease. Maternal investigations should be carried out prior to and at the onset of pregnancy in order to gain baseline referral points.

Management

All pregnant women with heart disease should be managed in obstetric units via a multidisciplinary approach involving midwives, obstetricians, cardiologists and anaesthetists. The aim is to maintain a steady haemodynamic state and prevent complications, as well as promote physical and psychological well-being. Visits to a joint clinic run by a cardiologist and obstetrician are usually made every 2 weeks until 30 weeks' gestation and weekly thereafter until birth. At each visit functional grading is made according to the New York Heart Association classification and the severity of the heart lesion is assessed by clinical examination.

Evaluation of fetal well-being will include:

- ultrasound examination to confirm gestational age and congenital abnormality
- assessment of fetal growth and amniotic fluid volume, both clinically and by ultrasound
- monitoring the fetal heart rate by CTG
- measurement of fetal and maternal placental blood flow indices by Doppler ultrasonography.

Intrapartum care

The first stage of labour

Vaginal birth is preferred unless there is an obstetric indication for caesarean section. Optimal management involves monitoring the maternal condition closely. This will include the measurement of:

- temperature
- pulse
- respiration
- blood pressure
- urine output.

Pulse oximetry, insertion of a central venous pressure (CVP) catheter and ECG monitoring may be utilised.

Fluid balance

Women with significant heart disease require care to be taken concerning fluid balance in labour. Indiscriminate use of intravenous crystalloid fluids will lead to an increase in circulating blood volume, which women with heart disease will find difficult to cope with and they may easily develop pulmonary oedema.

Pain relief

It is important to consult a doctor before administering any form of pain-relieving drug to a woman with a heart condition. In the majority, an epidural would be the analgesia of choice.

Positioning

Cardiac output is influenced by the position of the labouring woman It is preferable for an upright or left lateral position to be adopted.

Preterm labour

If a woman with heart disease should go into labour prematurely then beta-sympathomimetic drugs are contraindicated.

Induction

The least stressful labour for a woman with cardiac disease will be spontaneous in onset; induction is considered safe only if the benefits outweigh the disadvantages.

The second stage of labour

This should be short without undue exertion on the part of the mother.

- The midwife should encourage the woman to breathe normally and follow her natural desire to push, giving several short pushes during each contraction.
- Forceps or ventouse may be used to shorten the second stage if the maternal condition deteriorates.
- Care should be taken when the woman is in the lithotomy position, as this produces a sudden increase in venous return to the heart, which may result in heart failure.

The third stage of labour

This is usually actively managed owing to the increased risk of post-partum haemorrhage (PPH).

- Oxytocin is the drug of choice but its use in the prevention of PPH must be balanced against the risk of oxytocin-induced hypotension and tachycardia in women with cardiovascular compromise.
- Ergot-containing preparations such as ergometrine are contraindicated.

Postnatal care

- During the first 48 hours following birth the heart must cope with the extra blood from the uterine circulation. Close observation should identify early signs of infection, thrombosis or pulmonary oedema.

- Breastfeeding is not contraindicated.
- Discharge planning is particularly important for women with heart disease. The woman and her partner will need to discuss the implications of a future pregnancy with the cardiologist and obstetrician.

Respiratory Disorders

Asthma

Pregnancy does not consistently affect the maternal asthmatic status; some women experience no change in symptoms whereas others have a distinct worsening of the disease.

Antenatal care

The main anxiety for women and those providing care is generated by the use of medication and the fear that this may harm the fetus.

- To date all medications commonly used in the treatment of asthma, including systemic steroids, are considered safe and it is crucial that therapy is maintained during pregnancy in order to prevent deterioration of the condition and precipitation of adverse pregnancy events.
- The lynchpin of management is the use of peak expiratory flow rates (PEFR) to monitor the level of resistance in the airways caused by inflammation or bronchospasm, or both.

Intrapartum care

- If an asthma attack does occur, it should be treated with the same rapidity and medication as an attack outside of pregnancy.
- Intravenous, intra-amniotic and transcervical prostaglandins should be avoided in pregnancy and labour because of their bronchospasmic action.

■ Any woman who has received corticosteroids in pregnancy should have increased doses for the stress of labour.

Postnatal care

■ Breastfeeding should be encouraged, particularly as it may protect infants from developing certain allergic conditions.

Cystic fibrosis

Cystic fibrosis (CF) is an autosomal recessive disorder affecting the exocrine glands that causes production of excess secretions with abnormal electrolyte concentrations, resulting in the obstruction of the ducts and glands.

Prepregnancy care

■ When planning a pregnancy, a woman with CF and her partner should have genetic counselling.

■ Although pregnancy appears to be well tolerated in women with pre-existing mild pulmonary dysfunction, morbidity and mortality are increased in women with pancreatic insufficiency or moderate–severe lung disease, or both.

Antenatal care

■ Once pregnancy is confirmed, a multidisciplinary approach combining midwifery, obstetric, dietetic, medical, nursing and physiotherapy expertise is essential.

Intrapartum care

■ During labour close monitoring of cardiorespiratory function will be required and an anaesthetist should be involved at an early stage.

■ Fluid and electrolyte management requires careful attention, as women with CF may easily become hypovolaemic from the loss of large quantities of sodium in sweat.

- Epidural analgesia is the recommended form of pain relief in labour and general anaesthesia should be avoided.

Postnatal care

- Women should be cared for in a high-dependency unit and should be closely monitored, as studies have highlighted that cardiorespiratory function often deteriorates following birth.

- Breastfeeding is not contraindicated; however, in order for this to be successful, women need to be well nourished and maintain an adequate calorie intake.

Pulmonary tuberculosis

Tuberculosis (TB) is caused by the tubercle bacillus, *Myobacterium tuberculosis*. The lungs are the organ most commonly affected, although the disease may involve any organ.

Management

Standard antituberculous therapy should be used to treat TB in pregnancy. TB is treated in two phases:

- In the first phase, rifampicin, isoniazid and pyrazinamide are given daily for the first 2 months.
- In the second (continuation) phase, rifampicin and isoniazid are taken for a further 4 months.

These drugs are considered to be safe and are not associated with human fetal malformations. Attention should also be given to rest, good nutrition and education with regard to preventing the spread of the disease. TB is usually rendered non-infectious after 2 weeks of treatment.

Postnatal care

- Babies born to mothers with infectious TB should be protected from the disease by the prophylactic use of isoniazid syrup 5 mg/kg/day for 6 weeks and should then be tuberculin-tested.

- If the tuberculin test is negative, BCG (bacille Calmette–Guérin) vaccination should be given and drug therapy discontinued.

- If the test is positive, the baby should be assessed for congenital or perinatal infection, and drug therapy should be continued if these are excluded.

- Breastfeeding is contraindicated only if the mother has active TB.

It is advisable for a woman with TB to avoid further pregnancies until the disease has been quiescent for at least 2 years. The woman needs to be aware that rifampicin reduces the effectiveness of oral contraception.

Renal Disease

Asymptomatic bacteriuria

A diagnosis of asymptomatic bacteriuria (ASB) is made when there are more than 100 000 bacteria per millilitre of urine. All women should be screened for bacteriuria using a clean voided specimen of urine at their first antenatal visit.

If ASB is not identified and treated with antibiotics, 20–30% of affected women will develop a symptomatic urinary tract infection such as cystitis or pyelonephritis. These infections represent a significant risk for both mother and fetus and there is evidence to suggest that they may play a role in the onset of preterm labour.

Pyelonephritis

Clinical presentation

See Box 13.4.

> **Box 13.4** Clinical presentation of pyelonephritis
>
> - Pyrexia, rigors and tachycardia
> - Nausea and vomiting; dehydration
> - Pain and tenderness over the loin area; muscle guarding
> - Urine cloudy; infecting organism often found to be *Escherichia coli*

Management

- Refer to a doctor; admit to hospital.
- Obtain a midstream specimen of urine (MSU) to test for culture and sensitivity.
- Give intravenous antibiotics followed by oral antibiotics once the pyrexia has settled.
- Record fluid balance; intravenous fluids may be required.
- Maintain 4-hourly observation of temperature and pulse.
- Monitor uterine activity.
- Prevent complications of immobility, e.g. deep vein thrombosis.
- Repeat cultures 2 weeks after completion of antibiotics and monthly until birth.

Chronic renal disease

In order to determine the impact of pregnancy on a woman with chronic renal disease, the following factors need to be considered:

- type of pre-existing renal disease
- general health status of the woman
- presence or absence of hypertension
- current renal function
- prepregnancy drug therapy.

If renal disease is under control, the maternal and fetal outcome is usually good. In some instances renal function may deteriorate and the chance of pregnancy complications subsequently rises.

Care and management

The aim of pregnancy care is to prevent deterioration in renal function. This will necessitate more frequent attendance for antenatal care and close liaison between the midwife, obstetrician and nephrologist.

- Renal function is assessed on a regular basis by measuring serum urate levels, serum electrolyte and urea, 24-hour creatinine clearance and serum creatinine.

- Screen for glycosuria, proteinuria, haematuria, urinary tract infection and anaemia.

- Monitor for the emergence and severity of hypertension and pre-eclampsia.

- Fetal surveillance includes fortnightly ultrasound scans from 24 weeks, Doppler flow studies and daily fetal activity charts.

The Anaemias

Anaemia may be caused by a decrease in red blood cell (RBC) production, or a reduction in haemoglobin (Hb) content of the blood, or a combination of these. Signs and symptoms are listed in Box 13.5. A low Hb concentration only indicates that anaemia is present; it does not reveal the cause.

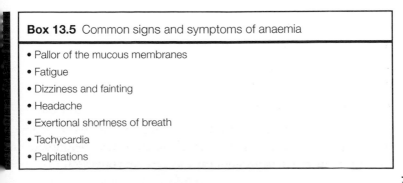

Box 13.5 Common signs and symptoms of anaemia

- Pallor of the mucous membranes
- Fatigue
- Dizziness and fainting
- Headache
- Exertional shortness of breath
- Tachycardia
- Palpitations

Physiological anaemia of pregnancy

During pregnancy the maternal plasma volume gradually expands by 50%, an increase of approximately 1200 ml by term. The total increase in RBCs is 25%, or approximately 300 ml. This relative haemodilution produces a fall in Hb concentration, which reaches a nadir during the second trimester of pregnancy and then rises again in the third trimester.

Iron deficiency anaemia

Iron deficiency anaemia in women is usually due to:

- reduced intake or absorption of iron; this includes dietary deficiency and gastrointestinal disturbances such as diarrhoea or hyperemesis

- excess demand, such as frequent, numerous or multiple pregnancies

- chronic infection, particularly of the urinary tract

- acute or chronic blood loss: for example, menorrhagia, bleeding haemorrhoids, or antepartum or postpartum haemorrhage.

Investigation

- Mean cell volume (MCV): normal value 80–95 femtolitres.

- Mean cell haemoglobin concentration (MCHC): normal value 32–36 g/dl.

- Serum iron levels: normal value 10–30 μmol/L.

- Total iron-binding capacity (TIBC): normal range 40–70 μmol/L.

- Serum ferritin: normal range 10–300 μg/L.

Management

- Identify the woman at risk through clinical observation and by taking an accurate medical, obstetric and social history.

- Give advice regarding the dietary intake of iron. The midwife needs to take into consideration how the intake of iron may be affected by social, religious and cultural preferences; she also needs to explain how iron is absorbed and identify the optimal sources of iron (bioavailability).

■ Iron supplements may be prescribed where the Hb level is outside the UK range (11 g/dl at first contact, 10.5 g/dl at 28 weeks) and iron deficiency anaemia has been diagnosed. Oral iron supplementation should continue postnatally, particularly if the woman is breastfeeding. In women who are unable to take, tolerate or absorb oral preparations, iron can also be given intramuscularly or intravenously.

Folic acid deficiency anaemia

Folic acid is needed for the increased cell growth of both mother and fetus but there is a physiological decrease in serum folate levels in pregnancy. The Medical Research Council Vitamin Study Research Group (1991) found a positive correlation between folate deficiency and the development of neural tube defects in the fetus.

Causes

■ A reduced dietary intake or reduced absorption, or a combination of these.

■ An excessive demand and loss of folic acid, e.g. haemolytic anaemia, multiple pregnancy.

■ Interference of some drugs with the utilisation of folic acid, e.g. anticonvulsants, sulphonamides and alcohol.

Investigation

Examination of the red cell indices will reveal that the red cells are reduced in number but enlarged in size.

Management

■ Advise on the correct selection and preparation of foods that are high in folic acid.

- Recommend folic acid supplements for all pregnant women, 400 μg/day (National Institute for Clinical Excellence 2003). Additional supplements may be prescribed for women considered at risk.

Haemoglobinopathies

This term describes inherited conditions where the haemoglobin is abnormal. Defective genes lead to the formation of abnormal Hb; this may be as a result of impaired globin synthesis (thalassaemia syndromes) or from structural abnormality of globin (Hb variants such as sickle cell anaemia). These conditions are found mainly in people whose families come from Africa, the West Indies, the Middle East, the eastern Mediterranean and Asia.

As these conditions are inherited and in the homozygous form can be fatal, screening of the population at risk should be carried out. If both parents are carriers (i.e. heterozygous), there is a 1 in 4 chance that the fetus will be homozygous for the condition.

Thalassaemia

Thalassaemia is most common in people of Mediterranean, African, Middle and Far Eastern origin. The basic defect is a reduced rate of globin chain synthesis in adult Hb. This leads to ineffective erythropoiesis and increased haemolysis with a resultant inadequate Hb content. The red cell indices show a low Hb and MCHC level, but raised serum iron level. Definitive diagnosis is obtained by electrophoresis. The severity of the condition depends on whether the abnormal genes are inherited from one parent or from both. There are also different types of thalassaemia, depending on whether the alpha or beta globin chain synthesis is affected:

- alpha thalassaemia major
- beta thalassaemia major
- alpha and beta thalassaemia minor.

Sickle-cell disorders

Sickle-cell disorders are found most commonly in people of African or West Indian origin. In these conditions defective genes produce abnormal Hb beta chains; the resulting Hb is called HbS.

- In sickle-cell anaemia (HbSS, or SCA) abnormal genes have been inherited from both parents.
- In sickle-cell trait (HbAS) only one abnormal gene has been inherited.

Maternal and fetal/neonatal risks are listed in Box 13.6.

All women in the at-risk population are screened in early pregnancy, and where possible their partners are screened too. Those who are diagnosed as having SCA should be referred to a specialist sickle-cell centre with trained haemoglobinopathy and genetic counsellors.

Sickle-cell trait

This is usually asymptomatic. The blood appears normal, although the sickle screening test is positive. There is no anaemia, even under the additional stress of pregnancy.

Box 13.6 Common risks and complications of sickle-cell disorders

Maternal risks
- Antenatal and postnatal pain crisis
- Infections
- Pulmonary complications
- Anaemia
- Pre-eclampsia
- Caesarean section

Fetal and neonatal complications
- Preterm birth
- Smallness for gestational age
- Neonatal jaundice

Diabetes Mellitus

The term 'diabetes mellitus' (DM) describes a metabolic disorder of multiple aetiology that affects the normal metabolism of carbohydrates, fats and protein.

Classification

See Box 13.7.

Diagnosis

Routine screening in pregnancy is not recommended. Increased thirst, increased urine volume, excessive tiredness, unexplained weight

---

Box 13.7 Classification of diabetes mellitus (DM)

Type 1 DM
- Occurs when beta cells in the islets of Langerhans in the pancreas are destroyed, stopping insulin production
- Insulin therapy is required in order to prevent the development of ketoacidosis, coma and death

Type 2 DM
- Results from a defect or defects in insulin action and insulin secretion
- Insulin therapy is not needed to survive
- The risk of developing this type of DM increases with age, obesity and lack of physical activity

Gestational diabetes mellitus (GDM)
- Carbohydrate intolerance resulting in hyperglycaemia of variable severity
- Onset or first recognition is during pregnancy

Impaired glucose regulation
- Includes *impaired glucose tolerance* (IGT) and *impaired fasting glycaemia* (IFG), metabolic states intermediate between normal glucose homeostasis and diabetes

loss and a family history require further investigations. The World Health Organization (WHO) criteria for diagnosis after a 75 g glucose load are:

- Two-hour venous glucose <7.8 mmol/L = Normal
- Two-hour venous glucose 7.8–11 mmol/L = Impaired glucose tolerance
- Two-hour venous glucose >11 mmol/L = Gestational diabetes.

However, these levels are based on a non-pregnant population and hence could lead to over-diagnosis.

Monitoring diabetes

The main objectives of diabetic therapy are:

- to maintain blood glucose levels as near to normal as possible
- to reduce the risk of long-term complications.

Long-term blood glucose control can be determined by undertaking a laboratory test to measure glycosylated haemoglobin (HbA1c). Between 5 and 8% of Hb in the red blood cells carries a glucose molecule and is said to be glycosylated. The degree of Hb glycosylation is dependent on the amount of glucose the red blood cells have been exposed to during their 120-day life. A random blood test measuring the percentage of Hb that is glycosylated will reflect the average blood glucose during the preceding 1–2 months. The higher the HbA1c, the poorer is the blood sugar control. Good diabetic control is defined as an HbA1c of <6.5%.

Carbohydrate metabolism in pregnancy

Pregnancy is characterised by several factors that produce a diabetogenetic state so that insulin and carbohydrate metabolism is altered in order to make glucose more readily available to the fetus. Women with DM do not have the capacity to increase insulin secretion in response to the altered carbohydrate metabolism in pregnancy and therefore glucose accumulates in the maternal and fetal system, leading to significant morbidity and mortality.

Prepregnancy care

- Assessment is made of current diabetic control, aiming for pre-meal glucose levels of <6 mmol/L and HbA1c of ≤7%.

- Insulin dosage is reviewed.

- Women with type 2 DM on oral hypoglycaemics will need to transfer to insulin to prevent the possibility of teratogenesis.

- Higher-dose folic acid supplementation is given.

- Smoking cessation support is arranged.

- Assessment and management is provided for diabetes complications.

Antenatal care

- Women and their partners should ideally be seen in a combined clinic by a team that includes a physician, an obstetrician with a special interest in diabetes in pregnancy, a specialist diabetes nurse, a specialist midwife and a dietitian. They will be seen as often as required in order to maintain good diabetic control and undertake relevant screening e.g. retinal examination.

- Blood glucose levels should be monitored frequently (four times a day using a reflectance meter) and insulin levels adjusted to achieve pre-meal blood sugar levels of 5.0–6.0 mmol/L and post-meal levels of <7.5 mmol/L. Additional estimations of blood glucose control, such as monthly HbA1c measurements, are also recommended.

- A diet that is high in fibre is beneficial, as carbohydrates are released slowly and therefore a more constant blood glucose level can be achieved.

- Advise women on early recognition of the signs and symptoms of urinary and vaginal infections.

- Anomaly ultrasound screening should be offered at 20 weeks' gestation and fetal echocardiography at 20–22 weeks to detect cardiac abnormalities. Serum screening for Down syndrome is altered with maternal diabetes and care should be taken when interpreting the results.

- There is an increased risk of growth restriction due to maternal vascular disease, pre-eclampsia, or a combination of both. A baseline measurement of the fetal abdominal circumference is taken at 20 weeks. This is followed by serial measurements every 2–4 weeks, commencing at 24 weeks. Serial ultrasound should also detect fetal macrosomia and whether polyhydramnios is present.

Intrapartum care

- Ideally, labour should be allowed to commence spontaneously at term for women with uncomplicated DM during pregnancy. Poor diabetic control or a deterioration in the maternal or fetal condition may necessitate earlier, planned birth. Induction of labour may also be considered where the fetus is judged to be macrosomic. Steroids such as dexamethasone may be used to aid lung maturation and surfactant production, but these will increase insulin requirements.

- The aim of intrapartum care is to maintain normoglycaemia in labour (i.e. $<7.0\,\text{mmol/L}$).

- Continuous electronic fetal monitoring is recommended and fetal blood sampling should be utilised if acidosis is suspected.

- Adequate pain relief, such as epidural analgesia, assists in regulating the blood sugar levels and preventing the development of metabolic acidosis. It is also useful if difficulties should arise with the birth of the shoulders or an operative birth is required.

Postpartum care

- Immediately after the third stage of labour the insulin requirements will fall rapidly to prepregnancy levels. The insulin infusion rate should be reduced by at least 50%.

- Women with type 2 DM who were previously on oral hypoglycaemics or dietary control need to be reviewed prior to recommencing therapy.

- Breastfeeding should be encouraged in all women with diabetes. An additional carbohydrate intake of 40–50 g is recommended and insulin therapy may need to be adjusted accordingly.

- All women should be offered contraceptive advice so that optimum metabolic control is achieved prior to planning the next pregnancy.

Neonatal care

The development of complications in the neonate is related to maternal hyperglycaemia during pregnancy leading to fetal hyperinsulinaemia. This will result in the following conditions: macrosomia, hypoglycaemia, polycythaemia and respiratory distress syndrome.

Macrosomia

This is defined as a fetal birth weight >4500 g. The increased fetal size may cause prolonged labour and predisposes the infant to shoulder dystocia and birth injuries. As a consequence, asphyxia is common and these infants are more likely than babies of normal weight to die from an intrapartum-related event.

Hypoglycaemia

Beta-cell hyperplasia causes the baby to continue to produce more insulin than required for up to 24 hours following birth. To prevent hypoglycaemia the neonatal blood glucose needs to be assessed 1–2 hours after birth and then every 4–6 hours for the first 24–48 hours

Regular feeding is encouraged to maintain a blood glucose of at least 2.6 mmol/L.

Polycythaemia

Fetal hyperinsulinaemia during pregnancy also leads to an increase in red cell production resulting in polycythaemia (venous haematocrit >65%). The rapid breakdown of the excess red blood cells, combined with the relative immaturity of the liver in the newborn, predisposes the baby to jaundice. This will be exacerbated if there is bruising as a result of birth trauma.

Respiratory distress syndrome

Hyperinsulinaemia is thought to impair the production of surfactant and delay lung maturation. Hence, babies born at term may display symptomatology of respiratory distress.

Observations of temperature, apex beat and respirations and monitoring of blood sugar levels are important in the first 24–48 hours. Clinical signs, together with symptomatology such as respiratory distress, apnoea or tachypnoea, cyanosis, jitteriness, irritability, seizures, feeding intolerance and temperature instability, may all be indicative of respiratory distress syndrome, polycythaemia and hypoglycaemia; these will require further investigation and treatment in a neonatal unit.

Gestational diabetes

Screening for GDM (including dipstick testing for glycosuria) is not a recommended intervention for *routine* antenatal care.

Diagnosis is based on the WHO recommendations. However, caution should be exercised if the following occur in the third trimester when glucose tolerance is known to be impaired:

- If the fasting venous plasma glucose is >7.0 mmol/L, *or*
- There is a fasting venous plasma glucose <7.0 mmol/L and a plasma glucose of >7.8 mmol/L 2 hours after a 75 g glucose load.

Treatment will depend on the blood glucose levels. Grossly abnormal results are likely to require insulin therapy, which will be discontinued immediately after the birth of the baby. It is recommended that a postnatal oral glucose tolerance test is performed at 6 weeks; if the results are abnormal, then appropriate referral should be made. Those with normal glucose levels require advice regarding the implications for future pregnancies and the development of type 1 or type 2 DM.

Epilepsy

The prevalence of epilepsy in the general population is 1 in 200 and it affects 0.3–0.5% of pregnant women.

An epileptic seizure results from abnormal electrical activity in the brain, which is manifest by brief sensory, motor and autonomic dysfunction. These disturbances recur spontaneously and are classified according to the parts of the brain affected. Seizures may be described as shown in Box 13.8.

Identification of the type of epilepsy is important in the treatment of epilepsy. The aim of treatment is to identify the cause of the seizure and provide appropriate therapy to prevent recurrence. The control

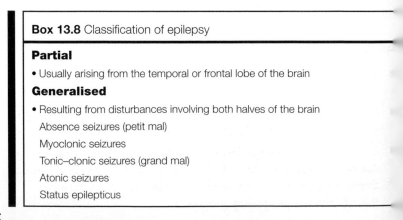

Box 13.8 Classification of epilepsy

Partial
• Usually arising from the temporal or frontal lobe of the brain

Generalised
• Resulting from disturbances involving both halves of the brain
  Absence seizures (petit mal)
  Myoclonic seizures
  Tonic–clonic seizures (grand mal)
  Atonic seizures
  Status epilepticus

of seizures can be achieved for the majority of people through the use of antiepileptic drugs (AEDs).

Prepregnancy care

- Women on AEDs become folic acid-deficient and may develop macrocytic anaemia. Folic acid deficiency has also been associated with neural tube defects and other congenital malformations.

- There is a 1–2% risk of neural tube defects if a woman is taking sodium valproate (Epilim) or carbamazepine (Tegretol) in pregnancy. Of the other older AEDs, phenytoin gives rise to a combination of malformations termed 'fetal hydantoin syndrome', which comprises craniofacial dysmorphic features, digital defects, microcephaly and growth retardation. Preconception advice is therefore essential for women with epilepsy.

- AED therapy may be withdrawn gradually prior to pregnancy in order to reduce the risk of teratogenicity when women suffer from seizures that are unlikely to harm the fetus, such as absence, partial or myoclonic seizures, or have been seizure-free for over 2 years.

- Folic acid supplementation (5 mg/day) should be commenced before pregnancy and continued throughout pregnancy.

Antenatal care

- Antenatal care should include a detailed anomaly scan at 18–22 weeks.

- Abnormalities are more common if AEDs are prescribed in high concentration and particularly if more than one is used.

- Some women may experience an increase in seizures; this is often due to non-compliance with the drug regimen, sleep deprivation during pregnancy and the decline in plasma concentrations of the AED as the pregnancy progresses.

- Particular emphasis should also be placed on the first aid measures that should be adopted following an epileptic seizure in order to prevent aspiration, and the dangers of hot baths inducing fainting and consequent drowning.

Intrapartum care

- Care during labour and childbirth is not likely to be different from that of other mothers.

- Seizures are more likely to occur in conditions such as sleep deprivation, hypoglycaemia, anaemia, stress or hyperventilation — all of which may arise during labour. AEDs should therefore be maintained throughout labour.

Postnatal care

- Safety precautions in the home are important. The mother is given advice about how to minimise risks when feeding, bathing, changing and transporting the baby.

- AED therapy should be reviewed 6 weeks postnatally and the dosage adjusted to prepregnancy levels.

Effect of epilepsy on the fetus and neonate

The majority of women with epilepsy will have uncomplicated pregnancies with normal births and healthy children.

When status epilepticus occurs, one-third of mothers and half of the fetuses do not survive. Convulsive status epilepticus is a medical emergency. AEDs cross the placenta freely and decrease production of vitamin K, leading to the risk of haemorrhagic disease of the newborn. This can be prevented by routine administration of vitamin K to the mother from 36 weeks' gestation and to the baby shortly after birth. The rate of clearance of AEDs varies according to the drug. Newborn infants may therefore suffer harmful effects from the AED level and, as a group, tend to be less efficient at feeding and gain weight more slowly. A minority will suffer withdrawal symptoms such as tremor, excitability and convulsions. AEDs pass into the breast milk in relatively small quantities and therefore breastfeeding is recommended. Some AEDs, such as phenobarbital, primidone or benzodiazepines, may have a sedative effect, in which case bottle feeding or mixed feeding may be advised.

Autoimmune Disease

Autoimmune disease arises from a disruption in the function of the immune system of the body, resulting in the production of anti-bodies against the body's own cells. Antigens normally present on the body's cells stimulate the development of autoantibodies, which, unable to distinguish the self antigens from non-self or foreign anti-gens, act against the body's cells to cause localised and systemic reac-tions. The cause of this condition is unknown but it is thought to be multifactorial with genetic, environmental, hormonal and viral influ-ences. Many autoimmune diseases are more prevalent in women, particularly between puberty and the menopause, which suggests that female hormonal factors may play a role. They broadly fall into two groups:

- multisystem disease, such as systemic lupus erythematosus (SLE)
- tissue- or organ-specific disorders, such as autoimmune thyroid disease.

These disorders are characterised by periods of remission interrupted by periods of crisis, which may require hospitalisation. Treatment is aimed at lessening the severity of the symptoms rather than effecting a cure.

- Mild cases usually respond to anti-inflammatory drugs.
- More severe illnesses may require steroids or immunosuppressant therapy.

Systemic lupus erythematosus

SLE, or lupus, is an inflammatory disorder of the connective tissue, which forms the fibrous, elastic, fatty or cartilaginous matrix that connects and supports other tissues.

- The initial manifestation of SLE is often arthritis accompanied by fever, fatigue, malaise, weight loss, photosensitivity and anaemia.

- A wide range of skin lesions are seen and an erythematous facial 'butterfly' rash is characteristic of the disorder.

- Depending on the organs involved, inflammatory conditions such as pleuritis, pericarditis, glomerulonephritis, neuritis and gastritis may arise.

- Renal disease and neurological abnormalities are the most serious manifestations of the disease.

Most people with SLE have a normal life expectancy and serious complications are rare. Infection is the major cause of mortality.

Diagnosis

The diagnosis of SLE is based on a collection of the signs and symptoms, particularly when joint pain, skin conditions and fatigue occur in combination or evolve over time. Blood tests are used to confirm the diagnosis and comprise:

- full blood count
- erythrocyte sedimentation rate (ESR)
- testing for antinuclear antibody (ANA).

There is often normochromic normocytic anaemia, the ESR is elevated even when the disease is in remission and more than 95% of people with SLE will have ANA. Antiphospholipid syndrome (APS) is found in conjunction with SLE in 30% of cases. A blood test will detect antiphospholipid antibodies (aPL), lupus anticoagulant and anticardiolipin antibodies (anti-Ro and anti-La) if APS is present

This will identify a group of people with SLE at particular risk of thromboembolic disorders and a high rate of fetal loss.

Effects of SLE on pregnancy

The effect of SLE on pregnancy is variable, although worsening of SLE symptoms is common and may occur at any trimester of pregnancy and in the postpartum period. The frequency of the 'flares' is, however, lower in women with mild and well-controlled disease. Women with SLE should be counselled about planning a pregnancy and the importance of being in remission for at least 6 months before conception. Overall, pregnancies in SLE women have an increased incidence of adverse pregnancy outcome. Approximately one-third of pregnancies will result in fetal wastage owing to spontaneous abortion, therapeutic abortion, intrauterine death or stillbirth. The rate of preterm birth and intrauterine growth restriction is closely related to the incidence of pre-eclampsia.

Neonatal lupus syndrome is rare but may occur as a result of the transplacental passage of maternal anti-Ro/La antibodies.

Antenatal care

Women should be referred as soon as possible to a centre that specialises in the care of people with lupus disorders.

- Baseline haematological and immunological blood tests are performed at the first antenatal visit.

- A baseline 24-hour urine collection for creatinine clearance and total protein to assess renal function is also recommended.

- An early first trimester scan is undertaken to confirm fetal viability and an anomaly scan is performed at 18–20 weeks. Women with SLE and APS are offered a fetal cardiac anomaly scan at 24 weeks' gestation and echocardiography to detect congenital heart block.

- Serial ultrasound examinations for fetal growth, placental size and quality, and amniotic fluid volume should begin at 28–32 weeks.

- Doppler flow studies are performed at 20 and 24 weeks and thereafter according to fetal growth and well-being.

The aim is to control disease activity and achieve clinical remission whilst keeping drug therapy to a minimum.

- Women who have a mild form of the disease or are in remission require minimal to no medication.

- Avoidance of emotional stress and the promotion of a healthy lifestyle may play a part in reducing the likelihood of flares or exacerbations of SLE arising during pregnancy.

- If treatment is required, simple analgesics such as paracetamol and co-dydramol are used for symptomatic relief.

- Mild flares with joint pain, skin lesions and fatigue respond well to low-dose steroid therapy such as prednisone or prednisolone.

- Antimalarial drugs are effective as maintenance therapy in women with frequent flares and hydroxychloroquine is considered safe to use in pregnancy.

- Advanced renal disease requires immunosuppressants.

- Women with SLE and APS have associated recurrent miscarriage, thrombosis and thrombocytopenia and it is recommended that treatment with low-dose aspirin (75 mg daily) and heparin (5000 IU every 12 hours given subcutaneously) is commenced as soon as these women have a positive pregnancy test.

Intrapartum care

- The timing of birth depends on current activity of the disease and whether there are any complications.

- Women with SLE are particularly prone to infection, hypertension, thrombocytopenia and thromboembolic disorders. Close monitoring of the maternal condition is required to evaluate cardiac, pulmonary and renal function. Blood tests should be undertaken to screen for haematological conditions, which may lead to clotting disorders. Comfort measures and thromboembolitic D (TED) stockings can reduce pressure sores and the development of deep vein thrombosis. Women who have been on long-term steroid therapy will require parenteral steroid cover during labour.

- As SLE may compromise the uteroplacental circulation, continuous fetal monitoring in conjunction with fetal blood gas estimation is recommended.

Postpartum care

- During the immediate postpartum period the midwife should observe closely for signs of SLE flares that may occur as a result of the stress of labour. In addition, she should watch for signs and symptoms of infection, pre-eclampsia, renal disease, thrombosis and neurological changes.

- Careful consideration needs to be given to breastfeeding, as most of the drugs used to treat SLE are excreted in breast milk. Large doses of aspirin should be avoided and non-steroidal anti-inflammatory drugs (NSAIDs) are contraindicated when breast-feeding jaundiced neonates; paracetamol is the drug of choice for postpartum analgesia. Low-dose steroids such as prednisone and prednisolone and the antimalarial hydroxychloroquine are considered safe to use when breastfeeding. Immuno-suppressive therapy is contraindicated and should be avoided.

- The choice of contraceptives for a woman with SLE may be limited.

Thyroid Disease

In pregnancy, thyroid function is affected by three factors that increase the basal metabolic rate by 20%:

- Oestrogen stimulates the production of thyroid-binding globulin (TBG), which binds more of the thyroid hormones resulting in a doubling of the total serum levels of *thyroxine* (T_4) and *triiodothyronine* (T_3).

- Human chorionic gonadotrophin (HCG) secreted by the placenta appears to stimulate the thyroid gland directly as *thyroid-stimulating hormone* (TSH) levels fall in early pregnancy and then increase in the second and third trimesters, with a corresponding rise and then fall in the level of HCG.

- A rise in the glomerular filtration rate in pregnancy leads to increased renal clearance of iodine, resulting in an increase in dietary iodine requirement.

Clinical assessment of thyroid dysfunction is difficult, as pregnancy-related symptoms are similar to hyperthyroidism and hypothyroidism. Thyroid function can be assessed by biochemical tests that measure total T_4, free thyroxine (FT_4), total T_3 and TSH. It is important to remember that thyroid function tests may appear abnormal in pregnancy despite normal activity of the thyroid gland.

Hyperthyroidism

The most common cause of hyperthyroidism in pregnancy is *Graves disease*, which is an autoimmune disorder that results in antibody activation of the thyroid gland. The gland becomes enlarged and secretes an increased amount of thyroid hormone. The metabolic processes of the body are accelerated, resulting in fatigue, heat intolerance, palpitations, diarrhoea and mood lability. Clinical diagnosis may be difficult, as the physiological signs and symptoms that pregnant women normally exhibit may mask this condition.

- The disease should be suspected in any woman who loses weight despite a good appetite.

- Other symptoms include an enlarged thyroid gland (goitre), exophthalmos, eyelid lag and persistent tachycardia.

A serious complication of untreated or poorly controlled hyperthyroidism is *thyroid storm*. This may occur spontaneously or be precipitated by infection or stress. It is characterised by signs and symptoms associated with a high metabolic rate:

- hyperthermia (temperature >41°C), leading to:
- dehydration
- tachycardia
- acute respiratory distress
- cardiovascular collapse.

This is a medical emergency requiring oxygen, cooling, hydration, antibiotics and drug therapy to stop the production and reduce the effect of thyroid hormone.

Hyperthyroidism in pregnancy is associated with an increase in the incidence of pre-eclampsia, preterm birth, low birth weight and fetal death.

Management

Treatment of hyperthyroidism is achieved through the use of antithyroid drugs.

- Propylthiouracil and carbimazole may be used in pregnancy. Propylthiouracil is the drug of choice, as less of it crosses the placenta and only small amounts are found in breast milk.
- The aim of management is to use the lowest dose possible, as these drugs may cause goitre and hypothyroidism in the fetus.
- During the antenatal period the pregnant woman should be seen monthly by the endocrinologist for clinical evaluation and monitoring of her thyroid levels.
- Factors that may precipitate thyroid storm include infection, the stress of labour and caesarean section.

Hypothyroidism

The most common cause of hypothyroidism in pregnancy is *autoimmune thyroiditis* (*Hashimoto's disease*). Slowing of the body's metabolic processes may occur, giving rise to mental and physical lethargy, excessive weight gain, constipation, cold intolerance and dryness of the skin. However, the symptoms may be non-specific and the condition can be difficult to diagnose. Hypothyroidism in pregnancy will result in reduced availability of the hormone for fetal requirements, leading to subsequent poor neurological development. Women should be encouraged to increase their dietary iodine intake during pregnancy and hypothyroidism should be treated with daily thyroxine. Following birth, the neonate's thyroid status should be checked to identify whether neonatal hypothyroidism is present. There is no contraindication to breastfeeding but the dose of thyroxine may need adjustment postpartum because of maternal weight loss following childbirth.

Postpartum thyroiditis

This is an autoimmune disorder and is a form of Hashimoto's thyroiditis, which occurs in 5% of women during the first year following childbirth. It is a transient thyroid disorder, characterised by a period of mild hyperthyroidism occurring a few months after birth and followed by a phase of hypothyroidism. In both phases the disorder presents with fatigue and a painless goitre; the condition may also mimic postpartum depression. Treatment is not required, as recovery is usually spontaneous.

Chapter 14

Hypertensive Disorders of Pregnancy

Hypertension is the commonest medical condition encountered in pregnancy, complicating approximately 5% of all pregnancies; it is a significant cause of maternal and fetal/neonatal morbidity and mortality. Pregnancy may induce hypertension in women who have been normotensive prior to pregnancy, or may aggravate existing hypertensive conditions.

Definition and Classification

The definition and classification of the hypertensive disorders are complex (Box 14.1). It is important to recognise the distinction between:

- a woman whose hypertension antedates pregnancy (pre-existing or chronic hypertension)
- a woman who develops an increased blood pressure during pregnancy (gestational hypertension).

An incremental rise in blood pressure is not included in this classification system. However, it is considered that women who have a rise

Box 14.1 Classification and definition of hypertensive disorders in pregnancy

Chronic hypertension

- Hypertension before pregnancy or a diastolic blood pressure of 90 mmHg or more before 20 weeks' gestation, and persisting 6 weeks after delivery

Gestational hypertension

- Development of hypertension without other signs of pre-eclampsia
- Diagnosed when, after resting, the woman's blood pressure rises above 140/90 mmHg, on at least two occasions, no more than 1 week apart after the 20th week of pregnancy in a woman known to be normotensive
- Hypertension diagnosed for the first time in pregnancy, which does not resolve postpartum, is also classified as gestational hypertension

Pre-eclampsia

- Diagnosed on the basis of hypertension with proteinuria, when proteinuria is measured as >1+ on dipstick or >0.3 g/L of protein in a random clean catch specimen or an excretion of 0.3 g protein/24 hours
- In the absence of proteinuria, pre-eclampsia is suspected when hypertension is accompanied by symptoms including:

  headache

  blurred vision

  abdominal/epigastric pain, *or*

  altered biochemistry: specifically, low platelet counts, abnormal liver enzyme levels

- These signs and symptoms, together with blood pressure above 160 mmHg systolic or above 110 mmHg diastolic and proteinuria of 2+ or 3+ on a dipstick, demonstrate the more severe form of the disease

Eclampsia

- The new onset of convulsions during pregnancy or postpartum, unrelated to other cerebral pathological conditions, in a woman with pre-eclampsia

Pre-eclampsia superimposed on chronic hypertension

- This may occur in women with pre-existing hypertension (under 20 weeks' gestation) who develop:

  new proteinuria (>0.3 g/24 hours)

  sudden increases in pre-existing hypertension and proteinuria

  thrombocytopenia (platelet count $<100 \times 10^9$/L)

  abnormal liver enzymes

of 30 mmHg systolic or 15 mmHg diastolic blood pressure require close observation especially if proteinuria and hyperuricaemia (raised uric acid level) are also present.

Pathological Changes

Blood

Hypertension, together with endothelial cell damage, affects capillary permeability. Plasma proteins leak from the damaged blood vessels, causing a decrease in the plasma colloid pressure and an increase in oedema within the extracellular space. The reduced intravascular plasma volume causes hypovolaemia and haemoconcentration, which is reflected in an elevated haematocrit. In severe cases the lungs become congested with fluid and pulmonary oedema develops, oxygenation is impaired and cyanosis occurs. With vasoconstriction and disruption of the vascular endothelium the coagulation cascade is activated.

Coagulation system

Increased platelet consumption produces thrombocytopenia. Disseminated intravascular coagulation (DIC) is characterized by low platelets and fibrinogen and prolonged prothrombin time. As the process progresses, fibrin and platelets are deposited, which will occlude blood flow to many organs, particularly the kidneys, liver, brain and placenta.

Kidneys

In the kidney, hypertension leads to vasospasm of the afferent arterioles, resulting in a decreased renal blood flow, which produces hypoxia and oedema of the endothelial cells of the glomerular capillaries. Glomeruloendotheliosis (glomerular endothelial damage) allows plasma proteins to filter into the urine, producing proteinuria.

Renal damage is reflected by reduced creatinine clearance and increased serum creatinine and uric acid levels. Oliguria develops as the condition worsens, signifying severe and renal vasoconstriction.

Liver

Vasoconstriction of the hepatic vascular bed will result in hypoxia and oedema of the liver cells. In severe cases oedematous swelling of the liver causes epigastric pain and can lead to intracapsular haemorrhages and, in very rare cases, rupture of the liver. Altered liver function is reflected by falling albumin levels and a rise in liver enzyme levels.

Brain

Hypertension, combined with cerebrovascular endothelial dysfunction, increases the permeability of the blood–brain barrier, resulting in cerebral oedema and microhaemorrhaging characterised by the onset of headaches, visual disturbances and convulsions. Where the mean arterial pressure (MAP — i.e. the systolic blood pressure plus twice the diastolic pressure divided by 3) exceeds 125 mmHg, the autoregulation of cerebral flow is disrupted, resulting in cerebral vasospasm, cerebral oedema and blood clot formation. This is known as *hypertensive encephalopathy*; if left untreated, it can progress to cerebral haemorrhage and death.

Fetoplacental unit

In the uterus, vasoconstriction caused by hypertension reduces the uterine blood flow which can result in placental abruption and placental scarring. The amount of oxygen that diffuses through the cells of the syncytiotrophoblast and cytotrophoblast into the fetal circulation within the placenta is diminished, the placental tissue becomes ischaemic, the capillaries in the chorionic villi thrombose and infarctions occur, leading to fetal growth restriction.

The Midwife's Role in Assessment and Diagnosis

As the hypertensive disorders are unlikely to be prevented, early detection and appropriate management can minimise the severity of the condition. A comprehensive history will identify:

- adverse social circumstances or poverty, which could prevent the woman from attending for regular antenatal care
- the mother's age and parity
- primipaternity and partner-related factors
- a family history of hypertensive disorders
- a past history of pre-eclampsia
- the presence of underlying medical disorders: for example, renal disease, diabetes, SLE and thromboembolic disorders.

The two essential features of pre-eclampsia, hypertension and proteinuria, are assessed for at regular intervals throughout pregnancy. Diagnosis is usually based on the rise in blood pressure and the presence of proteinuria after 20 weeks' gestation.

Blood pressure measurement

The mother's blood pressure is taken early in pregnancy to compare with all subsequent recordings, taking into account the normal pattern in pregnancy. It is important to consider several factors in assessing blood pressure.

- Blood pressure machines should be calibrated for use in pregnancy and regularly maintained.
- Blood pressure can be overestimated as a result of using a sphygmomanometer cuff of inadequate size relative to the arm circumference. The length of the bladder should be at least 80% of the arm circumference. Two cuffs should be available with inflation bladders of 35 cm for normal use and 42 cm for large arms.

- Rounding off of blood pressure measurements should be avoided and an attempt should be made to record the blood pressure as accurately as possible to the nearest 2 mmHg.

- The use of Korotkoff V (disappearance of sound) as a measure of the diastolic blood pressure has been found to be easier to obtain, more reproducible and closer to the intra-arterial pressure; therefore this reading should be used unless the sound is near zero, in which case Korotkoff IV (muffling sound) should be used instead.

Urinalysis

Proteinuria in the absence of urinary tract infection is indicative of glomerular endotheliosis. The amount of protein in the urine is frequently taken as an index of the severity of pre-eclampsia. A significant increase in proteinuria, coupled with diminished urinary output, indicates renal impairment. A 24-hour urine collection for total protein measurement will be required to be certain about the presence or absence of proteinuria and to provide an accurate quantitative assessment of protein loss.

- A finding of >300 mg/24 hours is considered to be indicative of mild–moderate pre-eclampsia.

- A finding of >3 g/24 hours is considered to be severe.

Oedema and excessive weight gain

These used to be included in the diagnostic criteria for pre-eclampsia but both are variable findings and nowadays are usually considered only when a diagnosis of pre-eclampsia has been made based on other criteria. The sudden severe widespread appearance of oedema is suggestive of pre-eclampsia or some underlying pathology and further investigations are necessary. This oedema pits on pressure and may be found in non-dependent anatomical areas such as the face, hands, lower abdomen, and vulval and sacral areas.

> **Box 14.2** Laboratory findings in pre-eclampsia
>
> - Increased Hb and haematocrit levels
> - Thrombocytopenia
> - Prolonged clotting times
> - Raised serum creatinine and urea levels
> - Raised serum uric acid level
> - Abnormal liver function tests, particularly raised transaminases

Laboratory tests

The alterations in the haematological and biochemical parameters listed in Box 14.2 are suggestive of pre-eclampsia.

Care and Management

The aim of care is to monitor the condition of the woman and her fetus and, if possible, to prevent the hypertensive disorder worsening by using appropriate interventions and treatment. The ultimate aim is to prolong the pregnancy until the fetus is sufficiently mature to survive, while safeguarding the mother's life.

Antenatal care

Rest

It is preferable for the woman to rest at home and to be visited regularly by the midwife or GP. When proteinuria develops in addition to hypertension, the risks to the mother and fetus are considerably increased. Admission to hospital is required to monitor and evaluate the maternal and fetal condition.

Diet

There is little evidence to support dietary intervention for preventing or restricting the advance of pre-eclampsia.

Weight gain

The value of routine weighing during antenatal visits has been questioned and in many areas has now been abandoned. However, weight gain may be useful for monitoring the progression of pre-eclampsia in conjunction with other parameters.

Blood pressure and urinalysis

The blood pressure is monitored daily at home or every 4 hours when in hospital. Urine should be tested for protein daily. If the woman or midwife identifies protein in a midstream specimen of urine, a 24-hour urine collection is instigated in order to determine the amount of protein. The level of protein indicates the degree of vascular damage. Reduced kidney perfusion is indicated by:

- proteinuria
- reduced creatinine clearance
- increased serum creatinine and uric acid.

Abdominal examination

This is carried out daily. Any discomfort or tenderness may be a sign of placental abruption. Upper abdominal pain is highly significant and indicative of HELLP syndrome (see p. 223) associated with fulminating (rapid-onset) pre-eclampsia.

Fetal assessment

It is advisable to undertake a biophysical profile in order to determine fetal health and well-being. This is done by the use of:

- kick charts
- CTG monitoring
- serial ultrasound scans to check for fetal growth

- assessment of liquor volume and fetal breathing movements or Doppler flow studies, or both, to determine placental blood flow.

Laboratory studies

These include:

- a full blood count, platelet count and clotting profile
- urea and electrolytes
- creatinine and liver function tests, including albumin levels.

In severe pre-eclampsia blood samples should be taken every 12–24 hours.

Antihypertensive therapy

The use of antihypertensive therapy as prophylaxis is controversial, as this shows no benefit in significantly prolonging pregnancy or improving maternal or fetal outcome. Its use is, however, advocated as short-term therapy in order to prevent an increase in blood pressure and the development of severe hypertension, thereby reducing the risk to the mother of cerebral haemorrhage.

- Methyldopa is the most widely used drug in women with mild to moderate gestational hypertension and appears to be safe and effective for both mother and fetus.
- Alpha and beta blockers such as labetalol are considered safe in pregnancy. Atenolol used over the long term is not recommended as it may cause significant fetal growth restriction.

Antithrombotic agents

Early activation of the clotting system may contribute to the later pathology of pre-eclampsia; as a result the use of anticoagulants or antiplatelet agents has been considered for the prevention of pre-eclampsia and fetal growth restriction. Aspirin is thought to inhibit the production of the platelet-aggregating agent, thromboxane A_2.

Intrapartum care

It is essential to monitor the maternal and fetal condition carefully.

Vital signs

- Blood pressure is measured half-hourly, or every 15–20 minutes in severe pre-eclampsia.

- Because of the potentially rapid haemodynamic changes in pre-eclampsia, a number of authors recommend the measurement of the MAP. MAP reflects the systemic perfusion pressure, and therefore the degree of hypovolaemia, whereas manual measurement of diastolic pressure alone is a better indicator of the degree of hypertension.

- Observation of the respiratory rate (>14/min) will be complemented with pulse oximetry in severe pre-eclampsia; this gives an indication of the degree of maternal hypoxia.

- Temperature should be recorded as necessary.

- In severe pre-eclampsia, examination of the optic fundi can give an indication of optic vasospasm. Cerebral irritability can be assessed by the degree of hyperreflexia or the presence of clonus (significant if more than 3 beats).

Fluid balance

The reduced intravascular compartment in pre-eclampsia, together with poorly controlled fluid balance, can result in circulatory overload, pulmonary oedema, acute respiratory distress syndrome and ultimately death. In severe pre-eclampsia a central venous pressure (CVP) line may be considered; measurements are taken hourly.

- If the value is >10 mmHg, then 20 mg furosemide should be considered. Intravenous fluids are administered using infusion pumps; the total recommended fluid intake in severe pre-eclampsia is 85 ml/h.

- Oxytocin should be administered with caution, as it has an antidiuretic effect.

- Urinary output should be monitored and urinalysis undertaken every 4 hours to detect the presence of protein, ketones and glucose.

- In severe pre-eclampsia a urinary catheter should be in situ and urine output is measured hourly; a level >30 ml/h reflects adequate renal function.

Plasma volume expansion

Although women with pre-eclampsia have oedema, they are hypovolaemic. The blood volume of women with pre-eclampsia is reduced, as shown by a high Hb concentration and a high haematocrit level. This results in movement of fluid into the extravascular compartment, causing oedema. The oedema initially occurs in dependent tissues, but as the disease progresses oedema occurs in the liver and brain.

Pain relief

Epidural analgesia may procure the best pain relief, reduce the blood pressure and facilitate rapid caesarean section, should the need arise. It is important to ensure a normal clotting screen and a platelet count >100 × 10^9/L prior to insertion of the epidural.

Fetal condition

The fetal heart rate should be monitored closely. Deviations from the normal must be reported and acted upon.

Birth plan

When the second stage commences, the obstetrician and paediatrician should be notified. A short second stage may be prescribed, depending on the maternal and fetal conditions.

- If the maternal or fetal condition shows significant deterioration during the first stage of labour, a caesarean section will be undertaken.

- Oxytocin is the preferred agent for the management of the third stage of labour.

- Ergometrine and syntometrine will cause peripheral vasoconstriction and increase hypertension; they should therefore not normally be used in the presence of any degree of pre-eclampsia, unless there is severe haemorrhage.

Postpartum care

The maternal condition should continue to be monitored at least every 4 hours for the next 24 hours or more following childbirth, as there is still a potential danger of the mother developing eclampsia.

Signs of impending eclampsia

See Box 14.3.

Box 14.3 Signs of impending eclampsia

- A sharp rise in blood pressure
- Diminished urinary output
- Increase in proteinuria
- Headache, which is usually severe, persistent and frontal in location
- Drowsiness or confusion
- Visual disturbances, such as blurring of vision or flashing lights
- Epigastric pain
- Nausea and vomiting

The aim of care at this time is to preclude death of the mother and fetus by controlling hypertension, inhibiting convulsions and preventing coma.

HELLP Syndrome

The syndrome of haemolysis (H), elevated liver enzymes (EL) and low platelet count (LP) is generally thought to represent a variant of the pre-eclampsia/eclampsia syndrome. Pregnancies complicated by this syndrome have been associated with significant maternal and perinatal morbidity and mortality.

Clinical presentation

HELLP syndrome typically manifests itself between 32 and 34 weeks' gestation and 30% of cases will occur postpartum.

- The woman often complains of malaise, epigastric or right upper quadrant pain, and nausea and vomiting.
- Some will have non-specific viral syndrome-like symptoms.
- Hypertension and proteinuria may be absent or slightly abnormal.

Diagnosis

Pregnant women presenting with the above symptoms should have a full blood count, platelet count and liver function tests, irrespective of maternal blood pressure. The diagnosis of HELLP syndrome may be assisted by confirming:

- haemolysis
- elevated lactate dehydrogenase (LDH)
- raised bilirubin levels
- low ($<100 \times 10^9$/L) or falling platelets

■ elevated liver transaminases (aspartate aminotransferase, alanine transaminase and gamma-glutamyl transferase — AST, ALT and GGT).

Complications

Subcapsular haematoma or rupture of the liver, or both together, is a rare but potentially fatal complication of the HELLP syndrome. The condition usually presents with severe epigastric pain, which may persist for several hours. In addition women may complain of neck and shoulder pain.

Management

Women with the HELLP syndrome should be admitted to a consultant unit with intensive or high-dependency care facilities available.

■ In pregnancies of less than 32 weeks' gestation expectant management may be undertaken with appropriate safeguards and consent.

■ In term pregnancies, or where there is a deteriorating maternal or fetal condition, immediate delivery is recommended.

Eclampsia

Eclampsia is rarely seen in developed countries today; it has an incidence of 2.1 per 10 000 maternities in the UK.

Eclampsia is associated with increased risks of maternal and perinatal morbidity and mortality. Significant maternal life-threatening complications as a result of eclampsia include:

■ pulmonary oedema

■ renal and hepatic failure

- Placental abruption and haemorrhage
- DIC
- HELLP syndrome
- brain haemorrhage.

There can be a problem in the prevention and treatment of eclampsia. A significant finding is that hypertension is not necessarily a precursor to the onset of eclampsia but will almost always be evident following a seizure. Detecting and managing imminent eclampsia is also made more difficult in that, unlike other types of seizure, warning symptoms are not always present before onset of the convulsion.

Care of a woman with eclampsia

The aims of immediate care are to:

- summon medical aid
- clear and maintain the mother's airway – this may be achieved by placing the mother in a semiprone position in order to facilitate the drainage of saliva and vomit
- administer oxygen and prevent severe hypoxia
- prevent the mother from being injured.

The midwife must remain with the mother constantly and provide assistance with medical treatment. In the first instance all effort is devoted to the preservation of the mother's life; the well-being of the baby is secondary. The woman will require intensive/high-dependency care, as she may remain comatose for a time following the seizure or may be sleepy. Recordings should be carried out, as previously mentioned for severe pre-eclampsia. The midwife must observe for periodic restlessness associated with uterine contraction, which indicates that labour has commenced. It is usual to expedite delivery of the baby when eclampsia occurs. In this instance caesarean section is the usual mode of delivery.

Anticonvulsant therapy

Magnesium sulphate is now the recommended drug of choice for routine anticonvulsant management of women with eclampsia; it is administered intravenously according to a protocol:

- A loading dose of 4 g is given over 5–10 minutes intravenously, followed by a maintenance dose of 5 g/500 ml normal saline given as an intravenous infusion at a rate of 1–2 g/h until 24 hours following delivery or the last seizure.

- Recurrent seizures should be treated with a further bolus of 2 g.

- Magnesium sulphate can be toxic and therefore the deep tendon reflexes should be monitored hourly. The respiratory rate and oxygen saturation levels are measured hourly and should remain >14/min and >95% respectively. In women with oliguria, serum magnesium levels should be monitored and maintained within the therapeutic range (2–3 mmol/L). Calcium gluconate is the antidote for magnesium toxicity and should be readily available.

Treatment of hypertension

Severe hypertension is defined as >160/110 mmHg or a MAP >125 mmHg.

- Intravenous hydralazine is the most useful agent to gain control of the blood pressure quickly; 5 mg should be administered slowly and the blood pressure measured at 5-minute intervals until the diastolic pressure reaches 90 mmHg. The diastolic blood pressure may be maintained at this level by titrating an intravenous infusion of hydralazine against the blood pressure.

- Labetalol may be used in preference to hydralazine, in which case 20 mg is given intravenously followed at 10-minute intervals by 40 mg, 80 mg and 80 mg up to a cumulative dose of 300 mg.

Fluid balance

Care must be taken not to overload the maternal system with intravenous fluids.

Anaesthesia

Both general and regional (epidural/spinal) anaesthesia carry a degree of risk in the eclamptic woman. In general, epidural is preferred in eclamptic women who are conscious, haemodynamically stable and cooperative.

Postnatal care

As almost half of eclamptic fits occur following childbirth, intensive surveillance of the woman is required in a high-dependency or intensive care unit. Parameters to monitor are:

- a return to normal blood pressure
- an increase in urine output and reduction in protein
- a reduction in oedema
- a return to normal laboratory indices.

Thromboelastic stockings should be worn to prevent deep vein thrombosis.

All the usual postpartum care is given, and as soon as the mother's condition permits, she should be taken to see her baby. Alternatively, if the baby's condition is good, he or she may be returned to the mother.

Chronic Hypertension

Chronic hypertension has the following possible causes:

- It may be a pre-existing disorder: for example, essential hypertension.
- It may be secondary to existing medical problems, such as renal disease, SLE, coarctation of the aorta, Cushing syndrome or phaeochromocytoma.

Diagnosis

Consistent blood pressure recordings of 140/90 mmHg or more, on two occasions more than 24 hours apart during the first 20 weeks of pregnancy, suggest that the hypertension is a chronic problem and unrelated to the pregnancy. The diagnosis may be difficult to make because of the changes seen with blood pressure in pregnancy. This is a particular problem in women who present late in their pregnancy with no baseline blood pressure measurement.

Investigation

Women with chronic hypertension tend to be older, parous and have a family or personal history of hypertension.

Accurate measurement of blood pressure is important. Serial blood pressure recordings should be made in order to determine the true pattern, as even normotensive women show occasional peaks.

There may be long-term effects of hypertension, such as retinopathy, ischaemic heart disease and renal damage. Renal function tests may be performed; however, it is important to realise the extent to which the alterations in the physiological norms may affect clinical interpretation in pregnancy. Blood urate levels may help to differentiate between chronic hypertension and pre-eclampsia; they do not rise in the former as they do in the latter.

Complications

The perinatal outcome in mild chronic hypertension is good. However

- The perinatal morbidity and mortality are increased in those women who develop severe chronic hypertension or superimposed pre-eclampsia.

- Other complications are independent of pregnancy and include renal failure and cerebral haemorrhage.

- Maternal mortality is high if phaeochromocytoma is not diagnosed and left untreated.

Management

Mild chronic hypertension

This is defined as a systolic blood pressure of <160 mmHg and a diastolic blood pressure of <110 mmHg. The woman is unlikely to need antenatal admission to hospital and may be cared for in the community. The woman's condition should be carefully monitored in order to identify any pre-eclampsia that develops.

Severe chronic hypertension

The systolic blood pressure is >160 mmHg and the diastolic blood pressure is >110 mmHg. Ideally, the woman will be cared for by the obstetric team in conjunction with the physician. Frequent antenatal visits are recommended in order to monitor the maternal condition. Monitoring includes:

- blood pressure monitoring
- urinalysis to detect proteinuria
- blood tests to measure the haematocrit and renal function.

Antihypertensive drug therapy is used in order to prevent maternal complications but has no proven benefit for the fetus, nor in the prognosis of the pre-eclamptic process.

- The most commonly used agent is methyldopa 1–4 g/day in divided doses. It has a sedative effect lasting 2–3 days and is generally considered safe for mother and fetus.
- Other drugs in common usage include labetalol, nifedipine and oral hydralazine.
- Sedative drugs may be given to reduce anxiety and help the woman to rest, but are rarely recommended.

Monitoring of fetal well-being and of placental function should be carried out assiduously because of the risk of fetal compromise. This would include using serial growth scans and placental blood flow studies by Doppler ultrasound. If the maternal or fetal condition causes concern, the woman will be admitted to hospital. The timing of the birth is planned according to the needs of mother and fetus. If early delivery is deemed necessary, induction of labour is preferred to caesarean section.

Renal function should be reassessed postnatally and the woman should be seen by the physician with a view to long-term management of persistent hypertension. Antihypertensive therapy may be required.

Chapter 15

Sexually Transmissible and Reproductive Tract Infections in Pregnancy

Trends in Sexual Health

The rates of sexually transmitted infections (STIs) in the UK have risen sharply since 1995 and the number of new episodes seen at genitourinary medicine (GUM) clinics now stands at over a million a year. Recent trends of particular concern are the high rates of and increase in STI diagnoses found in the 16–24-year age group. The highest rates of gonorrhoea and chlamydia are found in women aged 16–19 and men aged 20–24. Young people are particularly at risk from STIs, as they are more likely to have high numbers of sexual partners, partner change and unprotected sexual intercourse. Young women may also be vulnerable to sexual exploitation and coercion through lack of skills and confidence to negotiate safer sex.

Multidisciplinary team work

Joint management between an obstetrician and a GUM physician during pregnancy is essential for women with infections that are serious, life threatening, or both, such as human immunodeficiency virus (HIV); in addition, a paediatrician is required in the care and management of the neonate infected through vertical transmission. The midwife plays a vital role in caring for the mother and her family in the provision of individualised care throughout pregnancy, labour and the puerperium, and especially in health education and promotion. The psychological aspects of some STIs will require the expertise of specially trained counsellors. This is particularly important for those diagnosed with an STI during pregnancy and those who will have the extra burden of worrying about the welfare of their babies.

Infections of the Vagina and Vulva

There are three main types of vaginal and vulval infection:

- trichomoniasis
- bacterial vaginosis
- candidiasis.

Trichomoniasis

Trichomoniasis is almost exclusively sexually transmissible. It is caused by infection with the parasite *Trichomonas vaginalis*, a round or oval flagellated protozoan. Common symptoms include:

- vaginal discharge
- vulval pruritus
- inflammation.

However, 10–50% of women are asymptomatic. Vaginal discharge is present in up to 70% of cases and may vary in consistency from thin and scanty to profuse and thick. A classic frothy yellow–green discharge occurs in 10–30% of women. Dyspareunia, mild dysuria and lower abdominal pain may also be experienced.

Trichomoniasis in pregnancy

Trichomoniasis has been linked with a small risk of preterm birth and low birth weight, and an increase in the risk of HIV via sexual intercourse. Trichomoniasis may be acquired perinatally.

Diagnosis

In women:

- 95% of cases can be diagnosed by cultures
- 40–80% of cases by microscopic examination of a wet-film or acridine orange-stained slide from the posterior fornix.

Treatment

- The recommended treatment is metronidazole daily for 5–7 days or in a single dose. Although it is contraindicated, meta-analyses have concluded that there is no evidence of teratogenicity from its use in women during the first trimester of pregnancy.

- Clotrimazole pessaries daily for 7 days can be used in early pregnancy. High single-dose regimens should be avoided during pregnancy and breastfeeding.

- It is usual to treat the partner(s) and advise against sexual intercourse until the treatment is completed.

- In addition, patients should be advised not to take alcohol during the treatment and for at least 48 hours afterwards, as this may cause nausea and vomiting.

Bacterial vaginosis (BV)

BV is the most common cause of vaginal discharge in women of childbearing age. It can arise and remit spontaneously in sexually active and non-sexually active women. It often coexists with other STIs. It is more common in:

- black women
- those with an IUCD
- those who smoke.

The incidence of BV is high in women with pelvic inflammatory disease (PID) and some populations of women undergoing elective termination of pregnancy (TOP). It is also associated with post-TOP endometritis.

In this condition the normal lactobacilli-predominant vaginal flora are replaced with a number of anaerobic bacteria. The vaginal epithelium is not inflamed; hence the term 'vaginosis' rather than 'vaginitis'. The main symptom is a malodorous and greyish watery vaginal discharge, although approximately 50% of women are asymptomatic. The odour is usually more pronounced following sexual intercourse owing to the release of amines by the alkaline semen. Vulval irritation may occur in about one-third of women.

BV in pregnancy

BV is present in up to 20% of women during pregnancy, although the majority of these cases will be asymptomatic. BV during pregnancy is associated with preterm birth, low birth weight, preterm premature rupture of membranes, intra-amniotic infection and post partum endometritis.

Diagnosis

A diagnosis of BV is confirmed if three of the following criteria are present:

- a thin, white to grey, homogenous discharge
- 'clue cells' on microscopy (squamous epithelial cells covered with adherent bacteria)
- a vaginal pH of >4.7

■ the release of a fishy odour when potassium hydroxide is added to a sample of the discharge.

A Gram-stained vaginal smear is another diagnostic technique.

Treatment

Antibiotic therapy is highly effective at eradicating infection and improving the outcome of pregnancy for women with a past history of preterm birth.

■ The treatment regimen is the same as for trichomoniasis.

■ Alternative treatments include oral clindamycin, intravaginal clindamycin cream or metronidazole gel.

■ All these treatments have been shown in controlled trials to achieve cure rates of 70–80% after 4 weeks, but recurrences of infection are common.

■ Women should be advised to avoid vaginal douching, use of shower gel and use of antiseptic agents or shampoo in the bath.

Candidiasis

Candidiasis is a common cause of vulvitis, vaginitis and vaginal discharge. The causative organism is usually *Candida albicans*, a fungal parasite. It is a commensal and is found in the flora of the mouth, gastrointestinal tract and vagina. Colonisation of the vagina and vulva may be introduced from the lower intestinal tract or through sexual intercourse. During the reproductive years 10–20% of women may harbour *Candida* species but remain asymptomatic and do not require treatment. Predisposing factors that encourage *C. albicans* to convert from a commensal to a parasitic role are listed in Box 15.1.

The signs and symptoms of candidiasis include:

■ intense vulval pruritus and soreness

■ often, a thick, white curdy discharge (not always present)

■ erythema and oedema of the vulva, vagina and cervix may be erythematous and oedematous

> **Box 15.1** Factors that provoke the conversion of *Candida albicans* from a commensal to a parasite
>
> - Local changes to the vaginal immunity (e.g. vaginal douches)
> - Immunosuppressant disease or treatment (e.g. acquired immunodeficiency syndrome (AIDS), chemotherapy)
> - Drug therapy (e.g. antibiotics)
> - Endocrine disease (e.g. diabetes mellitus)
> - Physiological changes (e.g. pregnancy)
> - Miscellaneous disorders (e.g. iron deficiency)

■ white plaques of the vulva, vagina and cervix

■ dyspareunia.

Candidiasis in pregnancy

Vaginal candidiasis is found 2–10 times more frequently in pregnant than in non-pregnant women and it is more difficult to eradicate.

Diagnosis

Vaginal culture is the most sensitive method currently available for detecting *Candida* cells.

Treatment

Candidiasis is treated primarily with antifungal pessaries or cream inserted high into the vagina at night. Preparations that may be given include:

■ clotrimazole pessaries

■ nystatin pessaries or gel

■ oral fluconazole (Diflucan).

Diflucan is available from chemists without a prescription but this form of treatment has not been tested in pregnancy and it cannot be assumed to be safe. It should also be used with caution whilst breast-feeding owing to toxic effects in high doses.

Recurrence is common. This may be due to resistant cases or failure to complete the treatment. It is usual to treat the partner and advise against sexual intercourse until the treatment is completed. Vaginal douches or irritants such as perfumed products should be avoided. The wearing of tight-fitting synthetic clothing should be discouraged.

Bacterial Infections

Chlamydia

Chlamydia trachomatis is an intracellular bacterium. It is the most common cause of sexually transmitted bacterial infection and a leading cause of PID.

- Serotypes D–K are sexually transmitted and are important causes of morbidity in both sexes.
- Serotypes A, B and C cause trachoma and blindness
- Serotypes L1–L3 cause the genital disease lymphogranuloma venereum.

Chlamydial infection is asymptomatic in approximately 80% of cases. Some women may have a purulent vaginal discharge, postcoital or intermenstrual bleeding, lower abdominal pain, mucopurulent cervicitis and/or contact bleeding. Chlamydial infection of the cervix is found in 15–30% of women attending GUM clinics, and concurrently in 35–40% of women with gonorrhoea. Specific high-risk groups include:

- women aged less than 25
- those with a new sexual partner or more than one sexual partner in recent years
- those not using barrier contraception

- those using oral contraception
- those presenting for termination of pregnancy.

Chlamydial infection has been estimated to account for 40% of ectopic pregnancies.

Chlamydia in pregnancy

It can cause amnionitis and postpartum endometritis.

Fetal and neonatal infections

The major risk to the infant is from passing through an infected cervix during birth. Up to 70% of babies born to mothers with chlamydial infection will become infected, with 30–40% developing conjunctivitis and 10–20% a characteristic pneumonia. The incubation period of chlamydial ophthalmia is 6–21 days. Chlamydial pneumonia usually occurs between the 4th and 11th weeks of life. It affects about half the babies who develop conjunctivitis but is not always preceded by it. The pharynx, middle ear, rectum and vagina are also targets for infection, with a delay of up to 7 months before cultures become positive.

Diagnosis

Nucleic acid amplification (NAA) tests should be used to screen women for genital chlamydial infection.

Treatment

Genital chlamydial infections are sensitive to three classes of antibiotic:

- the tetracyclines
- macrolides (e.g. erythromycin)
- the fluorinated quinolones, especially ofloxacin.

The tetracyclines and the fluoroquinolones are currently contraindicated in pregnancy. Erythromycin has long been the preferred treatment for cervical chlamydial infection despite its gastrointestin effects. Erythromycin is also used for chlamydial infections in infants, young children and pregnant and lactating women. Single-dose azithromycin is expensive but gaining favour because of its effectiveness, low incidence of adverse gastrointestinal effects and enhanced compliance.

Gonorrhoea

Gonorrhoea is caused by *Neisseria gonorrhoeae*, a Gram-negative diplococcus. Transmission is by sexual contact. This organism adheres to mucous membranes and has a preference for columnar rather than squamous epithelium. The primary sites of infection are therefore the mucous membranes of the urethra, endocervix, rectum, pharynx and conjunctiva. Gonorrhoea may coexist with other genital mucosal pathogens, notably *T. vaginalis*, *C. albicans* and *C. trachomatis*. Gonorrhoea is a major cause of PID. The sequelae of PID include:

- infertility
- ectopic pregnancy
- chronic pelvic pain.

Although uncommon, gonorrhoea may also cause disseminated systemic disease and arthritis.

- The most common symptom is an increased or altered vaginal discharge, although up to 50% of women are asymptomatic.
- Lower abdominal pain, dysuria, intermenstrual uterine bleeding and menorrhagia may also be experienced, ranging in intensity from minimal to severe.

Gonorrhoea in pregnancy

The incidence of gonorrhoea in pregnancy is low but its presence has been associated with:

- spontaneous abortion
- very low birth weight

- prelabour rupture of the membranes
- chorioamnionitis
- preterm birth
- postpartum endometritis
- pelvic sepsis.

Fetal and neonatal infections

N. gonorrhoeae can be transmitted from the mother's genital tract to the newborn during birth, or occasionally in utero when there is prolonged rupture of the membranes. The risk of transmission from an infected mother is between 30 and 47%. Infection usually manifests as gonococcal ophthalmia neonatorum, a notifiable condition. A profuse, purulent discharge is usually evident within a few days of birth. It can be diagnosed by microscopy and culture of an eye swab. The eyes may be cleaned with saline but systemic antibiotics are required. If left untreated, the condition will eventually lead to blindness, and occasionally the neonate may develop further infection such as gonococcal arthritis.

Diagnosis

Culture on antibiotic-containing medium has long been considered to be the 'gold standard' for detecting *N. gonorrhoeae*. The sensitivity is almost 100% in specialised clinics, but isolation rates are lower in non-specialised settings.

Treatment

- The antibiotic regimen of penicillin and probenicid remains effective. Oral, single-dose preparations are now most commonly given.
- In the case of penicillin allergy or penicillin-resistant organisms, spectinomycin or ceftriaxone are also effective.

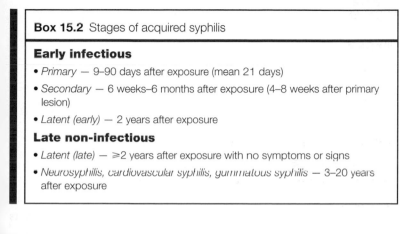

Box 15.2 Stages of acquired syphilis

Early infectious

- *Primary* — 9–90 days after exposure (mean 21 days)
- *Secondary* — 6 weeks–6 months after exposure (4–8 weeks after primary lesion)
- *Latent (early)* — 2 years after exposure

Late non-infectious

- *Latent (late)* — ≥2 years after exposure with no symptoms or signs
- *Neurosyphilis, cardiovascular syphilis, gummatous syphilis* — 3–20 years after exposure

Syphilis

Syphilis is caused by the bacterium *Treponema pallidum*, a spiral organism (spirochaete), and is usually acquired by sexual contact. It can also be congenitally transmitted. It is a complex systemic disease that can involve virtually any organ in the body.

Acquired syphilis is divided into the stages shown in Box 15.2.

Syphilis in pregnancy

Although sequelae are dependent on the stage of infection in the mother, untreated syphilis in pregnancy may result in:

- spontaneous abortion
- preterm birth
- stillbirth
- neonatal death
- significant infant or later morbidity.

Vertical transmission may occur at any time during pregnancy, but is more likely if the mother has primary, secondary or early latent syphilis. The infection does not usually occur before the 4th month of pregnancy because treponemes from the maternal circulation are unable to pass through the Langhans cell layer of the early placenta. Once this layer begins to atrophy during the 4th month of pregnancy, the fetus is exposed to the first risk of infection, although this is most likely after the 6th month when complete atrophy has taken place. A pregnant woman found to have early syphilis is likely to be suffering from early infectious syphilis and early treatment prevents most cases of congenital syphilis. In pregnant women with untreated early syphilis, up to one-third of cases will result in stillbirth.

Congenital syphilis

Approximately two-thirds of live-born infected infants do not have any signs or symptoms at birth, but they present over the following weeks, months or years. Lesions develop only after the 4th month when immunological competence becomes established. Serology at birth is unreliable owing to passive transfer from the mother and the treponemal-specific IgM test is prone to false positive and negative results.

Diagnosis

Women in the UK are screened for syphilis at antenatal booking and treated if need be. However, this does not detect women who acquire the infection during pregnancy, or women who are incubating syphilis at the time of serological testing. A range of serological tests is used for screening (Box 15.3).

If syphilis is suspected on the basis of clinical findings, dark-field microscopic examination or fluorescent antibody staining of a specimen taken from a lesion should be undertaken.

Treatment

- The preferred treatment is intramuscular penicillin.
- In the case of penicillin allergy, the alternative is erythromycin, as tetracycline is contraindicated in pregnancy.
- The poor placental transfer of erythromycin does not reliably cure the fetus and as a precaution the baby may be given a course of penicillin at birth.

> **Box 15.3** Serological tests for syphilis
>
> • Venereal Diseases Research Laboratory (VDRL)
> • Rapid plasma reagin test (RPR)
> • *Treponema pallidum* haemagglutination assay (TPHA)
> • *Treponema pallidum* particle agglutination assay (TPPA)
> • Fluorescent treponemal antibody absorption test (FTA-abs)
> • Treponemal enzyme immunoassay (EIA)

Group B streptococcus (GBS)

GBS (*Streptococcus agalactiae*) is a Gram-positive bacterium that naturally colonises the body. It is harboured primarily in the gastrointestinal tract, with approximately 30% of adults asymptomatically carrying the organism at any one time. It also colonises the vagina in up to 25% of women.

GBS in pregnancy

In pregnant women colonised with GBS, high-risk factors associated with vertical transmission include:

- preterm birth
- prolonged rupture of membranes
- maternal pyrexia during labour
- GBS cultured in a urine sample
- known carriage of GBS
- a history of a GBS infection in a previous pregnancy.

GBS is able to infiltrate the amniotic cavity, whether or not the membranes are intact, and infects the fetus through the lung epithelium. Postpartum endometritis and postcaesarean wound infection may also occur in the mother.

Fetal and neonatal infections

GBS is the commonest cause of overwhelming sepsis in newborns during the first days of life, occurring at a rate of approximately 1–2 per 1000 live births. The respiratory infection rapidly progresses to sepsis and shock and causes significant morbidity and mortality. GBS infection in the neonate may be:

- early onset, in which case the infection starts in utero
- late onset, which usually presents between 7 days and 3 months of age.

Diagnosis

- Vaginal and rectal swabs can detect colonisation with GBS, although higher rates are detected with a special enrichment culture medium. The degree of colonisation is extremely variable and the tendency for recolonisation after treatment makes control difficult.
- Swabs taken late in pregnancy at around 35 weeks are effective in predicting whether or not GBS will be carried during labour.

Treatment

Intrapartum antibiotic treatment of women colonised with GBS appears to reduce neonatal infection.

- The usual regimen is intravenous ampicillin during labour.
- Alternatives include benzyl penicillin or erythromycin.

Viral Infections

Genital warts

Genital warts are caused by human papillomavirus (HPV) types 6 an 11. Transmission is most often by sexual contact, although infants an young children may develop laryngeal papillomas after being infected from maternal genital warts at birth.

In pregnancy genital warts may dramatically increase in size and appear as cauliflower-like masses, although they usually diminish in size following the birth. Occasionally they can obstruct a vaginal birth; therefore a caesarean section would be indicated.

Genital warts are difficult and time-consuming to treat.

- They are usually treated initially with locally applied caustic agents such as podophyllum. However, this is contraindicated in pregnancy because of possible teratogenic effects.
- It is recommended that no treatment be offered during pregnancy, although there are alternatives such as trichloroacetic acid, cryotherapy or electrocautery.

Women presenting with genital warts should be fully investigated to exclude other STIs. In addition, colposcopy should be performed to exclude flat warts on the cervix. Most genital warts are benign, but cervical intraepithelial neoplasia (CIN) is strongly associated with HPV types 16, 18, 31, 33 and 35; therefore an annual cervical smear is recommended.

Hepatitis B virus (HBV)

HBV infection is a major public health problem worldwide; it is an important cause of morbidity and mortality from acute infection and chronic sequelae that include chronic active hepatitis, cirrhosis and primary liver cancer. HBV can be transmitted sexually or parenterally through infected blood or blood products. Body fluids such as saliva, menstrual and vaginal discharges, serous exudates, seminal fluid and breast milk have been implicated in the spread of infection, but infectivity is largely related to blood and body fluids contaminated with blood. It can be transmitted by means of unsterilised equipment, such as may be used when injecting drug-users share needles and syringes, or in tattooing or acupuncture, or as a consequence of needle-stick injury in health-care workers. Vertical transmission is a major mode of transmission, most frequently occurring perinatally. Acute HBV infection during pregnancy is associated with an increased rate of spontaneous abortion and preterm labour.

There are usually two phases of symptoms:

- the prodromal phase, characterised by flu-like symptoms
- the icteric phase, characterised by jaundice, anorexia, nausea and fatigue.

The infection may be asymptomatic in 10–50% of adults in the acute phase and in virtually all infants and children. If chronic infection occurs, there are often no physical signs but there may be signs of chronic liver disease.

In the acute early phase the hepatitis B surface antigen (HBsAg, formally called Australia antigen) is produced by the infected hepatocytes and appears in the sera of most patients. The presence of the hepatitis Be antigen (HBeAg) in the serum indicates viral activity, which can persist over days or weeks. IgM- and IgG-type antibodies to the core antigen develop. IgG antibodies may be detectable for many years after recovery. As the infection resolves, HBeAg becomes undetectable; once infection is cleared, the antibody to the surface antigen component, anti-HBs, appears, indicating immunity. I HBsAg remains detectable for more than 6 months, the patient i usually referred to as a hepatitis B virus carrier.

All pregnant women should be offered antenatal screening fo HBV and babies born to infected mothers should be vaccinated.

- The injections should be administered at birth and at 1 and 6 months.
- In addition, the babies of mothers who have become infected with HBV during pregnancy and those who do not have anti-HBe antibodies should also receive hepatitis B-specific immunoglobulin (HBIg) at birth. This should be injected at a different site to the vaccine (the anterolateral thigh is the preferred site in infants). This confers immediate immunity and reduces vertical transmission by 90%.

- Infected mothers should continue to breastfeed, as there is no additional risk of transmission.

Hepatitis C virus (HCV)

HCV infection is another type of viral hepatitis that occurs throughout the world.

- The principal route of transmission is by percutaneous inoculation, blood and blood products.
- The incidence of transmission by sexual contact is low.
- Vertical transmission is also low, occurring at 5% or less, but higher rates are seen if the mother is HIV- and HCV-positive.

At present, there is no known way of reducing the risk of vertical transmission. There is no firm evidence that breastfeeding constitutes an additional risk of transmission unless the mother is symptomatic with a high viral load.

Herpes simplex virus (HSV)

There are two types of HSV: HSV-1 and HSV-2.

- HSV-1 causes the majority of orolabial infections, and is often acquired during childhood through direct physical contact with oral secretions.
- HSV-2 is the most common cause of genital herpes and is sexually transmitted via genital secretions.

Infections may be primary or non-primary. Once infected, the virus remains in the individual for life, causing recurrent infection. Prior infection with HSV-1 modifies the clinical manifestations of first infection by HSV-2. The incidence of HSV infection depends on factors such as:

  age
  duration of sexual activity
  number of sexual partners

- socioeconomic status
- previous genital infections
- race.

In adults, HSV infection may be asymptomatic, but painful, vesicular or ulcerative lesions of the skin and mucous membranes occur frequently. Dysuria and vaginal or urethral discharge may also occur. There may be systemic symptoms of fever and myalgia. Symptoms are more common in primary infection.

Genital herpes infection

This is defined as:

- *First episode primary infection* — first infection with either HSV-1 or HSV-2 in an individual with no pre-existing antibodies to either type. The local symptoms tend to be severe and lesions may last for 2–3 weeks.

- *First episode non-primary infection* — first infection with either HSV-1 or HSV-2 in an individual with pre-existing circulating antibodies to the other type.

- *Recurrent infection* — recurrence of clinical symptoms due to reactivation of pre-existent HSV-1 or HSV-2 infection after a period of latency.

HSV in pregnancy

The most important complication of HSV infection in pregnancy is neonatal herpes, a rare but potentially very serious condition. Congenital infection, a consequence of primary infection early in pregnancy, can cause severe abnormalities that in the absence of vesicles are difficult to distinguish from similar syndromes caused by rubella, toxoplasmosis or cytomegalovirus. The risk of neonatal infection is about 40% with active primary infection, but less than 8% with recurrent infections at the time of delivery and rare with asymptomatic shedding.

Diagnosis

- Viral cultures from open lesions are one of the best methods of diagnosing infection but they have a significant false negative rate. Culture levels are normally available within 48–96 hours.

- Serological tests that demonstrate rising titres of HSV antibodies can be used for the diagnosis of primary infections only by confirming seroconversion. The presence of antibody titre in an initial specimen or the presence of a typical lesion is suggestive of non-primary first episode or recurrent disease.

- These tests cannot reliably distinguish between HSV-1 and HSV-2 except by using HSV-type specific glycoprotein G as the antigen.

Treatment

The treatment and management of genital HSV infection in pregnancy include:

- antiviral therapy
- saline bathing
- analgesia
- topical anaesthetic gels.

Primary infection acquired during the first or second trimester should be treated with oral or intravenous antiviral therapy, depending on the clinical condition. Aciclovir reduces viral shedding, reduces pain and promotes the healing of lesions. It is not licensed for use in pregnancy. The recommended dose is the same as for non-pregnant adults, but higher doses may be required for immunocompromised women. Continuous aciclovir in the last 4 weeks of pregnancy reduces the risk of clinical recurrence at term and delivery by caesarean section.

In the third trimester, women with active genital lesions after 34 weeks should be delivered by caesarean section, as the risk of viral shedding and vertical transmission is high. Recurrent HSV infection during pregnancy is also treated with aciclovir. Caesarean section is not indicated unless genital lesions or prodromal symptoms of an impending outbreak, such as vulval pain or burning, are present.

Cytomegalovirus (CMV)

Cytomegalovirus is a member of the herpes virus family. It is so named because it has the effect of enlarging the cells that it infects. Seroepidemiological studies show that CMV infection is common. Most CMV infections are subclinical. However, the clinical manifestations of CMV infection vary with age, route of transmission and the immune competence of the subject. Primary infection may cause generally mild mononucleosis-type symptoms such as malaise, myalgia and fever in immunocompetent adults, whereas it is particularly pathogenic among immunosuppressed individuals, recipients of organ transplants, premature infants and patients with AIDS.

CMV infection in pregnancy

Several studies have shown that primary infection occurs in all trimesters, with about 37% of neonates being born with congenital infection. As the majority of these do not develop the disease, it is not a sufficient criterion to recommend TOP.

Fetal and neonatal infections

CMV is the most common intrauterine infection, affecting from 0.4 to 2.3% of all live births. Unlike rubella, which has a teratogenic effect, CMV allows fetal organs to develop normally but causes disease by the secondary destruction of the cells. Up to 18% of infants born to mothers with primary infection may be symptomatic at birth. The prognosis is thus poor. More than 90% of all symptomatic patients develop sensorineural hearing loss, mental retardation, chorioretinitis and other more subtle complications in later years. In infants with subclinical infection the outlook is much better, but 5–15% will develop some sequelae that are generally less severe than in infants with symptomatic infection at birth.

Perinatal infections result from exposure to CMV in the maternal genital tract at birth or from breast milk. The majority of infants are asymptomatic; occasionally, however, perinatally acquired infection is associated with pneumonitis in preterm and sick full-term infants, neurological sequelae and psychomotor retardation.

Diagnosis

CMV infections can be diagnosed by direct methods such as:

- viral cultures (from urine, saliva, breast milk, cervical secretions, biopsy and autopsy specimens)
- polymerase chain reaction (PCR)
- antigen detection.

Treatment

Ganciclovir and foscarnet have been used with encouraging results in life-threatening CMV infections in immunocompromised hosts. Both drugs are, however, extensively toxic.

Human immunodeficiency virus (HIV)

There are two types of HIV: HIV-1 and HIV-2.

- HIV-1 is the cause of the worldwide spread of AIDS.
- HIV-2 is largely confined to West Africa.

The three principal means of HIV transmission are by:

- blood or blood products
- sexual contact
- passage from mother to child.

Two to six weeks after exposure to HIV, 50–70% of those infected develop a transient non-specific illness with fever, myalgia, malaise, lymphadenopathy and pharyngitis. Over 50% develop a rash. Oral and genital ulcers have also been reported. The illness begins abruptly and usually lasts for 1–2 weeks, but could be more protracted.

Seroconversion is usually followed by an asymptomatic period lasting on average 10 years without antiretroviral therapy. However, although the infection is latent clinically, there is intense viral and lymphocyte turnover with worsening immunodeficiency. Approximately one-third of patients will experience persistent generalised lymphadenopathy. The average time for progression from HIV to AIDS is about 10 years.

HIV in pregnancy

HIV-1 infection has become an important complication of pregnancy and is associated with poor pregnancy outcomes. The most serious effect of HIV-1 infection during pregnancy is vertical transmission. This can occur during pregnancy, in the intrapartum period or postnatally. In non-breastfed infants, up to 75% of transmission is thought to occur in late pregnancy and the period covering labour and birth. Transmission is influenced by a number of factors. The maternal plasma viral load is most important. The level of virus shed in cervical and vaginal secretions may also be a factor for perinatal HIV-1 transmission.

HIV-1 DNA is present in breast milk and so postnatal transmission can occur during breastfeeding. Avoidance of breastfeeding by HIV-1-infected women is therefore recommended if safe and affordable alternatives are available. Other factors associated with an increased risk of transmission are listed in Box 15.4.

Diagnosis

- Acute infection is accompanied by the development of serum antibodies in the case of core and surface proteins of the virus in 2–6 weeks. Over 90% of seroconversions occur within 3 months of infection. In a minority of cases seroconversion may be delayed to more than 6 months; therefore negative diagnostic tests need to be repeated 3 months after possible exposure and after 6–9 months where there has been a high risk of transmission. Following seroconversion, antibody persists indefinitely in the serum and forms a highly specific test for HIV

> **Box 15.4** Factors associated with an increased risk of transmission in HIV
>
> - Breastfeeding
> - Advanced clinical HIV disease
> - Impaired maternal immunocompetence
> - Maternal nutritional status
> - Resistant viral strains
> - Vaginal birth
> - Prolonged rupture of membranes
> - Invasive obstetric procedures
> - Maternal ulcerative genital infection
> - Recreational drug use during pregnancy
> - Promaturity
> - Low birth weight

infection. One or more enzyme immunoassays (EIAs) directed towards HIV-1 and HIV-2 are used as the initial screening tests.

■ Positive screening tests are confirmed by serum titre tests, a Western blot or immunofluorescence assay.

■ Primary infection in the neonatal period poses problems in the laboratory diagnosis of HIV. Tests for antibodies need to be repeated at intervals. However, rapid diagnosis during the early stages of infection, when anti-HIV antibodies may be absent, may be provided by detecting HIV viraemia using tests for HIV RNA or DNA (by PCR), p24 antigen or viral culture assays. These allow confirmation of HIV infection in 95% of infected infants by 1 month of age.

Treatment

■ In contrast to the increased mother-to-child transmission in developing countries, perinatal HIV infection has been reduced in many developed countries as a result of measures that include counselling, testing, antiretroviral treatment and infant formula feeding.

■ Zidovudine given orally to HIV-1-infected pregnant women starting at 14–34 weeks' gestation, intravenously during labour and orally to babies for 6 weeks, in the absence of breastfeeding, has been shown to lower the risk of perinatal HIV-1 transmission by two-thirds. So far there has been no evidence that high doses of zidovudine lead to teratogenicity or short-term adverse effects in the human fetus or newborn.

■ As well as the long-course zidovudine regimens, long-course combination antiretroviral therapy throughout pregnancy and short-course zidovudine regimens have been reported.

■ During labour and birth, measures can be taken to avoid situations known to predispose to vertical transmission of HIV. Amniotomy is contraindicated and labour should be augmented if contractions are either weak or absent to avoid a prolonged interval between membrane rupture and birth. Invasive techniques, such as direct CTG monitoring through scalp clips and fetal blood sampling, should be avoided and the restrictive use of episiotomy is recommended. Instrumental delivery should be avoided to minimise abrasions to both mother and baby.

■ Elective caesarean section has been found to reduce the likelihood of vertical transmission of HIV-1 by 50%. Breastfeeding should be avoided.

HIV antibody testing and counselling in pregnancy

Since 1999, an HIV test has been offered to all pregnant women. Post-test counselling will involve the giving of positive, negative or indeterminate results. Issues for discussion include the natural history of the infection, treatment options and safe sex to avoid transmission to an HIV-negative partner(s) and acquisition of other STIs. The diagnosis should be confirmed by a second test and an immediate referral should be made for specialist medical assessment. An important consideration for the woman is whether or not to continue with the pregnancy.

Chapter 16

Multiple Pregnancy

The term 'multiple pregnancy' is used to describe the development of more than one fetus in utero at the same time.

Twin Pregnancy

Types of twin pregnancy

Twins will be either monozygotic (MZ) or dizygotic (DZ) (Box 16.1). Of all twins born in the UK, two-thirds will be DZ and one-third MZ.

Superfecundation is the term used when twins are conceived from sperm from different men if a woman has had more than one partner during a menstrual cycle. It is not known how often this happens, but if suspected then paternity can be checked by DNA testing.

Superfetation is the term used for twins conceived as the result of two coital acts in different menstrual cycles. This is thought to be very rare.

Determination of zygosity and chorionicity

Determination of zygosity means determining whether or not the twins are identical.

■ In about one-third of all twins born this will be obvious, as the children will be of a different sex.

- At birth, identical twins tend to have a greater weight variation than non-identical ones.

- In approximately two-thirds of identical twins a monochorionic placenta will confirm monozygosity. If the babies have a single outer membrane, the chorion, they must be MZ.

- In one-third of identical twins the placenta will have two chorions and two amnions, and either fused placentae or two separate placentae (dichorionic); this situation is indistinguishable from that in non-identical twins. It occurs when the fertilised ovum splits within the first 3 or 4 days after fertilisation and while it is still in the uterine tube.

- When these entities are seen on an early scan they appear as two separate placentae and are dichorionic and diamniotic, exactly the same as non-identical twins.

- In about two-thirds of cases the division occurs up to approximately 10–12 days after fertilisation; these will be monochorionic and diamniotic.

Box 16.1 Monozygosity and dizygosity

Monozygotic or uniovular twins

- Also referred to as 'identical twins'
- Develop from the fusion of one ovum and one spermatozoon, which after fertilisation splits into two
- Are of the same sex and have the same genes, blood groups and physical features such as eye and hair colour, ear shapes and palm creases; may be of different sizes and sometimes have different personalities

Dizygotic or binovular twins

- Also referred to as 'non-identical twins'
- Develop from two separate ova that are fertilised by two different spermatozoa
- Are no more alike than any brother or sister and can be of the same or different sex

■ Monoamniotic twins occur in about 1% of cases, when the embryo divides after 12 days.

Monochorionic twin pregnancies have a 3–5 times higher risk of perinatal mortality and morbidity than dichorionic twin pregnancies.

Zygosity determination after birth

The most accurate method of determining zygosity is to compare DNA. DNA can be extracted from cells taken from a cheek swab from inside the mouth. Specific genetic markers extracted from different chromosomes are compared and the results are up to 99.99% accurate.

Zygosity determination should be routinely offered to all same-sex twins for the reasons listed in Box 16.2.

Diagnosis of twin pregnancy

This is usually through ultrasound examination. Diagnosis can be made as early as 6 weeks into the pregnancy, or later at the routine detailed structural scan between the 18th and 20th weeks. When a woman is being booked into the antenatal clinic, a family history of

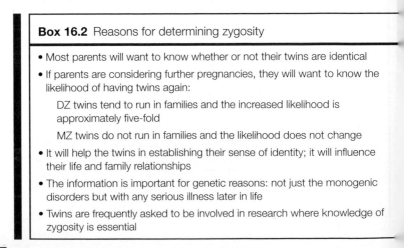

Box 16.2 Reasons for determining zygosity

- Most parents will want to know whether or not their twins are identical
- If parents are considering further pregnancies, they will want to know the likelihood of having twins again:

    DZ twins tend to run in families and the increased likelihood is approximately five-fold

    MZ twins do not run in families and the likelihood does not change

- It will help the twins in establishing their sense of identity; it will influence their life and family relationships
- The information is important for genetic reasons: not just the monogenic disorders but with any serious illness later in life
- Twins are frequently asked to be involved in research where knowledge of zygosity is essential

twins should alert the midwife to the possibility of a multiple pregnancy. If the pregnancy is diagnosed at 6 weeks the woman should have the 'vanishing twin syndrome' explained to her. Occasionally, one fetus may die in the second trimester and become a fetus papyraceous, which becomes embedded in the surface of the placenta and expelled with the placenta at delivery. This is very rare and probably occurs in 1 in 12 000 live births.

Since the advent of routine ultrasound scanning it is very rare for a woman to reach the birth with undiagnosed twins, but this will not apply in areas where this technology is unavailable or where the mother declines it.

Abdominal examination

See Box 16.3.

Box 16.3 Abdominal examination in the diagnosis of multiple pregnancy

Inspection

- The size of the uterus may be larger than expected for the period of gestation, particularly after the 20th week. The uterus may look broad or round
- Fetal movements may be seen over a wide area, although the findings are not diagnostic of twins
- Fresh striae gravidarum may be apparent
- Up to twice the amount of amniotic fluid is normal in a twin pregnancy but polyhydramnios is not an uncommon complication of a twin pregnancy, particularly with monochorionic twins

Palpation

- The fundal height may be greater than expected for the period of gestation
- The presence of two fetal poles (head or breech) in the fundus of the uterus may be noted; multiple fetal limbs may also be palpable
- The head may be small in relation to the size of the uterus
- Lateral palpation may reveal two fetal backs or limbs on both sides

(Continued)

> **Box 16.3** (Continued)
>
> - Pelvic palpation may give findings similar to those on fundal palpation, although one fetus may lie behind the other and make detection difficult
> - Location of three poles in total is diagnostic of at least two fetuses
>
> **Auscultation**
>
> - Hearing two fetal hearts is not diagnostic; however, if simultaneous comparison of the heart rates reveals a difference of at least 10 beats per minute, it may be assumed that two hearts are being heard

The pregnancy

A multiple pregnancy tends to be shorter than a single pregnancy. The average gestation for twins is 37 weeks, for triplets 34 weeks, and for quadruplets 33 weeks.

Effects of pregnancy

Exacerbation of common disorders

The presence of more than one fetus in utero and the higher level of circulating hormones often exacerbate the common disorders of pregnancy. Sickness, nausea and heartburn may be more persistent and more troublesome than in a singleton pregnancy.

Anaemia

Iron deficiency and folic acid deficiency anaemias are common. Early growth and development of the uterus and its contents make greater demands on the maternal iron stores; in later pregnancy (after the 28th week) fetal demands may lead to anaemia. However, recent research suggests that routine prescription of iron and folic acid supplements is not necessary.

Polyhydramnios

This is also common and is particularly associated with monochorionic twins and with fetal abnormalities. Polyhydramnios will add any discomfort that the woman is already experiencing. Acute poly-hydramnios can lead to miscarriage or premature labour.

Pressure symptoms

The increased weight and size of the uterus and its contents may be troublesome. Impaired venous return from the lower limbs increases the tendency to varicose veins and oedema of the legs. Backache is common and the increased uterine size may also lead to marked dyspnoea and to indigestion.

Other effects

There can be an increase in complications of pregnancy.

Antenatal screening

- Nuchal translucency for Down syndrome is accurate only if performed between 11 and 13 weeks.

- Serum screening is not usually performed in multiple pregnancy, as results are too complex to interpret.

- Chorionic villus sampling (CVS) is not usually recommended in multiple pregnancy, as loss rates are high.

- Amniocentesis can be performed in twin pregnancies, usually between 15 and 20 weeks. It should be performed in a specialist fetal medicine unit. Most obstetricians prefer to do a dual needle insertion so there is no chance of contamination between the two sacs.

- Chorionicity should be determined in the first trimester.

- All MZ twins should have echocardiography performed at approximately 20 weeks' gestation, as there is a much higher risk of cardiac anomalies in these babies.

Ultrasound examination

- Monochorionic twin pregnancies should be scanned every 2 weeks from diagnosis to check for discordant fetal growth and signs of twin-to-twin transfusion syndrome (TTTS).

- Dichorionic twin pregnancies should be scanned at 20 weeks for anomalies, and then usually every 4 weeks.

Antenatal preparation

Early diagnosis of a twin pregnancy and of chorionicity is extremely important in order to prepare the parents by giving them the specialist support and advice they will need.

Preparation for breastfeeding

Mothers will inevitably give a lot of thought to how they are going to feed their babies, not only from the nutritional but also from the practical point of view, because it will take up a large amount of their time during the first 6 months. Mothers should be advised right from the beginning not only that it is possible to breastfeed two, and in some cases three, babies, but also that, nutritionally, this is the best way for her to feed her babies; it can be a very rewarding experience for her, as well.

Labour and Birth

Onset of labour

The higher the number of fetuses the mother is carrying, the earlier the labour is likely to start. Term for twins is usually considered to be 37 weeks rather than 40, and approximately 30% of twins are born preterm. In addition to being preterm the babies may be small for gestational age and therefore prone to the associated complications of both conditions. If spontaneous labour begins very early, the chances of survival outside the uterus are small and the mother may be given drugs to inhibit uterine activity. Known causes of preterm labour must, if at all possible, be diagnosed and treated quickly; for example, urinary tract infection should be treated with antibiotics.

It is very unusual for a twin pregnancy to last more than 40 weeks; many obstetricians advise induction of labour at 38 weeks. If the first twin is in a cephalic presentation, labour is usually allowed to continue normally to a vaginal birth, but if the first twin is presenting in

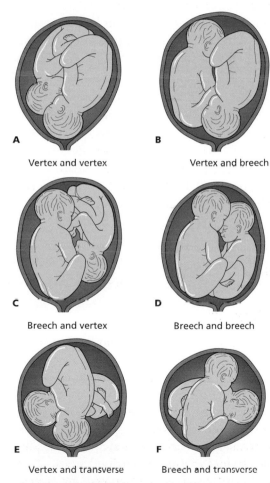

A — Vertex and vertex

B — Vertex and breech

C — Breech and vertex

D — Breech and breech

E — Vertex and transverse

F — Breech and transverse

Fig. 16.1 Presentation of twins before delivery.
(After Bryan 1984, with permission of Edward Arnold.)

any other way (Fig. 16.1), an elective caesarean section is usually recommended.

Management of labour

■ Induction of labour usually occurs around 38 weeks' gestation. The presence of complications such as pregnancy-induced hypertension, intrauterine growth restriction or twin-to-twin transfusion syndrome may be reasons for earlier induction.

■ The majority of women expecting twins will go into labour spontaneously. Theoretically, the duration of the first stage of labour should be no different from that of a single pregnancy. However, there is an increased incidence of dysfunctional labour in twin pregnancies, possibly because of overdistension of the uterus.

■ Labour in the mother of twins must be recognised as high-risk and so continuous fetal heart monitoring of both babies is advocated. This can be achieved:

with two external transducers, *or*

once the membranes are ruptured, with a scalp electrode on the presenting twin and an external transducer on the second.

■ If a 'twin monitor' is available, both heartbeats can be monitored simultaneously to give a more reliable reading. Uterine activity will also need to be monitored.

■ If CTG is not available, use of the Doptone or Sonicaid may give more accurate recordings of the fetal heart rates than a fetal stethoscope. If the latter has to be used, two people must auscultate simultaneously so that fetal heart rates are counted over the same minute.

■ Whilst in labour the woman should be encouraged to be mobile or to adopt whichever position she finds most comfortable. A foam rubber wedge under the side of the mattress will help to prevent supine hypotensive syndrome by giving a lateral tilt. It may be preferable for her to adopt a semiprone position, well supported by pillows or a beanbag. A birthing chair or a reclining chair, if available, may be more comfortable than a delivery bed.

- Regional epidural block provides excellent analgesia and, if necessary, allows easier instrumental deliveries and also manipulation of the second twin. The use of inhalation analgesia may be helpful, either before the epidural is in situ or during the second stage if the effect of the epidural is wearing off.

- If fetal compromise occurs during labour, delivery will need to be expedited, usually by caesarean section. Action may also need to be taken if the mother's condition gives cause for concern.

- If uterine activity is poor, the use of intravenous oxytocin may be required once the membranes have been ruptured.

- If the babies are expected to be premature and of low birth weight or known to have any other problems, the neonatal unit must be informed that the woman is in labour so that staff can make the necessary preparations to receive the babies. When the birth is imminent, the paediatric team should be summoned to be present when the babies are born.

Management of the births

- The second stage of labour may be confirmed by a vaginal examination. The obstetrician, paediatric team and anaesthetist should be present for the births because of the risk of complications.

If epidural analgesia has been used, it may be 'topped up'.

The possibility of emergency caesarean section is ever-present and the operating theatre should be ready to receive the mother at short notice.

Monitoring of both fetal hearts should continue.

Provided that the first twin is presenting by the vertex, the birth can be expected to proceed normally.

When the first twin is born, the time of birth and the sex are noted. This baby and cord must be labelled as 'twin one' immediately.

- The baby may be put to the breast because suckling stimulates uterine contractions.
- If the first baby requires active resuscitation, the paediatric team will take over his or her care once on the resuscitaire.
- After the birth of the first twin, abdominal palpation is carried out to ascertain the lie, presentation and position of the second twin and to auscultate the fetal heart:

    If the lie is not longitudinal, an attempt may be made to correct it by external cephalic version.

    If it is longitudinal, a vaginal examination is made to confirm the presentation.

    If the presenting part is not engaged, it should be guided into the pelvis by fundal pressure before the second sac of membranes is ruptured.

- The fetal heart should be auscultated again once the membranes are ruptured.
- If uterine activity does not recommence, intravenous oxytocin may be used to stimulate it.
- When the presenting part becomes visible, the mother should be encouraged to push with contractions to birth the second twin.
- The midwife should be aware that, owing to the reduced size of the placental site following the birth of the first twin, the second fetus may be somewhat deprived of oxygen.
- The birth of the second twin should be completed within 45 minutes of the first twin as long as there are no signs of fetal distress in the second twin; if there are, the birth must be expedite and the second twin may need to be delivered by caesarean section
- A uterotonic drug (usually Syntocinon or Syntometrine) is usually given intramuscularly or intravenously, depending on local policy, after the birth of the anterior shoulder.
- This baby and cord are labelled as 'twin two'. A note of the time of birth and the sex of the child is made.

■ The risk of asphyxia is greater for the second twin and the paediatric team may need to resuscitate this infant actively. The baby may need to be transferred to the neonatal unit; he or she should, however, be shown to the mother prior to transfer, and if at all possible, she may cuddle her child.

■ Once the uterotonic drug has taken effect, controlled cord traction is applied to both cords simultaneously and the placentae should be delivered without delay. Emptying the uterus enables bleeding to be controlled and postpartum haemorrhage (PPH) is prevented. An infusion of 40 IU of Syntocinon in 500 ml of normal saline should be prepared for prophylactic use in the management of PPH.

■ The placenta(e) should be examined and the number of amniotic sacs, chorions and placentae noted. Pathological examination of placenta and membranes may be needed to confirm chorionicity.

Complications associated with multiple pregnancy

The high perinatal mortality associated with twinning is largely due to complications of pregnancy, such as the premature onset of labour, intrauterine growth restriction and complications of delivery. The management of multiple pregnancy is concerned with the prevention, early detection and treatment of these complications.

Polyhydramnios

Acute polyhydramnios may occur as early as 18–20 weeks. It may be associated with fetal abnormality but it is more likely to be due to TTTS.

Twin-to-twin transfusion syndrome

Also known as fetofetal transfusion syndrome (FFTS), this can be acute or chronic. The acute form usually occurs during labour and is the result of a blood transfusion from one fetus (donor) to the other (recipient) through vascular anastomosis in a monochorionic placenta. Both fetuses may die of cardiac failure if not treated immediately.

Chronic TTTS can occur in up to 35% of monochorionic twin pregnancies and accounts for 15–17% of perinatal mortality in twins. The placenta in TTTS transfuses blood from one twin fetus to the other. These cases are characterised by one or more deep unidirectional arteriovenous anastomoses. This results in anaemia and growth restriction in the donor twin and polycythaemia with circulatory overload in the recipient twin (hydrops). The fetal and neonatal mortality is high but some infants may be saved by early diagnosis and prenatal treatment with either amnioreduction, which may have to be repeated regularly as fluid can reaccumulate rapidly or laser coagulation of communicating placental vessels. Selective fetocide is sometimes considered.

Fetal abnormality

This is particularly associated with MZ twins.

Conjoined twins

This extremely rare malformation of MZ twinning results from the incomplete division of the fertilised ovum. Delivery has to be by caesarean section. Separation of the babies is sometimes possible and will depend on how they are joined and which internal organs are involved.

Acardiac twins (twin reversed arterial perfusion — TRAP)

One twin presents without a well-defined cardiac structure and is kept alive through placental anastomoses to the circulatory system of the viable fetus.

Fetus-in-fetu (endoparasite)

Parts of one fetus may be lodged within another fetus; this can happen only in MZ twins.

Malpresentations

Although the uterus is large and distended, the fetuses are less mobile than may be supposed. They can restrict each other's movements, which may result in malpresentations, particularly of the second twin. After the birth of the first twin, the presentation of the second twin may change.

Premature rupture of the membranes

Malpresentations due to polyhydramnios may predispose to preterm rupture of the membranes.

Prolapse of the cord

This is associated with malpresentations and polyhydramnios and is more likely if there is a poorly fitting presenting part. The second twin is particularly at risk.

Prolonged labour

Malpresentations are a poor stimulus to good uterine action and a distended uterus is likely to lead to poor uterine activity and consequently prolonged labour.

Monoamniotic twins

Monoamniotic twins risk cord entanglement with occlusion of the blood supply to one or both fetuses. Delivery is usually at around 32–34 weeks and by caesarean section.

Locked twins

This is a rare but serious complication. There are two types; one occurs when the first twin presents by the breech and the second by the vertex, the other when both are vertex presentations (Fig. 16.2). In both instances the head of the second twin prevents the continued descent of the first.

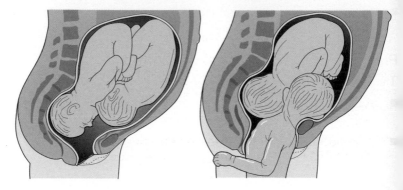

Fig. 16.2 Locked twins.

Delay in the birth of the second twin

After delivery of the first twin, uterine activity should recommenc
within 5 minutes. Birth of the second twin is usually complete
within 45 minutes of the first birth. In the past the birth interval wa
limited to 30 minutes in an attempt to minimise complication:
With the introduction of fetal heart rate monitoring the interv
time between babies is not so crucial as long as the fetal condition
monitored. Poor uterine action as a result of malpresentation may b
the cause of delay. The risks of delay are:

- intrauterine hypoxia
- birth asphyxia following premature separation of the placenta
- sepsis as a result of ascending infection from the first umbilical
  cord, which lies outside the vulva.

After the birth of the first twin the lower uterine segment begins
reform and the cervical canal may have to dilate fully again.

The midwife may need to 'rub up' a contraction and to put th
first twin to the mother's breast to stimulate uterine activity.

- If there appears to be an obstruction, medical aid is summoned
  and a caesarean section may be necessary.

- If there is no obstruction, oxytocin infusion may be commenced or forceps delivery considered.

Premature expulsion of the placenta

The placenta may be expelled before delivery of the second twin.

- In dichorionic twins with separate placentae, one placenta may be delivered separately.

- In monochorionic twins the shared placenta may be expelled. The risks of severe asphyxia and death of the second twin are then very high.

- Haemorrhage is also likely if one twin is retained in utero, as this prevents adequate retraction of the placental site.

Postpartum haemorrhage

Poor uterine tone as a result of overdistension or hypotonic activity is likely to lead to postpartum haemorrhage.

Undiagnosed twins

The possibility of an unexpected undiagnosed second baby should be considered if the uterus appears larger than expected after the birth of the first baby or if the baby is surprisingly smaller than expected. If a uterotonic drug has been given after the birth of the anterior shoulder of the first baby, the second baby is in great danger and delivery should be expedited. He or she will require active resuscitation because of severe asphyxia.

Postnatal Period

Care of the babies

Immediate care at delivery is the same as for a single baby. Identification of the infants should be clear and the parents should be given the opportunity to check the identity bracelets and cuddle their babies.

Nutrition

Both babies may be breastfed, either simultaneously or separately. The mother may choose to feed artificially. In the immediate post-natal days the mother may prefer to breastfeed the twins separately, as this gives her time with each baby.

- If the babies are small for gestational age or preterm, the paediatrician may recommend that the babies be 'topped up' after a breastfeed. Expressed breast milk is the best form of nutrition for these babies.

- If the babies are not able to suck adequately at the breast, then the mother should be encouraged to express her milk regularly for her babies.

- If she does not have sufficient milk for them, milk from a human milk bank can be used, which is much better for preterm babies than formula milk.

The more stimulation the breasts are given, the more plentiful is the milk supply.

Care of the mother

- Involution of the uterus will be slower because of its increased bulk. 'Afterpains' may be troublesome and analgesia should be offered.

- A good diet is essential, and if the mother is breastfeeding, she requires a high-protein, high-calorie diet. It is quite common for breastfeeding mothers to feel hungry between meals and they should be encouraged to keep sensible snacks to hand for such times.

- Once the mother is at home she must be encouraged to rest and catch up on her sleep during the day as much as possible, and eat a well-balanced diet in order to recover her strength and ability to cope with her family. Routine is the essence of coping with new babies.

■ Isolation can be a real problem for new mothers. The incidence of postnatal depression has been shown to be significantly higher in twin mothers.

Triplets and Higher-Order Births

The rapidly increasing number of surviving triplets and higher-order births will produce many more families needing special advice and support from health care workers.

A woman expecting three or more babies is at risk of all the same complications as one expecting twins, but more so. She is more likely to have a period in hospital resting before the babies are born and they will almost certainly be delivered prematurely. Perinatal mortality rates are higher for triplets than twins and the incidence of cerebral palsy is also increased.

The mode of delivery for triplets or more babies is usually by caesarean section. It is essential that the paediatric team be present. The special dangers associated with these births are:

■ asphyxia
■ intracranial injury
■ perinatal death.

The midwife must ensure that the mother's health visitor and, if necessary, a social worker are involved in her care. If the family need extra outside help, the organisation of this must start before the babies are born.

Disability and Bereavement

Perinatal mortality and long-term morbidity are both more common among multiple births than singletons. The perinatal mortality rate for twins is about four times that of singletons, and that of triplets 12 times higher.

The grief of parents following the death of one of a multiple set is often underestimated. The conflicting emotions the parents will feel — the need to grieve for the child who has died, whilst wanting to rejoice at the birth of the healthy twin — can be confusing. Addresses of organisations that offer support should be made available to the parents.

Where one or more of a multiple set has a disability, it is often the healthy child who needs special attention. He or she may feel guilt about doing something that caused the twin's disability and may be resentful of the attention that the other one needs, or of the loss of twinship.

Embryo Reduction

This is the reduction of an apparently healthy higher-order multiple pregnancy down to two or even one embryo so the chances of survival are much higher. The procedure may be offered to parents who have conceived triplets or more, whether spontaneously or as a result of infertility treatments, by the doctors who care for them.

The procedure is usually carried out between the 10th and 12th weeks of the pregnancy. Various techniques may be used, involving the insertion of a needle under ultrasound guidance either via the vagina or, more commonly, through the abdominal wall into the fetal thorax. Potassium chloride is usually used, although some doctors prefer saline. All embryos remain in the uterus until birth.

Selective Fetocide

This may be offered to parents with a multiple pregnancy when one of the babies has a serious abnormality. The affected fetus is injected as described in embryo reduction, so allowing the healthy fetus to grow and develop normally. The full impact of either of these procedures on the parents and their feelings of bereavement will often not be felt until the birth of their remaining baby (or babies) many weeks later. Moreover, unlike in the termination of a single pregnancy, the parents will be more aware of what could have been as they watch the survivor(s) grow up.

Sources of Help

In the UK the support provided by social services varies greatly, so it is always advisable for families with triplets to apply. Parents should be advised to contact organisations such as Home Start, or the local colleges with nursery training courses, both of which may be able to offer assistance.

- *Tamba (Twins and Multiple Births Association)*. The umbrella organisation for the 250 or so local twins clubs throughout the country. The clubs are run by parents of twins and are the best source of practical advice and support for parents expecting twins.

- *Multiple Births Foundation (MBF)*. Offers advice and support to families as soon as their multiple pregnancy is diagnosed, as well as to couples considering treatment for infertility. It offers information and support for couples and professionals.

Section 3

Labour

Chapter 17

The First Stage of Labour

The WHO defines normal labour as low-risk throughout, spontaneous in onset with the fetus presenting by the vertex, culminating in the mother and infant in good condition following birth. Normal labour occurs between 37 and 42 weeks' gestation. Where women are well supported throughout their birth experience, there are likely to be fewer interventions and greater satisfaction with their care and birth outcome.

Phases of the first stage
These are described in Box 17.1.

The Onset of Spontaneous Normal Labour

The onset of labour appears to be initiated by a combination of hormonal and mechanical factors.

- Levels of maternal oestrogen rise sharply during the last weeks of pregnancy, resulting in changes that overcome the inhibiting effects of progesterone.

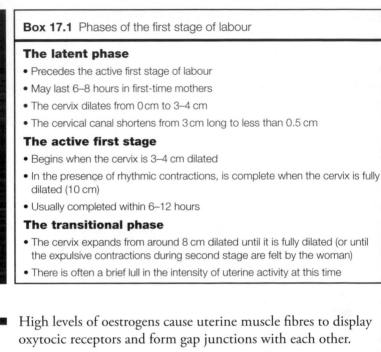

Box 17.1 Phases of the first stage of labour

The latent phase
- Precedes the active first stage of labour
- May last 6–8 hours in first-time mothers
- The cervix dilates from 0 cm to 3–4 cm
- The cervical canal shortens from 3 cm long to less than 0.5 cm

The active first stage
- Begins when the cervix is 3–4 cm dilated
- In the presence of rhythmic contractions, is complete when the cervix is fully dilated (10 cm)
- Usually completed within 6–12 hours

The transitional phase
- The cervix expands from around 8 cm dilated until it is fully dilated (or until the expulsive contractions during second stage are felt by the woman)
- There is often a brief lull in the intensity of uterine activity at this time

- High levels of oestrogens cause uterine muscle fibres to display oxytocic receptors and form gap junctions with each other.
- Oestrogen also stimulates the placenta to release prostaglandins that induce a production of enzymes that will digest collagen in the cervix, helping it to soften.

It is thought that both fetal and placental factors are involved in the process. Uterine activity may also result from mechanical stimulation of the uterus and cervix, brought about by overstretching or pressure from a presenting part that is well applied to the cervix.

The onset of labour is a process, not an event; therefore it is very difficult to pinpoint exactly when the painless (or sometimes painful) contractions of prelabour develop into the progressive rhythmic contractions of established labour.

Diagnosing the onset of labour is extremely important since it is on the basis of this finding that decisions are made that will affect care in labour. Contact with the midwife should be made when regular, rhythmic, uterine contractions are experienced, and these are perceived by the woman as uncomfortable or painful.

When the woman is in labour, contractions will often be accompanied or preceded by a blood-stained mucoid 'show'; this results from the operculum, which formed the cervical plug during pregnancy, being lost when the cervix dilates.

Occasionally the membranes will rupture; this should always be reported to the midwife, who will check that there are no changes in the fetal heart rate and that meconium is not present in the liquor.

Spurious labour

Many women experience contractions before the onset of labour; these may be painful and may even be regular for a time, causing a woman to think that labour has started. The two features of true labour that are absent here are:

- effacement of the cervix
- dilatation of the cervix (see below).

Physiological Processes

Uterine action

Fundal dominance (Fig. 17.1)

Each uterine contraction starts in the fundus near one of the cornua and spreads across and downwards. The contraction lasts longest in the fundus where it is also most intense, but the peak is reached simultaneously over the whole uterus and the contraction fades from all parts together and is weakest in the lower segment.

Polarity

Polarity is the neuromuscular harmony that prevails between the two poles or segments of the uterus throughout labour. During each uterine contraction:

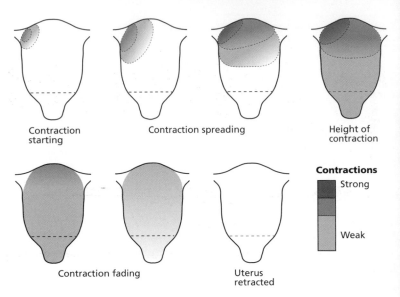

Fig. 17.1 Fundal dominance during uterine contractions.

- the upper pole contracts strongly and retracts to expel the fetus
- the lower pole contracts slightly and dilates to allow expulsion to take place.

If polarity is disorganised, then the progress of labour is inhibited.

Contraction and retraction

Retraction is when muscle fibres retain some of the shortening of the contraction instead of becoming completely relaxed (Fig. 17.2). It assists in the progressive expulsion of the fetus; the upper segment of the uterus becomes gradually shorter and thicker and its cavity diminishes.

Before labour becomes established, uterine contractions may occur every 15–20 minutes and may last for about 30 seconds; they may be imperceptible to the mother. By the end of the first stage they

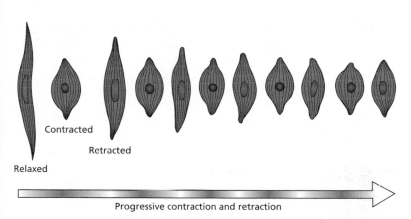

Contracted

Retracted

Relaxed

Progressive contraction and retraction

Fig. 17.2 How uterine muscle retains some shortening after each contraction.

occur at 2–3-minute intervals, last for 50–60 seconds and are very powerful.

Formation of upper and lower uterine segments

By the end of pregnancy, the body of the uterus is described as having divided into two anatomically distinct segments:

- The upper uterine segment is formed from the body of the uterus.
- The lower uterine segment is formed from the isthmus and the cervix, and is about 8–10 cm in length.

The muscle content reduces from the fundus to the cervix, where it is thinner. When labour begins, the retracted longitudinal fibres in the upper segment pull on the lower segment, causing it to stretch; this is aided by the force applied by the descending presenting part. A ridge forms between the upper and lower uterine segments; this is known as the *physiological retraction ring*.

Cervical effacement

'Effacement' refers to the inclusion of the cervical canal into the lower uterine segment (Fig. 17.3).

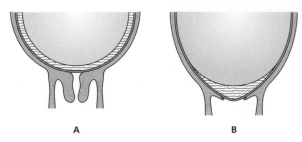

Fig. 17.3 (A) The cervix before effacement. (B) The cervix after effacement. The cervical canal is now part of the lower uterine segment.

Effacement may occur late in pregnancy, or it may not take place until labour begins.

- In the nulliparous woman the cervix will not usually dilate until effacement is complete.

- In the parous woman effacement and dilatation may occur simultaneously and a small canal may be felt in early labour. This is often referred to as a 'multips os'.

Cervical dilatation

Dilatation of the cervix is the process of enlargement of the os uteri from a tightly closed aperture to an opening large enough to permit passage of the fetal head.

- Dilatation is measured in centimetres and full dilatation at term equates to about 10 cm.

- Dilatation occurs as a result of uterine action and the counterpressure applied by either the intact bag of membranes or the presenting part, or both.

- A well-flexed fetal head closely applied to the cervix favours efficient dilatation.

- Pressure applied evenly to the cervix causes the uterine fundus to respond by contraction and retraction.

Mechanical factors

Formation of the forewaters

As the lower uterine segment forms and stretches, the chorion becomes detached from it; the increased intrauterine pressure causes this loosened part of the sac of fluid to bulge downwards into the internal os. The well-flexed head fits snugly into the cervix and cuts off the fluid in front of the head, the 'forewaters', from that which surrounds the body, the 'hindwaters'.

General fluid pressure

While the membranes remain intact, the pressure of the uterine contractions is exerted on the fluid and, as fluid is not compressible, the pressure is equalised throughout the uterus and over the fetal body; it is known as 'general fluid pressure'. Preserving the integrity of the membranes optimises the oxygen supply to the fetus and helps to prevent intrauterine and fetal infection.

Rupture of the membranes

- The optimum physiological time for the membranes to rupture spontaneously is at the end of the first stage of labour after the cervix becomes fully dilated and no longer supports the bag of forewaters.

- The uterine contractions are also applying increasing force at this time.

- Membranes may sometimes rupture days before labour begins or during the first stage.

  If there are no other signs of labour but the history of ruptured membranes is convincing or obvious liquor is draining, then digital examination should be avoided owing to an increased risk of ascending infection.

  If the diagnosis is not obvious, then one sterile speculum examination should be performed to try to visualise pooling of liquor in the posterior fornix; endocervical swabs may also be taken at this time.

- The majority of women will labour spontaneously within 48 hours. After 48 hours an obstetrician may consider augmentation of labour.

- Women with prelabour ruptured membranes should have their temperature recorded and be monitored for signs of fetal compromise associated with infection.

- Occasionally, the membranes do not rupture, even in the second stage, and appear at the vulva as a bulging sac covering the fetal head as it is born; this is known as the 'caul'.

Fetal axis pressure

During each contraction the uterus rises forward and the force of the fundal contraction is transmitted to the upper pole of the fetus and down the long axis of the fetus, and applied by the presenting part to the cervix. This is known as 'fetal axis pressure' and becomes much more significant after rupture of the membranes and during the second stage of labour.

Observations and Care in Labour

Maternal well-being

Women must be enabled to be in control throughout labour, with the midwife providing evidence-based information, listening to the woman and ensuring consent is given before any intervention.

Past history and reaction to labour

Factors of particular relevance at the onset of labour are listed in Box 17.2.

> **Box 17.2** Important factors in the history at the onset of labour
>
> - The birth plan — whatever choices the woman makes, she must be the focus of the care, and should be able to feel she is in control of what is happening to her and able to make decisions about her care
> - Parity and age
> - Character and outcomes of previous labours
> - Weights and condition of previous babies
> - Attendance at any specialist clinics
> - Any known problems — social or physical
> - Blood results, including Rhesus isoimmunisation and Hb

Pulse rate

This is recorded every 1–2 hours during early labour and every 30 minutes when labour is more advanced. If the rate increases to more than 100 beats per minute it may be indicative of:

■ anxiety

■ pain

■ infection

■ ketosis

■ haemorrhage.

Temperature

This is recorded at least every 4 hours in normal labour. Pyrexia is indicative of infection or ketosis, or may be associated with epidural analgesia.

Blood pressure

This is measured every 2–4 hours, unless it is abnormal. The blood pressure must be monitored very closely following epidural or spinal anaesthetic. Hypotension may be caused by:

■ the supine position

■ shock

■ epidural anaesthesia.

Urinalysis and bladder care

The woman should be encouraged to empty her bladder every 1–2 hours during labour. The urine passed should be tested for glucose, ketones and protein.

- A low level of ketones is very common during labour and is not thought to be significant.

- A trace of protein may be a contaminant following rupture of the membranes or a sign of a urinary infection, but more significant proteinuria may indicate pre-eclampsia.

A full bladder may prevent the fetal head from entering the pelvic brim and can increase the risk of postpartum haemorrhage. If the bladder is incompletely emptied or the woman is unable to void for some hours, it may become necessary to pass a catheter.

Fluid balance

A record should be kept of all urine passed and fluids administered.

Abdominal examination

This is undertaken at the initial assessment and then repeated at intervals throughout labour to assess the length, strength and frequency of contractions and the descent of the presenting part. Contractions that are unduly long or very strong and coming in quick succession should give cause for concern. Hyperstimulation should be considered if oxytocin is being infused. Descent of the presenting part is usually described in terms of fifths of the head, which can still be palpated above the brim.

Vaginal examination and progress in labour

Although it is not essential to examine the woman vaginally at frequent intervals, it may be useful to do so when progress is in doubt or another indication arises. The features that are indicative of progress are:

- effacement and dilatation of the cervix
- descent, flexion and rotation of the fetal head.

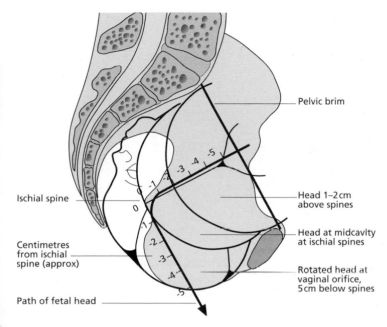

Pelvic brim

Head 1–2 cm above spines

Head at midcavity at ischial spines

Rotated head at vaginal orifice, 5 cm below spines

Ischial spine

Centimetres from ischial spine (approx)

Path of fetal head

Fig. 17.4 Stations of the fetal head in relation to the pelvic canal.

Progressive dilatation is monitored as labour continues and charted on either the partograph or the cervicograph.

The level or station of the presenting part is estimated in relation to the ischial spines; during normal labour the head descends progressively (Fig. 17.4). Moulding or a large caput will give a false impression of the level of the fetal head.

In vertex presentations, progress depends partly on increased flexion. Flexion is assessed by the position of the sutures and fontanelles:

- If the head is fully flexed, the posterior fontanelle becomes almost central (Fig. 17.5).
- If the head is deflexed, both anterior and posterior fontanelles may be palpable.

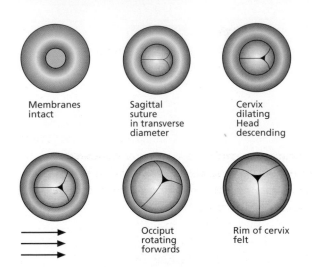

Membranes
intact

Sagittal
suture
in transverse
diameter

Cervix
dilating
Head
descending

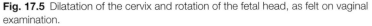

Occiput
rotating
forwards

Rim of cervix
felt

Fig. 17.5 Dilatation of the cervix and rotation of the fetal head, as felt on vaginal examination.

Rotation is assessed by noting changes in the position of the fetus between one examination and the next. The sutures and fontanelles are palpated in order to determine position.

Under no circumstances should a midwife make a vaginal examination if there is any frank bleeding, unless the placenta is positively known to be in the upper uterine segment.

Nutrition

In normal labour women may take a low-fat, low-residue diet according to appetite. The vigorous muscle contractions of the uterus during labour demand a continuous supply of glucose. If this is not obtained from the diet, the body will start to metabolise protein and fat stores in an effort to provide glucose (gluconeogenesis). This relatively inefficient method of producing glucose results in the occurrence of ketoacidosis.

In an effort to reduce gastric volume and decrease the gastric acidity of the labouring woman, prophylactic antacids may be administered

Prevention of infection

Invasive procedures should be kept to a minimum. Personal hygiene is important for both the woman and her attendants. The midwife must wash her hands before and after examining the mother, and wear gloves when handling used sanitary pads, blood-stained linen or body fluids.

The fetal membranes should be preserved intact unless there is a positive indication for their rupture that would outweigh the advantage of their protective functions. Women whose labours are prolonged are at particular risk of infection and are often subjected to a number of invasive procedures. The midwife should ensure that she has a sound reason before embarking on any procedure.

Some women will need specialised care, especially women with any transmissible infection such as gastroenteritis, hepatitis or HIV infection.

Bowel preparation

If there has been no bowel action for 24 hours or the rectum feels loaded on vaginal examination, the woman should be consulted and asked if she would like an enema or suppositories. This is never done as a routine procedure.

Position and mobility

Midwives must be flexible in their approach to positions that women adopt, as well as considering their own safety. Mobility in labour should be encouraged, as it lessens the need for pharmacological analgesia.

Pain management

The biological, psychological, social, spiritual, cultural and educational dimensions of each woman have an impact on how she expresses herself and how she perceives pain during labour.

Midwives should work with women to encourage them to maintain control and be as mobile as possible throughout labour.

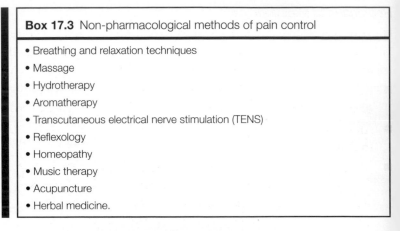

Box 17.3 Non-pharmacological methods of pain control

- Breathing and relaxation techniques
- Massage
- Hydrotherapy
- Aromatherapy
- Transcutaneous electrical nerve stimulation (TENS)
- Reflexology
- Homeopathy
- Music therapy
- Acupuncture
- Herbal medicine.

Non-pharmacological methods of pain control

These are listed in Box 17.3.

Pharmacological methods of pain control

Opiate drugs

Three systemic opioids are commonly used for pain relief in labour:

- *pethidine*, the most frequently used in England: usually administered intramuscularly in doses of 50–150 mg; takes about 20 minutes to have an effect
- *diamorphine*: usual dosage 10 mg given via intramuscular injection
- *meptazinol*: usually given in doses of 100–150 mg intramuscularly.

Inhalation analgesia

The most commonly used inhalation analgesia in labour is a premixed gas made up of 50% nitrous oxide and 50% oxygen administered through a piped system or via the Entonox apparatus. It takes effect within 20 seconds, maximum efficacy occurring after about 45–5 seconds.

Regional (epidural) analgesia

- A local anaesthetic is administered via a catheter into the epidural space of the lumbar region, usually between vertebrae L1 and L2, or between L2 and L3, or between L3 and L4.

- Bolus injections of bupivacaine (Marcain) or continuous infusion of dilute bupivacaine and opioids (usually fentanyl) may be used.

- An intravenous infusion of crystalloid fluids is commenced prior to siting the epidural.

- After the administration of the first dose of bupivacaine and any subsequent top-up doses of local anaesthetic, the blood pressure and pulse should be measured and recorded every 5 minutes for 20–30 minutes, and then every 30 minutes. The fetal heart is usually monitored electronically.

- The mother may sit up in bed once it has been established that her blood pressure is stable, but should be tilted to one side to prevent aortocaval compression.

- The spread of the block is checked regularly by the midwife.

Table 17.1 shows contraindications to regional analgesia and Table 17.2 lists the advantages and disadvantages of epidural analgesia.

Fetal well-being

Fetal condition during labour can be assessed by obtaining information about:

- the fetal heart rate and patterns
- the pH of the fetal blood
- the amniotic fluid.

The fetal heart

Women with an uncomplicated pregnancy should have intermittent auscultation with a Pinard stethoscope or handheld Doppler device.

Table 17.1 Contraindications to regional analgesia, with associated risks

Contraindication	Risk
Uncorrected anticoagulation or coagulopathy	Vertebral canal haematoma
Local or systemic sepsis (pyrexia above 38ºC not treated with antibiotics)	Vertebral canal abscess
Hypovolaemia or active haemorrhage	Cardiovascular collapse secondary to sympathetic blockade
Patient refusal	Legal action
Lack of sufficient trained midwives for continuous care and monitoring of mother and fetus for the duration of the epidural blockade	Maternal collapse, convulsion, respiratory arrest; fetal compromise

Table 17.2 Advantages and disadvantages of epidural analgesia

Disadvantages	Advantages
Ineffective blocks	Effective pain relief
More frequent monitoring of vital signs	Tendency to lower blood pressure can be advantage in cases of pregnancy-induced hypertension
Lengthens first stage of labour Mother less able to adopt different birth positions	If labour is prolonged, gives effective pain relief, allowing mother to rest
Less sensation of expulsive efforts and lengthens second stage of labour. Increase in instrumental vaginal delivery	Does not depress respiratory centre of fetus

There is no evidence to support an admission CTG; it should therefore not be done as routine.

For women with problems in their pregnancy or other risk factors including the use of oxytocin or epidural analgesia, electronic fetal monitoring (EFM) is appropriate.

The use of a CTG may limit the choice of position.

Intermittent monitoring

The heart rate should be counted over a complete minute.

- The baseline rate should be between 110 and 160 beats per minute (bpm).
- Variability of more than 5 bpm should be maintained throughout labour.

If decelerations are heard in the first stage of labour with a Pinard or Doppler instrument, then electronic monitoring may be indicated to assess their extent.

Continuous EFM

Continuous recording usually combines a fetal cardiograph and a maternal tocograph in a CTG apparatus. This presents a graphic record of the response of the fetal heart to uterine activity, as well as information about its rate and variability.

Findings

The CTG provides information on:

- baseline fetal heart rate
- baseline variability
- accelerations
- decelerations
- uterine activity.

Response of the fetal heart to uterine contractions

The fetal heart rate will normally remain steady or accelerate during uterine contractions during the first stage of labour. Compression of the umbilical cord or fetal head will result in some decelerations, particularly if the membranes are not intact. These would be early or variable decelerations lasting less than 3 minutes, with good recovery to predeceleration rate.

A late or variable deceleration lasting longer than 3 minutes begins during or after a contraction reaches its nadir (lowest point) after the peak of the contraction and has not recovered by the time that the contraction has ended. The *time lag* between the peak of the contraction and the nadir of the deceleration is more significant in terms of severity than the drop in the fetal heart rate.

Interpretation of CTG

'Darth Vader' is a useful acronym for thorough evaluation of a CTG (Box 17.4).

Only four variables are considered when interpreting a CTG:

- baseline rate
- baseline variability
- whether accelerations are present
- presence or absence of decelerations.

Box 17.4 The 'Darth Vader' mnemonic

D details (name, time, etc.)
A assess quality
R recorded fetal movements
T tocograph
H heart rate
V variability
A accelerations
D decelerations
E evaluation
R response

This makes a CTG interpretable using the three categories recommended by NICE in 2001 (Fig. 17.6):

- normal
- suspicious
- pathological.

All areas that use EFM should have ready 24-hour access to fetal blood sampling facilities.

All CTG traces should be secured in the notes.

Fetal blood sampling (FBS)

When the fetal heart rate pattern is suspicious or pathological and fetal acidosis is suspected, then FBS should be carried out unless the birth is imminent.

- A fetal blood sample result of 7.25 or below should be repeated usually within 30 minutes to an hour.
- An FBS below 7.20 indicates that the fetus should be delivered.

Amniotic fluid

- If the fetus becomes hypoxic, meconium may be passed, causing the amniotic fluid to be stained green.

- Amniotic fluid that is a muddy yellow colour or is only slightly green may signify a previous event from which the fetus has recovered; it is also common and of no significance in postdates babies.

- the breech is presenting, the fetus may pass meconium because of e compression of the abdomen or as a result of hypoxia.
- Bleeding of sudden onset at the time of rupture of the membranes ay be the result of ruptured vasa praevia and is an acute emergency.

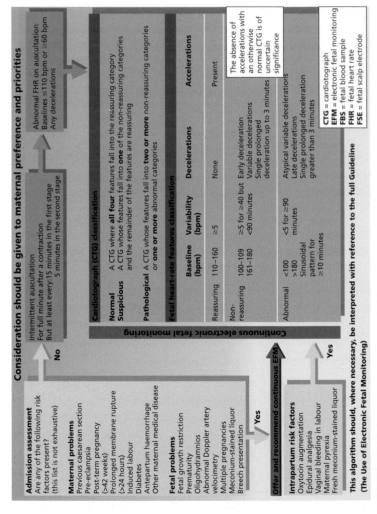

Consideration should be given to maternal preference and priorities

Admission assessment
Are any of the following risk factors present?
(this list is not exhaustive)

Maternal problems
Previous caesarean section
Pre-eclampsia
Post-term pregnancy
(>42 weeks)
Prolonged membrane rupture
(>24 hours)
Induced labour
Diabetes
Antepartum haemorrhage
Other maternal medical disease

Fetal problems
Fetal growth restriction
Prematurity
Oligohydramnios
Abnormal Doppler artery
velocimetry
Multiple pregnancies
Meconium-stained liquor
Breech presentation

Offer and recommend continuous EFM

Intrapartum risk factors
Oxytocin augmentation
Epidural analgesia
Vaginal bleeding in labour
Maternal pyrexia
Fresh meconium-stained liquor

No

Intermittent auscultation
For full minute after a contraction
But at least every:15 minutes in the first stage
5 minutes in the second stage

Abnormal FHR on auscultation
Baselines ≤110 bpm or ≥60 bpm
Any decelerations

Continuous electronic fetal monitoring

Cardiotograph (CTG) classification

Normal A CTG where **all four** features fall into the reassuring category
Suspicious A CTG whose features fall into **one** of the non-reassuring categories
and the remainder of the features are reassuring
Pathological A CTG whose features fall into **two or more** non-reassuring categories
or **one or more** abnormal categories

Fetal heart-rate features classification

	Baseline (bpm)	Variability (bpm)	Decelerations	Accelerations
Reassuring	110–160	≥5	None	Present
Non-reassuring	100–109 161–180	≥5 for ≥40 but <90 minutes	Early deceleration Variable decelerations Single prolonged deceleration up to 3 minutes	The absence of accelerations with an otherwise normal CTG is of uncertain significance
Abnormal	<100 >180 Sinusoidal pattern for ≥10 minutes	<5 for ≥90 minutes	Atypical variable decelerations Late decelerations Single prolonged deceleration greater than 3 minutes	

CTG = cardiotograph
EFM = electronic fetal monitoring
FBS = fetal blood sample
FHR = fetal heart rate
FSE = fetal scalp electrode

Yes

Yes

This algorithm should, where necessary, be interpreted with reference to the full Guideline
(The Use of Electronic Fetal Monitoring)

Fig. 17.6 Guidelines for fetal monitoring in labour.

Fetal compromise

Signs of fetal compromise resulting from oxygen deprivation are:

- fetal tachycardia
- a pathological CTG and corresponding poor FBS result
- fetal bradycardia or a severe change in fetal heart rate or decelerations related to uterine contractions, or both
- passage of meconium-stained amniotic fluid.

Midwife's management of fetal compromise

- Summon medical assistance.
- Stop oxytocin if it is being administered.
- Place the woman in a more favourable position, usually on her left side.
- In cases of maternal oxygen lack, give oxygen.
- Assist with arrangements to expedite the birth.

Preterm labour

Preterm labour is defined as labour commencing after 24 weeks' gestation and before the 37th completed week of pregnancy.

A woman who is at risk of giving birth preterm should be transferred to a unit with intensive neonatal facilities, preferably with the fetus in utero. Tocolytic drugs may be used in very early labour to try to delay the birth. Antenatal administration of steroids has been shown to reduce the incidence of hyaline membrane disease, intraventricular haemorrhage and necrotising enterocolitis in fetuses of 26–34 weeks' gestation. Two doses given over 24 hours last for at least 7 days.

Records

The record of labour is a legal document and must be kept meticulously. It provides current, comprehensive and concise information regarding:

■ the woman's observations

■ her physical, psychological and sociological state

■ any problem that arose

■ the midwife's response to that problem, including any interventions.

An accurate record during labour provides the basis on which clinical improvements, progress or deterioration of the mother or fetus can be judged. For this reason the notes should be kept in chronological order.

Key points for practice are summarised in Box 17.5.

Box 17.5 Key points for practice

• Women should be well informed and offered choice founded on evidence-based information where possible

• A competent woman can give or withhold consent for any procedure

• Another adult cannot consent or withhold consent on behalf of a competent woman

• Good communication between women and midwives and between professionals is a fundamental component of maternity services

• The latent phase of labour should be more widely acknowledged in hospital settings

• The use of strict time limits for first and second stages of labour should be reviewed in problem-free pregnancies

• Good record-keeping and care plans are an essential aspect of care

---

Chapter 18

The Second Stage of Labour

The Nature of Transition and Second-Stage Phases of Labour

The second stage of labour has traditionally been regarded as the phase between full dilatation of the cervical os and the birth of the baby. However, most midwives and labouring women are aware of a transitional period between the dilatation, or first stage of labour, and the time when active maternal pushing efforts begin. This period is typically characterised by maternal restlessness, discomfort, desire for pain relief, a sense that the process is never-ending and demands to attendants to get the birth over with as quickly as possible. Some women may experience the urge to push before the cervix is fully dilated, and others may have a lull in activity before the full expulsive nature of the second-stage contractions becomes evident. This latter phenomenon is termed the *resting phase* of the second stage of labour. The onset of the second stage of labour is traditionally confirmed with a vaginal examination to check for full cervical dilatation; however, there is an increasing movement not to undertake vaginal examinations unless there are observable maternal or fetal signs, or both, that the labour is not progressing as anticipated.

Uterine action

Contractions become stronger and longer but may be less frequent. The membranes often rupture spontaneously towards the end of the first stage or during transition to the second stage. Fetal axis pressure increases flexion of the head, which results in smaller presenting diameters, more rapid progress and less trauma to both mother and fetus. If the mother is upright during this time, these processes are optimised.

The contractions become expulsive as the fetus descends further into the vagina. Pressure from the presenting part stimulates nerve receptors in the pelvic floor (this is termed the 'Ferguson reflex') and the woman experiences the need to push. This reflex may initially be controlled to a limited extent but becomes increasingly compulsive, overwhelming and involuntary during each contraction. The mother's response is to employ her secondary powers of expulsion by contracting her abdominal muscles and diaphragm.

Soft tissue displacement

As the fetal head descends, the soft tissues of the pelvis become displaced.

- Anteriorly, the bladder is pushed upwards; this results in the stretching and thinning of the urethra so that its lumen is reduced.

- Posteriorly, the rectum becomes flattened into the sacral curve and the pressure of the advancing head expels any residual faecal matter.

- The levator ani muscles dilate, thin out and are displaced laterally, and the perineal body is flattened, stretched and thinned.

The fetal head becomes visible at the vulva, advancing with each contraction and receding between contractions until crowning takes place. The head is then born. The shoulders and body follow with the next contraction, accompanied by a gush of amniotic fluid and sometimes of blood. The second stage culminates in the birth of the baby.

Duration of the second stage

Once a woman has reached the transition stage of labour, she should not be left without a midwife in attendance. Accurate observation of progress and of maternal responses is vital. The time taken to complete the second stage will vary considerably. Although many maternity units do currently impose routine limits on the duration of the second stage, beyond which medical help should be called, these are not based on good evidence.

Maternal Response to Transition and the Second Stage

Pushing

The urge to push may come before the vertex is visible. Traditionally, in order to conserve maternal effort and allow the vaginal tissues to stretch passively, the mother is encouraged to avoid active pushing at this stage. It is now accepted that managed active pushing accompanied by breath-holding (the *Valsalva manœuvre*) has adverse consequences. Whenever active pushing commences, the woman should be encouraged to follow her own inclinations in relation to expulsive effort. Few women need instruction on how to push unless they are using epidural analgesia; the desire is so overwhelming that the response becomes involuntary and compelling. Some mothers vocalise loudly as they push. This may help a woman to cope with the contractions and she should feel free to express herself in this way.

Position

There is evidence to suggest that, if the mother lies flat on her back, then vena caval compression is increased, resulting in hypotension. This can lead to reduced placental perfusion and diminished fetal oxygenation. The efficiency of uterine contractions may be reduced and it may be difficult for a mother to direct her pushing efficiently unless she is well supported.

The mother's instinctive preference should always be a primary consideration:

- *Semirecumbent or supported sitting position, with the thighs abducted.* This is the posture most commonly used in Western cultures.

- *Squatting, kneeling, all fours or standing.* Radiological evidence demonstrates an average increase of 1 cm in the transverse diameter and 2 cm in the anteroposterior diameter of the pelvic outlet when the squatting position is adopted.

- *Left lateral position.* An assistant may be required to support the right thigh, which may not be ergonomic. It is an alternative position for women who find it difficult to abduct their hips.

The Mechanism of Normal Labour

As the fetus descends, soft tissue and bony structures exert pressure that lead to descent through the birth canal by a series of movements. Collectively, these movements are called the *mechanism of labour*. During vaginal birth, the fetal presentation, position and size will govern the exact mechanism, as the fetus responds to external pressures.

Principles common to all mechanisms are:

- Descent takes place.
- Whichever part leads and first meets the resistance of the pelvic floor will rotate forwards until it comes under the symphysis pubis.
- Whichever part emerges from the pelvis will pivot around the pubic bone.

During the mechanism of normal labour the fetus turns slightly to take advantage of the widest available space in each plane of the pelvis. The widest diameter of the pelvic brim is the transverse; at the pelvic outlet the greatest space lies in the anteroposterior diameter.

At the onset of labour, the most common presentation is the vertex and the most common position either left or right occipitoanterior. When these conditions are met, the way that the fetus is normally situated can be described as follows:

- The lie is longitudinal.
- The presentation is cephalic.
- The position is right or left occipitoanterior.
- The attitude is one of good flexion.
- The denominator is the occiput.
- The presenting part is the posterior part of the anterior parietal bone.

Main movements

Descent

Throughout the first stage of labour the contraction and retraction of the uterine muscles allow less room in the uterus, exerting pressure on the fetus to descend. Following rupture of the forewaters and the exertion of maternal effort, progress speeds up.

Flexion

Pressure exerted down the fetal axis will increase flexion, resulting in smaller presenting diameters that will negotiate the pelvis more easily.

- At the onset of labour the suboccipitofrontal diameter (10 cm) is presenting.
- With greater flexion the suboccipitobregmatic diameter (9.5 cm) presents.

The occiput becomes the leading part.

Internal rotation of the head

During a contraction the leading part is pushed downwards on to the pelvic floor. The resistance of this muscular diaphragm brings about rotation.

- In a well-flexed vertex presentation the occiput leads and meets the pelvic floor first and rotates anteriorly through one-eighth of a circle.
- This causes a slight twist in the neck of the fetus, as the head is no longer in direct alignment with the shoulders.
- The anteroposterior diameter of the head now lies in the widest (anteroposterior) diameter of the pelvic outlet.
- The occiput slips beneath the subpubic arch and crowning occurs when the head no longer recedes between contractions and the widest transverse diameter (biparietal) is born.
- Whilst flexion is maintained, the suboccipitobregmatic diameter (9.5 cm) distends the vaginal orifice.

Extension of the head

Once crowning has occurred, the fetal head can extend, pivoting on the suboccipital region around the pubic bone. The sinciput, face and chin sweep the perineum and are born.

Restitution

The twist in the neck of the fetus that resulted from internal rotation is corrected by a slight untwisting movement. The occiput moves one-eighth of a circle towards the side from which it started (Fig 18.1A and B).

Internal rotation of the shoulders

The anterior shoulder is the first to reach the levator ani muscle and it therefore rotates anteriorly to lie under the symphysis pubis. This movement can be clearly seen as the head turns at the same time (external rotation of the head) (Fig. 18.1C).

Lateral flexion

The anterior shoulder is usually born first, although it has been noted by midwives who commonly use upright or kneeling positions that the posterior shoulder is commonly seen first. In the former case the

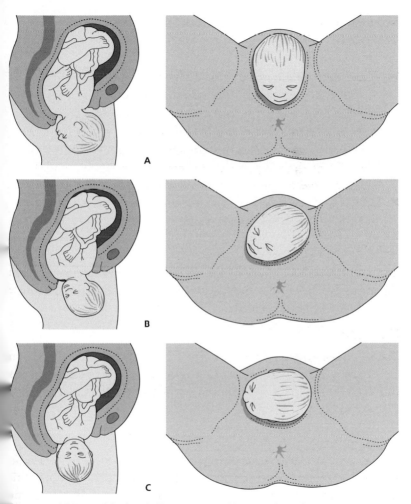

Fig. 18.1 (A) Birth of the head. (B) Restitution. (C) External rotation.

anterior shoulder slips beneath the subpubic arch and the posterior shoulder passes over the perineum. The remainder of the body is born by lateral flexion as the spine bends sideways through the curved birth canal.

Observations and Care During the Second Stage of Labour

Principles of care

See Box 18.1.

- Surgical gloves should be worn during the birth for the protection of both mother and midwife from infection. In some units, goggles or plain glasses are also advised to minimise the risk of transmission of infection through blood splashes to the eyes.

- A uterotonic agent (commonly Syntometrine 1 ml or oxytocin 5 or 10 units) may be prepared, either in readiness for the active management of the third stage if this is acceptable to the woman, or for use during an emergency.

- Neonatal resuscitation equipment should be thoroughly checked and readily accessible and blood bottles prepared if, for example, mother is Rhesus negative.

- A warm cot and clothes should be prepared for the baby.

Observations

At least five factors determine whether the second stage is continuing optimally, and these must be carefully observed:

- uterine contractions
- descent, rotation and flexion

Box 18.1 Principles of care during the second stage of labour

- Observation of progress
- Prevention of infection
- Emotional and physical comfort of the mother
- Anticipation of normal events
- Recognition of abnormal developments

- fetal condition
- suspicious/pathological changes in the fetal heart
- maternal condition.

Uterine contractions

The strength, length and frequency of contractions should be assessed continuously by observation of maternal responses, and regularly by uterine palpation.

Descent, rotation and flexion

If there is a delay in progress despite regular strong contractions and active maternal pushing, a vaginal examination may be performed:

- to confirm whether or not internal rotation of the head has taken place
- to assess the station of the presenting part
- to determine whether a caput succedaneum has formed.

In the absence of good rotation and flexion, or a weakening of uterine contractions, or both, then a change of position, nutrition and hydration, or use of optimal fetal positioning techniques may be considered. If there is evidence that either fetal or maternal condition is compromised, an experienced obstetrician must be consulted. A full bladder impedes progress.

Fetal condition

If the membranes are ruptured, the liquor amnii is observed to ensure that it is clear.

- Thick, fresh meconium is always ominous.

  Thin, old meconium staining is not always regarded as a sign of fetal compromise.

As the fetus descends, fetal oxygenation may be less efficient owing either to cord or head compression or to reduced perfusion at the placental site. A well-grown healthy fetus will not be compromised by this transitory hypoxia. This will tend to be manifest in early decelerations of the fetal heart, with a swift return to the normal baseline after a contraction. During the second stage the fetal heart is usually auscultated immediately after a contraction, with some readings being taken through a contraction if the woman can tolerate this.

Suspicious/pathological changes in the fetal heart

Signs for concern include:

- late decelerations
- lack of return to the normal baseline
- a rising baseline
- diminishing beat-to-beat variation.

If these are heard for the first time in second stage, they may be due to cord or head compression, which may be helped by a change in position. If they persist following such a change, then medical advice must be sought. If the labour is taking place in a unit that is distant from an obstetric unit, an episiotomy may be considered if the birth is imminent. Midwives who are trained and experienced in ventouse birth may consider expediting the birth at this point. Otherwise, transfer to an obstetric unit should be arranged.

Maternal condition

Monitoring includes an appraisal of the mother's ability to cope emotionally, as well as an assessment of her physical well-being. Maternal pulse rate is usually recorded every half-hour and blood pressure every hour, provided that these remain within normal limits. The woman should be encouraged to pass urine at the beginning of the second stage, unless she has recently done so.

Birth of the head

- Once the birth is imminent, the perineum may be swabbed and a clean pad placed under the woman on the bed or floor as appropriate.

- With each contraction the head descends. As it does so, the superficial muscles of the pelvic floor can be seen to stretch. The head recedes between contractions, which allows these muscles to thin gradually. The skill of the midwife in ensuring that the active phase is unhurried helps to safeguard the perineum from trauma. She must either watch the advance of the fetal head or control it with light support from her hand, or both.

- Once the head has crowned, the mother can achieve control by gently blowing or 'sighing' out each breath in order to minimise active pushing.

- The head is born by extension as the face appears at the perineum.

- During the resting phase before the next contraction, the midwife may check that the cord is not around the baby's neck.

If it is, then the usual practice is to slacken it to form a loop through which the shoulders may pass.

If the cord is very tightly wound around the neck, it is common practice to apply two artery forceps approximately 3 cm apart and to sever the cord between the two clamps.

Once severed, the cord may be unwound from around the neck.

The mother may now be able to see and touch her baby's head and assist in the birth of the trunk.

Birth of the shoulders

Restitution and external rotation of the head usually occurs, maximising the smooth birth of the shoulders and minimising the risk of perineal laceration.

- If the woman is in an upright position, the shoulders may be left to birth spontaneously with the help of gravity.

- During a water birth, it is important not to touch the emerging baby to avoid stimulating it to gasp underwater.

- If the midwife is to give physical aid in the birth of the shoulders and trunk, she should ensure that restitution has occurred fully; a hand is placed on each side of the baby's head, over the ears, and gentle downward traction is applied. The anterior shoulder escapes under the symphysis pubis. When the axillary crease is seen, the head and trunk are guided in an upward curve to allow the posterior shoulder to pass over the perineum. The midwife or mother may now grasp the baby around the chest to aid the birth of the trunk and lift the baby towards the mother's abdomen.

- The time of birth is noted.

- The cord is severed between two clamps and a cord clamp is applied close to the umbilicus.

- The baby is dried and placed in the skin-to-skin position with the mother, unless she requests otherwise.

- A warm cover is placed over the exposed areas of the baby to prevent cooling.

Episiotomy

As the perineum distends, a decision to undertake an episiotomy may very occasionally be necessary. This is an incision through the perineal tissues to enlarge the vulval outlet during the birth. The rationale for its use depends largely on the need to minimise the risk of severe spontaneous, maternal trauma and to expedite the birth when there evidence of fetal compromise. As this is a surgical incision, it is essential that the mother gives consent prior to the procedure.

- The perineum should be adequately anaesthetised prior to the incision. Lidocaine is commonly used, either 0.5% 10 ml or 1% 5 ml.
- The incision is made during a contraction when the tissues are stretched so that there is a clear view of the area and bleeding is less likely to be severe.
- Birth of the head should follow immediately and its advance must be controlled in order to avoid extension of the episiotomy.

Types of incision

- *Mediolateral.* Begins at the midpoint of the fourchette and is directed at a 45° angle to the midline towards a point midway between the ischial tuberosity and the anus (Fig. 18.2).
- *Median.* A midline incision that follows the natural line of insertion of the perineal muscles. It is associated with reduced blood loss but a higher incidence of damage to the anal sphincter.

Perineal trauma

Spontaneous trauma may be of the labia anteriorly, the perineum posteriorly, or both. A gentle, thorough examination must be carried out to assess the extent of the trauma accurately and to determine who should carry out the repair.

- *Anterior labial tears.* A suture may be necessary to secure haemostasis.
- *Posterior perineal trauma.* Spontaneous tears are usually classified in degrees (Box 18.2). Third- and fourth-degree tears should be repaired by an experienced obstetrician. A general anaesthetic or effective epidural or spinal anaesthetic is necessary.

Records

Records should include:

- details of any drugs administered
- duration and progress of labour

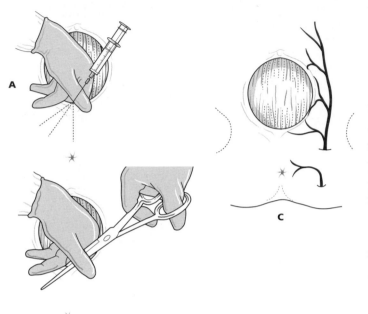

Fig. 18.2 (A) Infiltrating the perineum. (B) Performing an episiotomy. (C) Innervation of the vulval area and perineum.

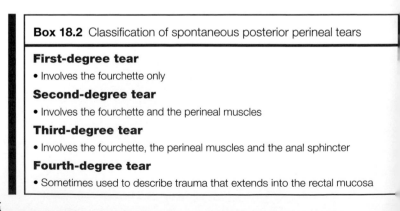

Box 18.2 Classification of spontaneous posterior perineal tears

First-degree tear
• Involves the fourchette only

Second-degree tear
• Involves the fourchette and the perineal muscles

Third-degree tear
• Involves the fourchette, the perineal muscles and the anal sphincter

Fourth-degree tear
• Sometimes used to describe trauma that extends into the rectal mucosa

---

Box 18.3 Key points for practice

- The transitional and second-stage phases of labour are emotionally intense and physically hard
- The vast majority of labours will progress physiologically
- Maternal behaviour is usually a good indication of progress during this time
- The core midwifery skill is to support the mother in the context of a sound knowledge of the physiology and the mechanisms of this phase of labour
- Support should be unobtrusive
- The woman is the central player
- Clear, comprehensive record-keeping is essential
- There are many gaps in the research evidence in this area

- reason for performing an episiotomy
- perineal repair.

The birth notification must be completed within 36 hours of the birth.

See Box 18.3 for key points relating to the second stage of labour.

Chapter 19

The Third Stage of Labour

Physiological Processes

During the third stage of labour, separation and expulsion of the placenta and membranes occur as the result of an interplay of mechanical and haemostatic factors. The time at which the placenta actually separates from the uterine wall can vary. It may shear off during the final expulsive contractions accompanying the birth of the baby or remain adherent for some considerable time. The third stage usually lasts between 5 and 15 minutes, but any period up to 1 hour may be considered to be within normal limits.

Separation and descent of the placenta

Mechanical factors (Fig. 19.1)

Separation usually begins centrally so that a retroplacental clot is formed (Fig. 19.2).

Two methods of separation are described:

- Schultze (Fig. 19.3A)
- Matthews Duncan (Fig. 19.3B).

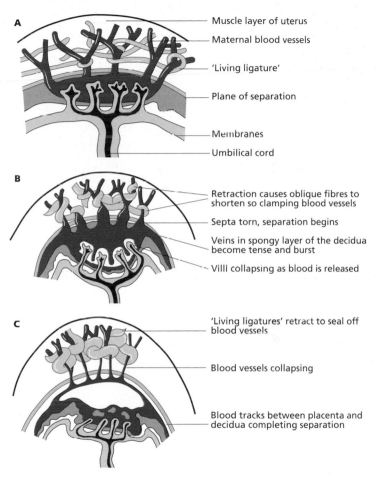

Fig. 19.1 The placental site during separation.
(A) Uterus and placenta before separation. (B) Separation begins. (C) Separation is almost complete.

Labels in figure:

A
- Muscle layer of uterus
- Maternal blood vessels
- 'Living ligature'
- Plane of separation
- Membranes
- Umbilical cord

B
- Retraction causes oblique fibres to shorten so clamping blood vessels
- Septa torn, separation begins
- Veins in spongy layer of the decidua become tense and burst
- Villi collapsing as blood is released

C
- 'Living ligatures' retract to seal off blood vessels
- Blood vessels collapsing
- Blood tracks between placenta and decidua completing separation

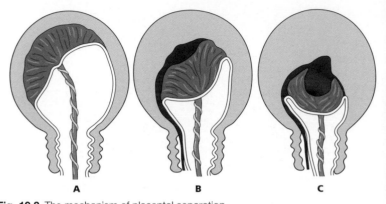

Fig. 19.2 The mechanism of placental separation.
(A) Uterine wall is partially retracted, but not sufficiently to cause placental separation.
(B) Further contraction and retraction thicken the uterine wall, reduce the placental site and aid placental separation. (C) Complete separation and formation of the retroplacental clot. *Note*: The thin lower segment has collapsed like a concertina following the birth of the baby.

Once separation has occurred, the uterus contracts strongly, forcing placenta and membranes to fall into the lower uterine segment and finally into the vagina.

Haemostasis

The three factors that are critical to control of bleeding are:

- *Retraction* of the oblique uterine muscle fibres in the upper uterine segment through which the tortuous blood vessels intertwine.

- The presence of vigorous uterine *contraction* following separation — this brings the walls into apposition so that further pressure is exerted on the placental site.

- The achievement of *haemostasis* — following separation, the placental site is rapidly covered by a fibrin mesh utilising 5–10% of the circulating fibrinogen.

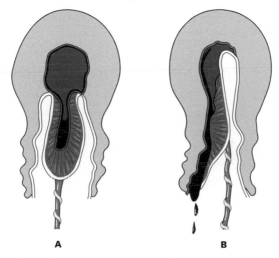

Fig. 19.3 Expulsion of the placenta.
(A) Schultze method. (B) Matthews Duncan method.

Management of the Third Stage

Uterotonics or uterotonic agents

These are drugs (e.g. syntometrine, syntocinon, ergometrine and prostaglandins) that stimulate the smooth muscle of the uterus to contract. They may be administered with crowning of the baby's head, at the time of birth of the anterior shoulder of the baby, at the end of the second stage of labour or following the delivery of the placenta.

Information related to the best available research information on the use of uterotonic drugs during the third stage of labour should be offered in an objective manner to the woman to enable her to make informed choices.

Expectant or physiological management

In the event of expectant management:

◀ routine administration of the uterotonic drug is withheld

- the umbilical cord is left unclamped until cord pulsation has ceased or the mother requests it to be clamped, or both
- the placenta is expelled by use of gravity and maternal effort.

With this approach, *therapeutic* uterotonic administration would be administered either to stop bleeding once it has occurred or to maintain the uterus in a contracted state when there are indications that excessive bleeding is likely to occur.

Active management

This is a policy whereby *prophylactic* administration of a uterotonic is applied, regardless of the assessed obstetric risk status of the woman. This is undertaken in conjunction with clamping of the umbilical cord shortly after birth of the baby and delivery of the placenta by the use of controlled cord traction.

One of the following uterotonic drugs is usually used:

- ergometrine
- oxytocin
- combined ergometrine and oxytocin.

Intravenous ergometrine 0.5 mg

- This drug acts within 45 seconds; therefore it is particularly useful in securing a rapid contraction where hypotonic uterine action results in haemorrhage.
- If a doctor is not present in such an emergency, a midwife may give the injection.

Combined ergometrine and oxytocin

(A commonly used brand is Syntometrine.)

- A 1 ml ampoule contains 5 IU of oxytocin and 0.5 mg ergometrine and is administered by intramuscular injection.
- The oxytocin acts within $2\frac{1}{2}$ minutes, and the ergometrine within 6–7 minutes.

- Their combined action results in a rapid uterine contraction enhanced by a stronger, more sustained contraction lasting several hours.

- It is usually administered as the anterior shoulder of the baby is born.

- *Caution*. No more than two doses of ergometrine 0.5 mg should be given, as it can cause headache, nausea and an increase in blood pressure; it is normally contraindicated where there is a history of hypertensive or cardiac disease.

Oxytocin

(A commonly used brand is Syntocinon.)

- Oxytocin can be administered as both an intravenous and an intramuscular injection. However, an intravenous bolus of oxytocin can cause profound, fatal hypotension, especially in the presence of cardiovascular compromise.

- No more than 5 IU should be given by slow intravenous injection.

Clamping of the umbilical cord

This may have been carried out during birth of the baby if the cord was tightly around the neck. Early clamping is carried out in the first 1–3 minutes immediately after birth, regardless of whether cord pulsation has ceased.

Proponents of late clamping suggest that no action be taken until cord pulsation ceases or the placenta has been completely delivered, thus allowing the physiological processes to take place without intervention.

Delivery of the placenta and membranes

Controlled cord traction (CCT)

This manoeuvre is believed to reduce blood loss and shorten the third stage of labour, therefore minimising the time during which

> **Box 19.1** Conditions for starting controlled cord traction
>
> - A uterotonic drug has been administered
> - It has been given time to act
> - The uterus is well contracted
> - Countertraction is applied
> - Signs of placental separation and descent are present*

the mother is at risk from haemorrhage. It is designed to enhance the normal physiological process. Before starting CCT check that the conditions listed in Box 19.1 have been met. At the beginning of the third stage, a strong uterine contraction results in the fundus being palpable below the umbilicus. It feels broad, as the placenta is still in the upper segment. As the placenta separates and falls into the lower uterine segment there is a small fresh blood loss, the cord lengthens, and the fundus becomes rounder, smaller and more mobile as it rises in the abdomen. (*Note**. There is a school of thought that does not believe it necessary to wait for signs of separation and descent *but* the uterus must be well contracted and care exerted with cord traction.)

It is important not to manipulate the uterus in any way, as this may precipitate incoordinate action. No further step should be taken until a strong contraction is palpable. If tension is applied to the umbilical cord without this contraction, uterine inversion may occur (see ch. 23).

When CCT is the preferred method of management, the following sequence of actions is usually undertaken:

- Once the uterus is found on palpation to be contracted, one hand is placed above the level of the symphysis pubis with the palm facing towards the umbilicus and exerting pressure in an upwards direction. This is countertraction.

- The other hand, firmly grasping the cord, applies traction in a downward and backward direction following the line of the birth canal.

- Some resistance may be felt but it is important to apply steady tension by pulling the cord firmly and maintaining the pressure. Jerky movements and force should be avoided.

- The aim is to complete the action as one continuous, smooth, controlled movement. However, it is only possible to exert this tension for 1 or 2 minutes, as it may be an uncomfortable procedure for the mother and the midwife's hand will tire.

- Downward traction on the cord must be released *before* uterine countertraction is relaxed, as sudden withdrawal of countertraction while tension is still being applied to the cord may also cause uterine inversion.

- If the manoeuvre is not immediately successful, there should be a pause before uterine contraction is again checked and a further attempt is made.

- Should the uterus relax, tension is temporarily released until a good contraction is again palpable.

- Once the placenta is visible, it may be cupped in the hands to ease pressure on the friable membranes.

- A gentle upward and downward movement or twisting action will help to coax out the membranes and increase the chances of delivering them intact. Great care should be taken to avoid tearing the membranes.

Expectant management

This management policy allows the physiological changes within the uterus that occur at the time of birth to take their natural course with minimal intervention; it excludes the administration of uterotonic drugs. The processes of placental separation and expulsion are quite distinct from one another and the signs of separation and descent must be evident before maternal effort can be used to expedite expulsion.

- If the mother is sitting or squatting at this stage, gravity will aid expulsion.

- If good uterine contractions are sustained, maternal effort will usually bring about expulsion. The mother simply pushes, as during the second stage of labour.

- Encouragement is important, as by now she may be exhausted and the contractions will feel weaker and less expulsive than those during the second stage of labour.

- Providing that fresh blood loss is not excessive, the mother's condition remains stable and her pulse rate normal, there need be no anxiety. This spontaneous process can take from 20 minutes to an hour to complete.

- It is important that the midwife monitors uterine action by placing a hand lightly on the fundus. She can thus palpate the contraction whilst checking that relaxation does not result in the uterus filling with blood.

- Vigilance is crucial, as it should be remembered that the longer the placenta remains undelivered, the greater is the risk of bleeding because the uterus cannot contract down fully whilst the bulk of the placenta is in situ.

- Early attachment of the baby to the breast may enhance these physiological changes by stimulating the release of oxytocin from the posterior lobe of the pituitary gland.

Asepsis

The need for asepsis is even greater now than in the preceding stage of labour. Laceration and bruising of the cervix, vagina, perineum and vulva provide a route for the entry of micro-organisms. The placenta site, a raw wound, provides an ideal medium for infection. Strict attention to the prevention of sepsis is therefore vital.

Cord blood sampling

This may be required:

- when the mother's blood group is Rhesus negative or her Rhesus type is unknown
- when atypical maternal antibodies have been found during an antenatal screening test
- where a haemoglobinopathy is suspected (e.g. sickle cell disease)
- to estimate pH of blood if there is an indication of fetal compromise.

The sample should be taken from the fetal surface of the placenta where the blood vessels are congested and easily visible.

Completion of the Third Stage

- Once the placenta is delivered, the midwife must first check that the uterus is well contracted and fresh blood loss is minimal.
- Careful inspection of the perineum and lower vagina is important.
- Blood loss is estimated; account must be taken of blood that has soaked into linen and swabs as well as measurable fluid loss and clot formation.
- A thorough inspection of the placenta or membranes must be carried out to make sure that no part has been retained.
- If there is any suspicion that the placenta or membranes are incomplete, they must be kept for inspection and a doctor informed immediately.

Immediate care

It is advisable for mother and infant to remain in the midwife's care for at least an hour after birth, regardless of the birth setting.

- The woman should be encouraged to pass urine because a full bladder may impede uterine contraction.

- Uterine contraction and blood loss should be checked on several occasions during this first hour.

- Throughout this same period the midwife should pay regard to the baby's general well-being. She should check the security of the cord clamp and observe general skin colour, respirations and temperature.

- The warmest place for a baby to be placed is in a direct skin-to-skin contact position with the mother or wrapped and cuddled, whichever she prefers.

- Most women intending to breastfeed will wish to put their babies to the breast during these early moments of contact.

Complications of the Third Stage of Labour

Postpartum haemorrhage

Postpartum haemorrhage (PPH) is defined as excessive bleeding from the genital tract at any time following the baby's birth up to 6 weeks after delivery.

- If it occurs during the third stage of labour or within 24 hours of delivery, it is termed *primary postpartum haemorrhage*.

- If it occurs subsequent to the first 24 hours following birth up until the 6th week postpartum, it is termed *secondary postpartum haemorrhage*.

Primary postpartum haemorrhage

A measured loss that reaches 500 ml or any loss that adversely affects the mother's condition constitutes a PPH.

There are several reasons why a PPH may occur, including:

- atonic uterus
- retained placenta
- trauma
- blood coagulation disorder.

Atonic uterus

This is a failure of the myometrium at the placental site to contract and retract, and to compress torn blood vessels and control blood loss by a living ligature action. Causes of atonic uterine action resulting in PPH are listed in Box 19.2.

There are, in addition, a number of factors that do not directly *cause* a PPH, but do increase the likelihood of excessive bleeding (Box 19.3).

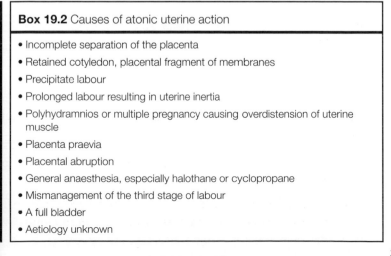

Box 19.2 Causes of atonic uterine action

- Incomplete separation of the placenta
- Retained cotyledon, placental fragment of membranes
- Precipitate labour
- Prolonged labour resulting in uterine inertia
- Polyhydramnios or multiple pregnancy causing overdistension of uterine muscle
- Placenta praevia
- Placental abruption
- General anaesthesia, especially halothane or cyclopropane
- Mismanagement of the third stage of labour
- A full bladder
- Aetiology unknown

> **Box 19.3** Predisposing factors which might increase the risks of postpartum haemorrhage
>
> • Previous history of postpartum haemorrhage or retained placenta
> • High parity, resulting in uterine scar tissue
> • Presence of fibroids
> • Maternal anaemia
> • Ketoacidosis

Signs of PPH

These may be obvious, such as:

- visible bleeding
- maternal collapse.

However, more subtle signs may present, such as:

- pallor
- rising pulse rate
- falling blood pressure
- altered level of consciousness; the mother may become restless or drowsy
- an enlarged uterus that feels 'boggy' on palpation (i.e. soft, distended and lacking tone); there may be little or no visible loss of blood.

Prophylaxis

- During the antenatal period, identify risk factors, e.g. previous obstetric history, anaemia.
- During labour, prevent prolonged labour and ketoacidosis.
- Ensure the mother does not have a full bladder at the start of the third stage.
- Give prophylactic administration of a uterotonic agent.
- If a woman is known to have a placenta praevia, keep 2 units of cross-matched blood available.

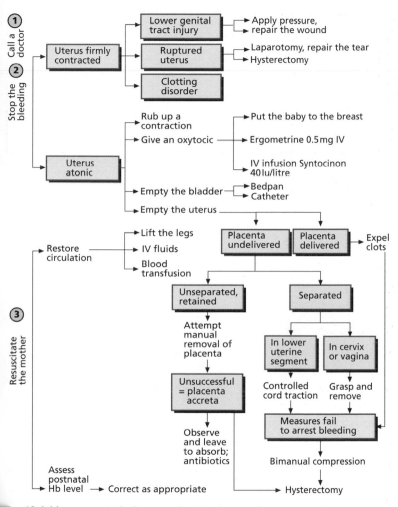

Fig. 19.4 Management of primary postpartum haemorrhage.

Management of PPH

Three basic principles of care should be applied immediately upon observation of excessive bleeding:

- Call for medical aid.
- Stop the bleeding:

  Rub up a contraction

  Give a uterotonic

  Empty the bladder

  Empty the uterus

  Apply pressure if there is trauma.
- Resuscitate the mother.

See Figure 19.4 for a summary of management; at the same time as taking these measures, check the blood is clotting.

Secondary postpartum haemorrhage

See chapter 25.

Chapter 20

Prolonged Pregnancy and Disorders of Uterine Action

Post-term or Prolonged Pregnancy

Risks and clinical implications of post-term pregnancy

- Post-term pregnancy is one that is in excess of 287 days (although 42 weeks is often considered acceptable).
- Accurate dating of a pregnancy is essential, as incorrect diagnosis that a pregnancy has gone beyond term may lead to inappropriate or unnecessary intervention.
- Post-term pregnancy is associated with an increase in perinatal mortality and neonatal morbidity rates.
- Possible fetal consequences include macrosomia or fetal compromise due to placental demise.
- Prolonged pregnancy is the largest single indication for induction of labour.

Management of post-term pregnancy

Two forms of care are offered:

expectant management with fetal surveillance

elective induction of labour after 41 weeks of gestation.

Antenatal surveillance

- *Biophysical profile.* A combined ultrasound assessment of fetal breathing, fetal movement, fetal tone, reactivity of the heart rate and amniotic fluid volume is used to predict fetal well-being in a high-risk pregnancy. A total score of 8–10 indicates the fetus is in good condition.

- *Doppler ultrasound of umbilical artery.*

- *CTG*, also known as non-stress testing (NST). This is carried out twice weekly.

- *Amniotic fluid measurement.*

Induction of Labour

Indications for induction

Induction is indicated when the benefits to the mother or the fetus outweigh those of continuing the pregnancy. It is associated with the maternal and fetal factors described in Box 20.1.

Contraindications to induction

These include:

- placenta praevia
- transverse or compound fetal presentation
- cord presentation or cord prolapse
- cephalopelvic disproportion
- severe fetal compromise
- active genital herpes.

If, in these circumstances, delivery is imperative, it should be effected by caesarean section.

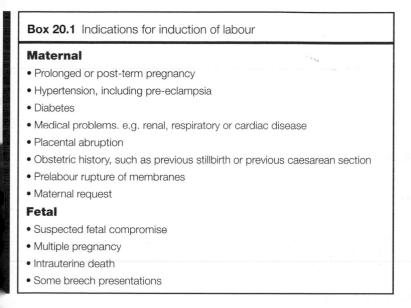

Box 20.1 Indications for induction of labour

Maternal
- Prolonged or post-term pregnancy
- Hypertension, including pre-eclampsia
- Diabetes
- Medical problems. e.g. renal, respiratory or cardiac disease
- Placental abruption
- Obstetric history, such as previous stillbirth or previous caesarean section
- Prelabour rupture of membranes
- Maternal request

Fetal
- Suspected fetal compromise
- Multiple pregnancy
- Intrauterine death
- Some breech presentations

Cervical ripening

Structural changes in ripening

Successful induction occurs when the cervix is favourable or so-called 'ripe'. The cervix is then more compliant, offering less soft-tissue resistance to the actions of the myometrium and the presenting part.

Prostaglandins

Pre-induction prostaglandin can be used to prime or mature the cervix for induction. A low-dose prostaglandin is administered to bring about effacement and dilatation without stimulating contractions.

Methods of inducing labour

Prostaglandins and induction

Prior to the prescription of the prostaglandin, the cervix is assessed using the Bishop's score (Table 20.1). PGE_2 preparations are available in gel or slow-release tablet form; they are inserted close to the cervix within the posterior fornix of the vagina. Fetal heart rate and uterine contractions should be monitored continuously for 30–60 minutes thereafter. The mother should remain recumbent or resting for 1 hour. Changes in the cervix can be assessed by an increase in the Bishop's score.

Recommended prescribed doses of PGE_2 are shown in Table 20.2.

Sweeping or stripping of membranes

Sweeping the membranes can be an effective method of inducing labour where there is an uncomplicated pregnancy. During a vaginal

Table 20.1 Modified Bishop's pre-induction pelvic scoring system

Inducibility features	0	1	2	3
Dilatation of cervix in cm	0	1–2	3–4	5–6
Consistency of cervix	Firm	Medium	Soft	–
Cervical canal length in cm	>2	1–2	0.5–1	<0.5
Position of cervix	Posterior	Mid	Anterior	–
Position of presenting part in cm above or below ischial spine	−3	−2	−1, 0	+1, +2

Table 20.2 Recommended prescribed doses of prostaglandin E_2

Form	Dose
Tablets	3 mg 6–8-hourly
	Maximum dose 6 mg
Gels	Nulliparous women with an unfavourable cervix: 2 mg
	All other women: 1 mg
	Repeat doses of 1–2 mg 6-hourly may be given
	Maximum dose 4 mg for nulliparous women with an unfavourable cervix; 3 mg for all other women

examination the clinician inserts a finger through the cervical os, and using a sweeping or circular movement releases the fetal membranes from the lower uterine segment. Prior to this procedure being undertaken, the woman should be made aware that it may cause some discomfort and bleeding.

Amniotomy

Amniotomy is the artificial rupture of the fetal membranes (ARM), resulting in drainage of liquor. It is performed to induce labour when the cervix is favourable or during labour to augment contractions. ARM may also be carried out to visualise the colour of the liquor or to attach a fetal scalp electrode for the purposes of continuous electronic monitoring of the fetal heart rate. A well-fitting presenting part is essential to prevent cord prolapse.

ARM is carried out using an amnihook or an amnicot. Procedures are shown in Box 20.2.

Box 20.2 Amniotomy procedures

Prior to intervention

- Informed maternal consent is obtained
- The reason for the amniotomy is clearly stated in the records
- Presentation and degree of engagement of the presenting part are confirmed by abdominal palpation
- The fetal heart rate is auscultated
- The presence of a low-lying placenta or cord is excluded

Following intervention

- Note the colour and quantity of liquor
- Check the presentation, position and station of the fetus
- Ensure no cord has prolapsed
- Auscultate the fetal heart rate

Hazards of ARM

These include:

- intrauterine infection
- early decelerations of the fetal heart
- cord prolapse
- bleeding from fetal vessels in the membranes (vasa praevia); friable vessels in the cervix; or a low-lying placental site (placenta praevia).

Oxytocin

Oxytocin is used in conjunction with amniotomy and may be commenced at the same time as ARM or after a delay of several hours.

Administration of oxytocin to induce labour

- Oxytocin is used intravenously, diluted in an isotonic solution such as normal saline.
- The infusion should be controlled through a pump to enable accurate assessment of volume and rate.
- Dosage should be recorded in milliunits per minute, with the suggested dilution being 30 IU in 500 ml of normal saline. The midwife should aim to administer the lowest dose required to maintain effective, well-spaced uterine contractions, with a maximum of 3–4 contractions every 10 minutes (Table 20.3).
- Oxytocin should not be started within 6 hours of the administration of prostaglandins.

Side-effects of oxytocin

- Hyperstimulation of the uterus, which could cause fetal hypoxia and uterine rupture.
- Water retention.
- Prolonged use may contribute to uterine atony postpartum.

Table 20.3 Suggested regimen for intravenous oxytocin in the presence of ruptured membranes

Time in minutes after starting	Dose delivery (milliunits per minute)	Notes
0	1	Most women should have
30	2	adequate contractions at 12
60	4	milliunits per minute
90	8	Maximum licensed dose is 20
120	12	milliunits per minute
150	16	If regular contractions are not
180	20	established after 5 IU (5 hours
210	24	on suggested regimen), then
240	28	induction should be stopped
270	32	

Responsibilities of the midwife and care of a mother in induction of labour

The role of the midwife is to monitor the well-being of the mother and fetus throughout the process of induction, assess progress in labour, and observe for signs of side-effects of oxytocin. The parameters listed in Box 20.3 should be monitored.

The midwife should be aware of the risk of uterine rupture associated with excessive use of oxytocin, particularly if there is a previous history of caesarean section.

Prolonged Labour

Prolonged labour is associated with the medical model of management of childbirth and for many women — and midwives — the attempts to place time limits on the physiological process of labour is problematic. However, prolonged labour is associated with increasing risks to mother and fetus.

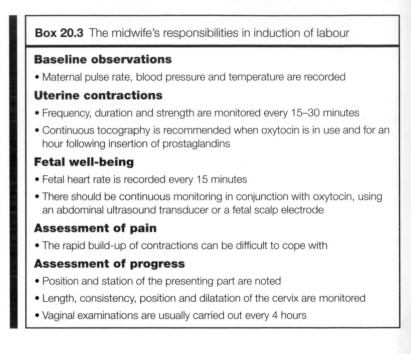

Box 20.3 The midwife's responsibilities in induction of labour

Baseline observations
- Maternal pulse rate, blood pressure and temperature are recorded

Uterine contractions
- Frequency, duration and strength are monitored every 15–30 minutes
- Continuous tocography is recommended when oxytocin is in use and for an hour following insertion of prostaglandins

Fetal well-being
- Fetal heart rate is recorded every 15 minutes
- There should be continuous monitoring in conjunction with oxytocin, using an abdominal ultrasound transducer or a fetal scalp electrode

Assessment of pain
- The rapid build-up of contractions can be difficult to cope with

Assessment of progress
- Position and station of the presenting part are noted
- Length, consistency, position and dilatation of the cervix are monitored
- Vaginal examinations are usually carried out every 4 hours

Prolonged labour is most common in primigravidae and may be caused by:

- ineffective uterine contractions
- cephalopelvic disproportion
- an occipitoposterior position.

Dystocia literally means 'difficult labour' and is associated with slowness or lack of progress in labour. This can be caused by problems with the contractions:

- not being effective in dilating and effacing the cervix
- being uncoordinated, where the two segments of the uterus fail to work in harmony
- giving inadequate involuntary expulsion.

Other causes of dystocia are abnormalities of presentation and position, of the bony pelvis and of the birth canal, including congenital abnormalities.

Prolonged latent phase

The latent phase of labour is still poorly understood and its duration difficult to define; therefore, a diagnosis of a prolonged latent phase may be arbitrary and result in inappropriate intervention.

Prolonged active phase

Slow progress may be defined either as total duration of hours in labour or as failure of the cervix to dilate at a fixed rate per hour. A rate of 1 cm per hour is most commonly taken as normal, but use of a standardised progress rate is now being questioned. A prolonged active phase is caused by a combination of factors, including the cervix, the uterus, the fetus and the mother's pelvis.

Inefficient uterine action

In the absence of effective contractions, descent of the presenting part and dilatation of the cervix may be delayed.

Factors that may affect uterine action

- Restricting food and fluids to mothers in labour may have a detrimental effect.
- Ambulation may promote more effective uterine activity.
- An upright position improves the application of the presenting part on to the cervix, and may trigger the neuroendocrine Ferguson reflex.
- Stress and psychosocial factors are known to affect contractions adversely.

Augmentation of labour

Augmentation of labour refers to intervention to correct slow progress in labour. Correction of ineffective uterine contractions includes amniotomy, administration of oxytocin and amniotomy, or administration of oxytocin in the presence of the previously ruptured membranes. Cephalopelvic disproportion should be excluded before attempts are made to speed up the contractions.

Incoordinate uterine activity

This may be hypertonic and also inefficient. Possible signs include the following:

- Fundal dominance is lacking.
- Polarity is reversed.
- Resting tone of the uterus is raised.
- Pain is intense and out of proportion to the effect of the contraction on the dilatation of the cervix.

Where coordination of the contractions is completely lacking, different areas of the uterus contract independently, causing a 'colicky' uterus. The mother suffers severe generalised pain. Fetal compromise may occur due to diminished placental perfusion.

Constriction ring dystocia

This is a localised spasm of a ring of muscle fibres that occurs at the junction of the upper and lower segments of the uterus. It is associated with the use of oxytocin.

Management of prolonged labour

When progress in labour is slow, attempts should be made to determine the cause before deciding on management. Hypotonic uterine activity may be corrected with amniotomy or oxytocin infusion, or both. If, however, there have been strong contractions and slow progress, a decision may be made to carry out a caesarean section. Obvious disproportion or malpresentation is an indication for caesarean section.

Principles of care are summarised in Box 20.4.

Box 20.4 Principles of care in prolonged labour

Comfort and analgesia
- Adequate analgesia should be offered
- An epidural block may be beneficial

Observations
- Temperature is recorded every 4 hours
- Vaginal swabs may be taken and broad-spectrum antibiotics commenced if infection is suspected
- Pulse and blood pressure recorded hourly, or more frequently if the woman's condition dictates this

Fluid balance
- Input and output should be recorded
- The mother should be encouraged to empty her bladder every 2 hours; a full bladder may affect the uterine action in labour
- Reduced urinary output and ketones may indicate dehydration

Assessment of progress
- Vaginal examination is usually carried out 4-hourly

Fetal well-being
- Fetal heart is monitored continuously
- The presence of meconium-stained liquor and an abnormal fetal heart tracing are suggestive of fetal hypoxia; FBS may be carried out
- A paediatrician may be required, and if the mother is in labour at home it may be necessary for her to be transferred into hospital

---

Prolonged second stage of labour

Provided that there is evidence of descent of the fetus and in the absence of fetal or maternal distress, there is no basis for placing a time limit on the duration of the second stage of labour.

Causes of delay in the second stage

These are listed in Box 20.5.

Box 20.5 Causes of delay in the second stage of labour

- Ineffective contractions
- Poor maternal effort
- Loss or absence of a desire to push caused by epidural analgesia
- A large fetus, malpresentation or malposition
- A full bladder or a full rectum
- A reduced pelvic outlet, in association with an occipitoposterior position — may result in deep transverse arrest

---

Management of a prolonged second stage of labour

- Confirm the position, attitude and station of the presenting part by vaginal examination.

- Auscultate the fetal heart after every contraction or use electronic monitoring.

- In the presence of inefficient uterine contractions, an infusion of oxytocin should be commenced.

- Where the mother is in labour at home, arrange for transfer to hospital or seek support from the supervisor of midwives.

- Birth may be expedited where the conditions alter and maternal or fetal well-being become compromised. Ventouse or forceps will be utilised where the pelvic outlet is adequate and vaginal birth can be safely carried out. Caesarean section may be necessary where there is evidence of cephalopelvic disproportion.

Cervical dystocia

This occurs rarely and is often acquired as a consequence of scarring of the cervix or a congenital structural abnormality. Despite effective contractions the cervix fails to dilate, although it may efface. Caesarean section is necessary to deliver the baby.

Overefficient Uterine Activity (Precipitate Labour)

The contractions are strong and frequent from the onset of labour. Resistance from the soft tissue is low, resulting in rapid completion of the first and second stages. The mother may be distressed by the intensity of the contractions and the unexpected speed of the birth. Soft tissue damage to the cervix or perineum may complicate the birth. The uterus may fail to retract during the third stage, leading to retained placenta or postpartum haemorrhage.

Fetal hypoxia and rapid moulding can occur. The speed of the birth may result in the baby being born in an inappropriate place and sustaining injury.

Precipitate labour tends to recur.

Trial of Labour

A trial of labour is offered to mothers when there is a minor degree of cephalopelvic disproportion. Review of place of birth may be necessary. If, despite good uterine contractions, cervical dilatation is slow and the head fails to descend, the outlook for vaginal birth is poor and the decision must be made whether to allow labour to continue.

If at any stage during this labour the mother or fetus is under stress, then a caesarean section will be performed. A trial of labour or vaginal birth may also be considered following previous caesarean section (VBAC).

Obstructed Labour

Labour is obstructed when there is no advance of the presenting part despite strong uterine contractions. The obstruction usually occurs at the pelvic brim but may occur at the outlet.

Causes of obstructed labour

- Cephalopelvic disproportion.
- Deep transverse arrest.
- Malpresentation, e.g. shoulder or brow presentation, or in persistent mentoposterior position.
- Pelvic mass, e.g. fibroids, ovarian or pelvic tumours.
- Fetal abnormalities, e.g. hydrocephalus, conjoined twins, locked twins.

Signs of obstructed labour

These are listed in Box 20.6.

Box 20.6 Signs of obstructed labour

Early signs

- The presenting part does not enter the pelvic brim despite good contractions (exclude full bladder, loaded rectum or excessive liquor)
- Cervical dilatation is slow; the cervix hangs loosely like 'an empty sleeve'
- Pressure may result in early rupture or formation of a large elongated sac of forewaters

Late signs

- The mother is dehydrated, ketotic and in constant pain
- The mother is pyrexial
- Urinary output is poor and haematuria may be present
- There is evidence of fetal distress
- The uterus becomes moulded round the fetus and fails to relax properly between contractions
- Contractions continue to build in strength and frequency until the uterus is in a continuous state of tonic contraction
- A visible retraction ring (Bandl's ring), similar in appearance to a full bladder, appears at an oblique angle across the abdomen
- In a primigravida, uterine contractions may cease for a while before recommencing with renewed vigour

---

On examination the vagina feels hot and dry; the presenting part is high and feels wedged and immovable. It may be difficult to assess the station of the presenting part accurately due to excessive moulding of the fetal skull and a large caput succedaneum.

Management of obstructed labour

- An intravenous infusion must be commenced to correct dehydration.
- Blood is taken for cross-matching in case a transfusion is needed.
- Antibiotics should be given to overcome any infection that may be present.
- If obstructed labour is recognised in the first stage of labour, delivery should be by caesarean section.
- In the second stage of labour, failure to progress and descend may be due to deep transverse arrest. If the obstruction cannot be overcome by rotation and assisted birth, caesarean section should be performed.
- If the mother is in labour at home, arrangements should be made to transfer her to the nearest maternity unit with facilities for an

---

Box 20.7 Complications of obstructed labour

Maternal

- There is trauma to the bladder, e.g. vesicovaginal fistula
- There is intrauterine infection due to prolonged rupture of membranes
- Neglected obstruction will result in rupture of the uterus, leading to haemorrhage and possible death of the mother and the fetus

Fetal

- Intrauterine asphyxia may result in a fresh stillbirth or, if the baby is born alive, permanent brain damage
- Ascending infection can cause neonatal pneumonia; this may also develop as a consequence of meconium aspiration

immediate caesarean section. The midwife should take blood for cross-matching and site an intravenous infusion prior to transfer.

- The paediatrician should be present at the birth.

Complications of obstructed labour

Complications are listed in Box 20.7.

Chapter 21

Malpositions of the Occiput and Malpresentations

Occipitoposterior Positions

Occipitoposterior positions are the most common type of malposition of the occiput and occur in approximately 10% of labours. A persistent occipitoposterior position results from a failure of internal rotation prior to delivery. The vertex is presenting, but the occiput lies in the posterior rather than the anterior part of the pelvis. As a consequence, the fetal head is deflexed and larger diameters of the fetal skull present.

Causes

The direct cause is often unknown, but it may be associated with an android- or anthropoid-shaped pelvis.

Antenatal diagnosis

Abdominal examination

Inspection

- There is a saucer-shaped depression at or just below the umbilicus.

Palpation

- The back is difficult to palpate, as it is well out to the maternal side.
- Limbs can be felt on both sides of the midline.
- The head is usually high.
- The occiput and sinciput are on the same level.

Auscultation

- The fetal heart can be heard in the midline or at the flank on the same side as the back.

Diagnosis during labour

- The woman may complain of continuous and severe backache worsening with contractions.
- Spontaneous rupture of the membranes may occur at an early stage of labour.
- Contractions may be incoordinate.
- There is slow descent of the head, even with good contractions.
- The woman may have a strong desire to push early in labour.

Vaginal examination

The findings will depend upon the degree of flexion of the head; locating the anterior fontanelle in the anterior part of the pelvis is diagnostic. The direction of the sagittal suture and location of the posterior fontanelle will help to confirm the diagnosis.

Management of labour

Labour with a fetus in an occipitoposterior position can be long and painful. The deflexed head does not fit well on to the cervix

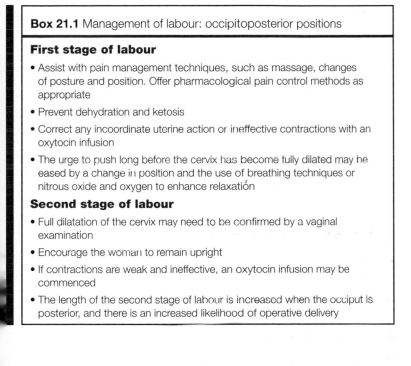

Box 21.1 Management of labour: occipitoposterior positions

First stage of labour

- Assist with pain management techniques, such as massage, changes of posture and position. Offer pharmacological pain control methods as appropriate
- Prevent dehydration and ketosis
- Correct any incoordinate uterine action or ineffective contractions with an oxytocin infusion
- The urge to push long before the cervix has become fully dilated may be eased by a change in position and the use of breathing techniques or nitrous oxide and oxygen to enhance relaxation

Second stage of labour

- Full dilatation of the cervix may need to be confirmed by a vaginal examination
- Encourage the woman to remain upright
- If contractions are weak and ineffective, an oxytocin infusion may be commenced
- The length of the second stage of labour is increased when the occiput is posterior, and there is an increased likelihood of operative delivery

and therefore does not produce optimal stimulation for uterine contractions.

Management is described in Box 21.1.

Mechanism of the right occipitoposterior position (long rotation)

See Figures 21.1–21.4 and Table 21.1.

- *Flexion*. Descent takes place with increasing flexion. The occiput becomes the leading part.
- *Internal rotation of the head*. The occiput reaches the pelvic floor first and rotates forwards three-eighths of a circle along the right side of the pelvis to lie under the symphysis pubis. The shoulders

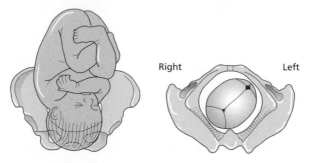

Fig. 21.1 Head descending with increased flexion.
Sagittal suture in right oblique diameter of the pelvis.

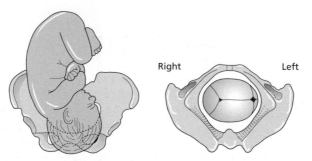

Fig. 21.2 Occiput and shoulders have rotated one-eighth of a circle forwards.
Sagittal suture in transverse diameter of the pelvis.

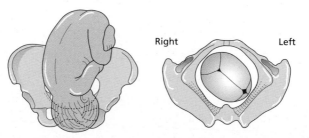

Fig. 21.3 Occiput and shoulders have rotated two-eighths of a circle forwards.
Sagittal suture in the left oblique diameter of the pelvis. The position is right
occipitoanterior.

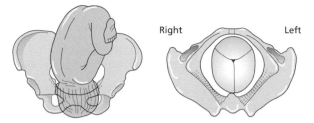

Fig. 21.4 Occiput has rotated three-eighths of a circle forwards.
Note the twist in the neck. Sagittal suture in the anteroposterior diameter of the
pelvis.

Table 21.1 Terminology for mechanisms of the right
occipitoposterior, left mentoanterior and left sacroanterior positions

	Right occipitoposterior	**Left mento-anterior**	**Left sacroanterior**
Lie	Longitudinal	Longitudinal	Longitudinal
Attitude	Deflexion of head	Extension of head and back	Complete flexion
Presentation	Vertex	Face	Breech
Denominator	Occiput	Mentum	Sacrum
Presenting part	Middle or anterior area of left parietal bone	Left malar bone	Anterior (left) buttock
Diameter	Occipitofrontal diameter (11.5 cm) lies in right oblique diameter of pelvic brim		Bitrochanteric diameter (10 cm) enters pelvis in the oblique diameter of brim
	Occiput points to right sacroiliac joint and sinciput to left iliopectineal eminence		Sacrum points to left iliopectineal eminence

follow, turning two-eighths of a circle from the left to the right oblique diameter.

■ *Crowning*. The occiput escapes under the symphysis pubis and the head is crowned.

■ *Extension*. The sinciput, face and chin sweep the perineum and the head is born by a movement of extension.

■ *Restitution*. The occiput turns one-eighth of a circle to the right and the head realigns itself with the shoulders.

■ *Internal rotation of the shoulders*. The shoulders enter the pelvis in the right oblique diameter; the anterior shoulder reaches the pelvic floor first and rotates forwards one-eighth of a circle to lie under the symphysis pubis.

■ *External rotation of the head*. At the same time the occiput turns a further one-eighth of a circle to the right.

■ *Lateral flexion*. The anterior shoulder escapes under the symphysis pubis, the posterior shoulder sweeps the perineum and the body is born by a movement of lateral flexion.

Possible course and outcomes of labour

Long internal rotation

This is the most common outcome, with good uterine contractions producing flexion and descent of the head so that the occiput rotates forward three-eighths of a circle, as described above.

Short internal rotation (persistent occipitoposterior position)

This results from failure of flexion:

■ The sinciput reaches the pelvic floor first and rotates forwards.

■ The occiput goes into the hollow of the sacrum.

■ The baby is born facing the pubic bone (face to pubis).

Diagnosis

In the first stage of labour:

- There is slow descent with a deflexed head and fetal heart audible in the flank or in the midline.

In the second stage of labour:

- Delay is common.
- On vaginal examination the anterior fontanelle is felt behind the symphysis pubis.
- Dilatation of the anus and gaping of the vagina may occur while the fetal head is barely visible; there may also be excessive bulging of the perineum.

The birth

The sinciput will first emerge from under the symphysis pubis; the midwife maintains flexion to prevent it from escaping further than the glabella. The occiput sweeps the perineum and is born. The head is then extended to bring the face down from under the symphysis pubis. An episiotomy may be required to prevent excessive perineal trauma.

Deep transverse arrest

- This occurs when the occiput begins to rotate forwards but flexion is not maintained; the occipitofrontal diameter becomes caught at the narrow bispinous diameter of the outlet.
- Arrest may be due to weak contractions, a straight sacrum or a narrowed outlet.

Diagnosis

On vaginal examination:

- The sagittal suture is in the transverse diameter of the pelvis and both fontanelles are palpable.
- The head is at the level of the ischial spines and there is no advance.

Management

Pushing may not resolve the problem, though a change of position and sighing out slowly (SOS) breathing may help to overcome the urge to bear down.

An operative delivery may be required, either by vacuum extraction or the obstetrician may use forceps to rotate the head to an occipitoanterior position before delivery. Adequate analgesia or anaesthesia should be given.

Conversion to face or brow presentation

- This occurs when the head is deflexed at the onset of labour and extension occurs instead of flexion.

- Complete extension results in a face presentation; incomplete extension leads to a brow presentation.

Complications

- Prolonged labour with increased likelihood of instrumental delivery.

- Obstructed labour.

- Maternal perineal trauma.

- Neonatal trauma/cerebral haemorrhage.

- Cord prolapse.

Face Presentation

This occurs when the attitude of the head is one of complete extension. It may be primary (presents before labour) or secondary (develops during labour). The denominator is the mentum and the presenting diameters are the submentobregmatic (9.5 cm) and the bitemporal (8.2 cm) (Figs 21.5–21.10).

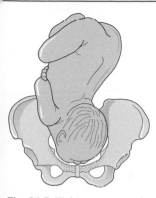

Fig. 21.5 Right mentoposterior.

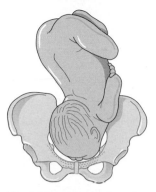

Fig. 21.6 Left mentoposterior.

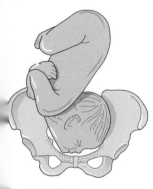

Fig. 21.7 Right mentolateral.

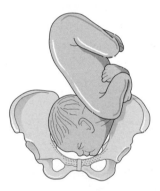

Fig. 21.8 Left mentolateral.

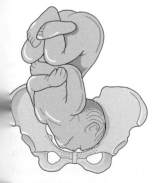

Fig. 21.9 Right mentoanterior.

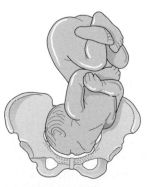

Fig. 21.10 Left mentoanterior.

Causes

- Anterior obliquity of the uterus.
- Contracted pelvis.
- Polyhydramnios.
- Congenital abnormality, e.g. anencephaly.

Diagnosis during labour

Abdominal palpation

Face presentation may be difficult to diagnose, especially if the mentum is anterior.

- The occiput feels prominent, with a groove between head and back.
- The limbs may be palpated on the side opposite to the occiput.
- The fetal heart is best heard through the fetal chest on the same side as the limbs. In a mentoposterior position the fetal heart is difficult to hear.

Vaginal examination

- The presenting part is high, soft and irregular.
- The orbital ridges, eyes, nose and mouth may be felt.
- As labour progresses the face becomes oedematous, making it more difficult to distinguish from a breech presentation.
- Care must be taken not to injure or infect the eyes with the examining finger.

Mechanism of the left mentoanterior position

See Table 21.1 (p. 351).

- *Extension*. Descent takes place with increasing extension. The mentum becomes the leading part.

- *Internal rotation of the head.* This occurs when the chin reaches the pelvic floor and rotates forwards one-eighth of a circle. The chin escapes under the symphysis pubis.

- *Flexion.* Flexion takes place when the sinciput, vertex and occiput sweep the perineum; the head is born.

- *Restitution.* This occurs when the chin turns one-eighth of a circle to the woman's left.

- *Internal rotation of the shoulders.* The shoulders enter the pelvis in the left oblique diameter, and the anterior shoulder reaches the pelvic floor first and rotates forwards one-eighth of a circle along the right side of the pelvis.

- *External rotation of the head.* This occurs simultaneously. The chin moves a further one-eighth of a circle to the left.

- *Lateral flexion.* The anterior shoulder escapes under the symphysis pubis, the posterior shoulder sweeps the perineum and the body is born by a movement of lateral flexion.

Possible course and outcomes of labour

Prolonged labour

This is due to an ill-fitting presenting part and facial bones that do not mould. The fetal axis pressure is directed to the chin and the head is extended almost at right angles to the spine, increasing the diameters to be accommodated in the pelvis.

Mentoanterior positions

With good uterine contractions, descent and rotation of the head occur and labour progresses to a spontaneous birth.

Mentoposterior positions

If the head is completely extended and the contractions are effective, the mentum will rotate forwards and the position becomes anterior.

Persistent mentoposterior position

If the head is incompletely extended and the sinciput reaches the pelvic floor first and rotates forwards one-eighth of a circle, bringing the chin into the hollow of the sacrum, no further mechanism is possible and labour becomes obstructed.

Management of labour

See Box 21.2.

Box 21.2 Management of labour: face presentations

First stage of labour

- Inform the obstetrician
- Do not apply a fetal scalp electrode and take care not to infect or injure the eyes during vaginal examinations
- Following rupture of the membranes, exclude cord prolapse
- Observe descent of the head by abdominal palpation
- Assess cervical dilatation and descent of the head by vaginal examination every 2–4 hours. In mentoposterior positions, note whether the mentum is lower than the sinciput. If the head remains high in spite of good contractions, caesarean section is likely

Birth of the head

- When the face appears at the vulva, maintain extension by holding back the sinciput and permitting the mentum to escape under the symphysis pubis before the occiput is allowed to sweep the perineum. In this way the submentovertical diameter (11.5 cm), instead of the mentovertical diameter (13.5 cm), distends the vaginal orifice
- Because the perineum is also distended by the biparietal diameter (9.5 cm), an elective episiotomy may be performed
- If the head does not descend in the second stage and is in a mentoanterior position, it may be possible for the obstetrician to deliver the baby with forceps; when rotation is incomplete, or the position remains mentoposterior, a rotational forceps delivery may be feasible
- If the head has become impacted, or there is any suspicion of disproportion, a caesarean section will be necessary

---

Complications

- Obstructed labour.
- Cord prolapse.
- Facial bruising/oedema.
- Cerebral haemorrhage.
- Maternal perineal and vaginal trauma.

Brow Presentation

Here the fetal head is partially extended with the frontal bone, which is bounded by the anterior fontanelle and the orbital ridges, lying at the pelvic brim. The presenting diameter is the mentovertical (13.5 cm).

Causes

These are the same as for a secondary face presentation; during the process of extension from a vertex presentation to a face presentation, the brow will present temporarily and in a few cases this will persist.

Diagnosis

Brow presentation is not usually detected before the onset of labour.

Abdominal palpation

- The head is high, appears unduly large and does not descend into the pelvis despite good uterine contractions.

Vaginal examination

- The presenting part is high.

  The anterior fontanelle may be felt on one side of the pelvis and the orbital ridges, and possibly the root of the nose, at the other.

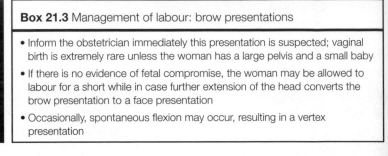

Box 21.3 Management of labour: brow presentations

- Inform the obstetrician immediately this presentation is suspected; vaginal birth is extremely rare unless the woman has a large pelvis and a small baby
- If there is no evidence of fetal compromise, the woman may be allowed to labour for a short while in case further extension of the head converts the brow presentation to a face presentation
- Occasionally, spontaneous flexion may occur, resulting in a vertex presentation

■ A large caput succedaneum may mask these landmarks if the woman has been in labour for some hours.

Management

Management of brow presentations is summarised in Box 21.3.

Complications

These are the same as in a face presentation, except that obstructed labour requiring caesarean section is the probable rather than a possible outcome.

Breech Presentation

Here the fetus lies longitudinally with the buttocks in the lower pole of the uterus. There are six positions for a breech presentation (Fig. 21.11–21.16).

Types of breech presentation position

■ Breech with extended legs (frank breech) (Fig. 21.17).
■ Complete breech (Fig. 21.18).
■ Footling breech (Fig. 21.19).
■ Knee presentation (Fig. 21.20).

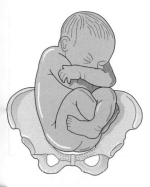

Fig. 21.11 Right sacroposterior.

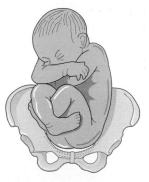

Fig. 21.12 Left sacroposterior.

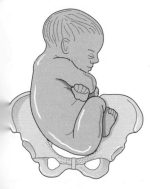

ig. 21.13 Right sacrolateral.

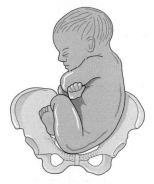

Fig. 21.14 Left sacrolateral.

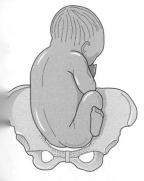

g. 21.15 Right sacroanterior.

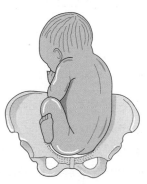

Fig. 21.16 Left sacroanterior.

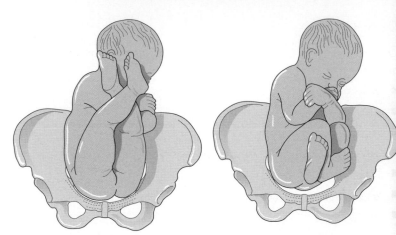

Fig. 21.17 Frank breech.

Fig. 21.18 Complete breech.

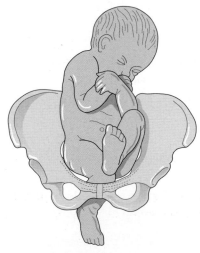

Fig. 21.19 Footling presentation.

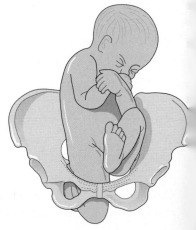

Fig. 21.20 Knee presentation.

Causes

Often no cause is identified, but the following circumstances favour breech presentation:

- extended legs
- preterm labour
- multiple pregnancy
- polyhydramnios
- hydrocephaly
- uterine abnormalities
- placenta praevia.

Antenatal diagnosis

Abdominal examination

Palpation

- The lie is longitudinal with a soft presentation, which is more easily felt using Pawlik's grip.
- The head can usually be felt in the fundus as a round hard mass, which may be made to move independently of the back by ballottement with one or both hands.
- If the legs are extended, the feet may prevent such nodding.
- When the breech is anterior and the fetus well flexed, it may be difficult to locate the head, but use of the combined grip, in which the upper and lower poles are grasped simultaneously, may aid diagnosis.

The woman may complain of discomfort under her ribs, especially at night, owing to pressure of the head on the diaphragm.

Auscultation

When the breech has not passed through the pelvic brim, the fetal heart is heard most clearly above the umbilicus.

- When the legs are extended, the breech descends into the pelvis easily. The fetal heart is then heard at a lower level.

Ultrasound examination

- This may be used to demonstrate a breech presentation.

X-ray examination

- Although largely superseded by ultrasound, X-ray has the added advantage of allowing pelvimetry to be performed at the same time.

Diagnosis during labour

Abdominal examination

- Breech presentation may be diagnosed on admission in labour.

Vaginal examination

- The breech feels soft and irregular with no sutures palpable.
- The anus may be felt and fresh meconium on the examining finger is usually diagnostic.
- If the legs are extended (Fig. 21.21), the external genitalia are very evident but it must be remembered that these become oedematous
- If a foot is felt (Fig. 21.22), the midwife should differentiate it from the hand.

Presentation may be confirmed by ultrasound scan or X-ray.

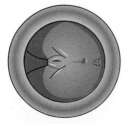

Fig. 21.21 No feet felt; the legs are extended.

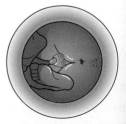

Fig. 21.22 Feet felt; complete breech presentation.

Antenatal management

If the midwife suspects or detects a breech presentation at 36 weeks' gestation or later, she should refer the woman to an obstetrician. There are differing opinions amongst obstetricians as to the management of breech presentation during pregnancy and a decision on management is usually deferred until near term.

External cephalic version

External cephalic version (ECV) is the use of external manipulation on the mother's abdomen to convert a breech to a cephalic presentation. ECV may be offered at term by a practitioner skilled and experienced in the procedure, and should only be undertaken in a unit where there are facilities for emergency delivery. Contraindications include:

- pre-eclampsia or hypertension
- multiple pregnancy
- oligohydramnios
- ruptured membranes
- a hydrocephalic fetus
- any condition that would require delivery by caesarean section.

Persistent breech presentation

At 37 weeks' gestation a discussion of the available options should take place between the mother and an experienced practitioner, and a decision made as to whether to perform an elective caesarean section or to attempt a vaginal birth.

Assessment for vaginal birth

Any doubt as to the capacity of the pelvis to accommodate the fetal head must be resolved before the buttocks are delivered and the head attempts to enter the pelvic brim.

Fetal size

This, especially in relation to maternal size, can be assessed on abdominal palpation but is more accurately judged in association with an ultrasound examination.

Pelvic capacity

This can be judged on vaginal assessment. This will show the shape of the sacrum and give accurate measurements of the anteroposterior diameters of the pelvic brim, cavity and outlet. In a multigravida, information about the type of birth and the size of previous babies when compared with the size of the present fetus can be helpful.

Mechanism of the left sacroanterior position

This is described in Table 21.1 (p. 351).

- *Compaction*. Descent takes place with increasing compaction, owing to increased flexion of the limbs.
- *Internal rotation of the buttocks*. The anterior buttock reaches the pelvic floor first and rotates forwards one-eighth of a circle along the right side of the pelvis to lie underneath the symphysis pubis. The bitrochanteric diameter is now in the anteroposterior diameter of the outlet.
- *Lateral flexion of the body*. The anterior buttock escapes under the symphysis pubis, the posterior buttock sweeps the perineum and the buttocks are born by a movement of lateral flexion.
- *Restitution of the buttocks*. The anterior buttock turns slightly to the mother's right side.
- *Internal rotation of the shoulders*. The shoulders enter the pelvis in the same oblique diameter as the buttocks, the left oblique. The anterior shoulder rotates forwards one-eighth of a circle along the right side of the pelvis and escapes under the symphysis pubis, the posterior shoulder sweeps the perineum and the shoulders are born.

- *Internal rotation of the head.* The head enters the pelvis with the sagittal suture in the transverse diameter of the brim. The occiput rotates forwards along the left side and the suboccipital region (the nape of the neck) impinges on the undersurface of the symphysis pubis.

- *External rotation of the body.* At the same time the body turns so that the back is uppermost.

- *Birth of the head.* The chin, face and sinciput sweep the perineum and the head is born in a flexed attitude.

Management of labour

Vaginal birth should be presented to the woman as the norm for breech presentation, provided there are no complications, although it should be made clear that there is a possibility of delivery by caesarean section.

Careful assessment should be made at the start of labour and anticipated labour management should be reviewed (Box 21.4). A consultant obstetrician should be informed of a breech presentation in labour.

Types of vaginal birth

- *Spontaneous breech birth.* The birth occurs with little assistance from the attendant.

- *Assisted breech birth.* The buttocks are born spontaneously, but some assistance is necessary for delivery of extended legs or arms and the head.

- *Breech extraction.* This is a manipulative delivery carried out by an obstetrician and is performed to hasten delivery in an emergency situation such as fetal compromise.

Management of breech birth

When the buttocks are distending the perineum, the woman is upright or in the lithotomy position. The bladder must be empty

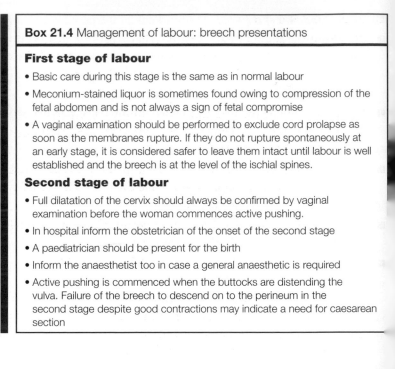

Box 21.4 Management of labour: breech presentations

First stage of labour

- Basic care during this stage is the same as in normal labour
- Meconium-stained liquor is sometimes found owing to compression of the fetal abdomen and is not always a sign of fetal compromise
- A vaginal examination should be performed to exclude cord prolapse as soon as the membranes rupture. If they do not rupture spontaneously at an early stage, it is considered safer to leave them intact until labour is well established and the breech is at the level of the ischial spines.

Second stage of labour

- Full dilatation of the cervix should always be confirmed by vaginal examination before the woman commences active pushing.
- In hospital inform the obstetrician of the onset of the second stage
- A paediatrician should be present for the birth
- Inform the anaesthetist too in case a general anaesthetic is required
- Active pushing is commenced when the buttocks are distending the vulva. Failure of the breech to descend on to the perineum in the second stage despite good contractions may indicate a need for caesarean section

and it is usually catheterised at this stage. If epidural analgesia is not being used, the perineum is infiltrated with up to 10 ml of 0.5% plain lidocaine if an episiotomy is to be performed. (Pudendal block is sometimes used by an obstetrician.)

- The buttocks are born spontaneously.

- If the legs are flexed, the feet disengage at the vulva and the baby is born as far as the umbilicus.

- A loop of cord may be gently pulled down to avoid traction on the umbilicus.

- The midwife should feel for the elbows, which are usually on the chest. If so, the arms will escape with the next contraction. If the arms are not felt, they are extended.

Birth of the shoulders

- The shoulders should rotate into the anteroposterior diameter of the outlet. (It is helpful to wrap a small towel around the baby's hips, which preserves warmth and improves the grip on the slippery skin).

- Grasp the baby by the iliac crests with thumbs held parallel over the sacrum and tilt the baby towards the maternal sacrum in order to free the anterior shoulder.

- When the anterior shoulder has escaped, the buttocks are lifted towards the mother's abdomen to enable the posterior shoulder and arm to pass over the perineum.

- The head enters the pelvic brim and descends through the pelvis with the sagittal suture in the transverse diameter.

- The back must remain lateral until this has happened but afterwards will be turned uppermost. If the back is turned upwards too soon, the anteroposterior diameter of the head will enter the anteroposterior diameter of the brim and may become extended. The shoulders may then become impacted at the outlet and the extended head may cause difficulty.

Birth of the head

- When the back has been turned, the infant is allowed to hang from the vulva without support.

- The baby's weight brings the head on to the pelvic floor on which the occiput rotates forwards. The sagittal suture is now in the anteroposterior diameter of the outlet.

- If rotation of the head fails to take place, two fingers should be placed on the malar bones and the head rotated.

- The baby can be allowed to hang for 1 or 2 minutes.

- Gradually the neck elongates, the hair-line appears and the suboccipital region can be felt.

Controlled birth of the head is vital to avoid any sudden change in intracranial pressure and subsequent cerebral haemorrhage. There are three methods:

- forceps delivery
- Burns Marshall method (if the head is flexed)
- Mauriceau–Smellie–Veit manoeuvre (jaw flexion and shoulder traction).

Forceps delivery

Most breech births are performed by an obstetrician, who will apply forceps to the after-coming head to achieve a controlled delivery.

Burns Marshall method

- Stand facing away from the mother and, with the left hand, grasp the baby's ankles from behind with forefinger between the two (Fig. 21.23A).
- The baby is kept on the stretch with sufficient traction to prevent the neck from bending backwards and being fractured.
- The suboccipital region, and not the neck, should pivot under the apex of the pubic arch or the spinal cord may be crushed.
- The feet are taken up through an arc of 180° until the mouth and nose are free at the vulva.
- The right hand may guard the perineum in order to prevent sudden escape of the head. The mother should be asked to take deliberate, regular breaths that allow the vault of the skull to escape gradually (Fig. 21.23B).

Mauriceau–Smellie–Veit manoeuvre

This is mainly used when there is delay in descent of the head because of extension.

- The baby is laid astride the right arm with the palm supporting the chest. Two fingers are placed on the malar bones.

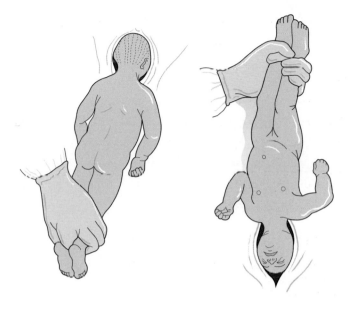

A   **B**

Fig. 21.23 Burns Marshall method of delivering the after-coming head of a breech presentation.
(A) The baby is grasped by the feet and held on the stretch. (B) The mouth and nose are free. The vault of the head is delivered slowly.

- Two fingers of the left hand are hooked over the shoulders, with the middle finger pushing on the occiput to aid flexion.

- Traction is applied to draw the head out of the vagina and, when the suboccipital region appears, the body is lifted to assist the head to pivot around the symphysis pubis.

- The speed of delivery of the head must be controlled so that it does not emerge suddenly.

Alternative positions

When the woman has chosen to birth in an alternative position, it is the upright or supported squat that is the most suitable. The techniques described above will be adapted accordingly and the midwife will observe and encourage the spontaneous mechanism of birth.

Use of uterotonics for third stage

These are withheld until the head is born.

Delivery of extended legs

- Delay may occur at the outlet because the legs splint the body and impede lateral flexion of the spine.
- When the popliteal fossae appear at the vulva, two fingers are placed along the length of one thigh with the fingertips in the fossa.
- The leg is swept to the side of the abdomen (abducting the hip) and the knee is flexed by the pressure on its undersurface. As this movement is continued, the lower part of the leg will emerge from the vagina (Fig. 21.24).

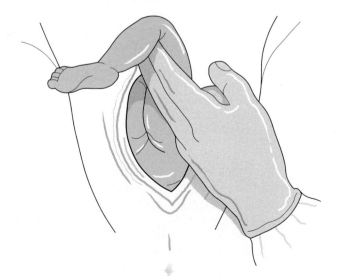

Fig. 21.24 Assisting delivery of extended leg by pressure on the popliteal fossa.

- Repeat to deliver the second leg. The knee is a hinge joint, which bends in one direction only. If the knee is pulled forwards from the abdomen, severe injury to the joint can result.

Delivery of extended arms

Extended arms are diagnosed when the elbows are not felt on the chest after the umbilicus is born. This may be dealt with by using the Løvset manœuvre (Figs 21.25 and 21.26). This is a combination of rotation and downward traction to deliver the arms, whatever position they are in. The direction of rotation must always bring the back uppermost and the arms are delivered from under the pubic arch.

- When the umbilicus is born and the shoulders are in the anteroposterior diameter, the baby is grasped by the iliac crests with the thumbs over the sacrum.

- Downward traction is applied until the axilla is visible.

- Maintaining downward traction throughout, the body is rotated through a half-circle, 180°, starting by turning the back uppermost. The friction of the posterior arm against the pubic bone as the shoulder becomes anterior sweeps the arm in front of

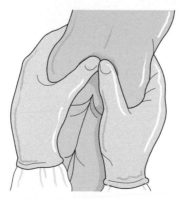

Fig. 21.25 Correct grasp for Løvset manœuvre.

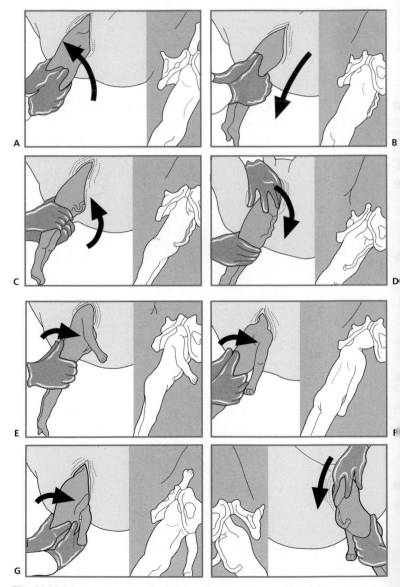

Fig. 21.26 Løvset manœuvre for delivery of extended arms (see text).

the face. The movement allows the shoulders to enter the pelvis in the transverse diameter.

- The first two fingers of the hand that is on the same side as the baby's back are used to splint the humerus and draw it down over the chest as the elbow is flexed.

- The body is now rotated back in the opposite direction and the second arm delivered in a similar fashion.

Delay in birth of the head

- *Extended head.* If, when the body has been allowed to hang, the neck and hair-line are not visible, it is probable that the head is extended. This may be dealt with by the use of forceps or the Mauriceau–Smellie–Veit manœuvre.

- *Posterior rotation of the occiput.* This malrotation of the head is rare and is usually the result of mismanagement. To deliver the head with the occiput posterior, the chin and face are permitted to escape under the symphysis pubis as far as the root of the nose, and the baby is then lifted up towards the mother's abdomen to allow the occiput to sweep the perineum.

Complications

Apart from those difficulties already mentioned, other complications can arise, most of which affect the fetus. Many of these can be avoided by allowing only an experienced operator, or a closely supervised learner, to deliver the baby:

- impacted breech
- cord prolapse
- birth injury:
    - superficial tissue damage
    - fractures of humerus, clavicle or femur or dislocation of shoulder or hip

Erb's palsy

trauma to internal organs

damage to the adrenals

spinal cord damage or fracture of the spine

intracranial haemorrhage

fetal hypoxia

premature separation of the placenta

maternal trauma.

The maternal complications of a breech delivery are the same as those found in other operative vaginal deliveries.

Shoulder Presentation

When the fetus lies with its long axis across the long axis of the uterus (*transverse lie*) the shoulder is most likely to present. Occasionally the lie is oblique but this does not persist, as the uterine contractions during labour make it longitudinal or transverse. Before term, transverse or oblique lie may be transitory.

Causes

Maternal

- Lax abdominal and uterine muscles.
- Uterine abnormality.
- Contracted pelvis.

Fetal

- Preterm pregnancy.
- Multiple pregnancy.
- Polyhydramnios.

- Macerated fetus.
- Placenta praevia.

Antenatal diagnosis

Abdominal palpation

- The uterus appears broad and the fundal height is less than expected for the period of gestation.
- On pelvic and fundal palpation, neither head nor breech is felt. The mobile head is found on one side of the abdomen and the breech at a slightly higher level on the other.

Ultrasound

- An ultrasound scan may be used to confirm the lie and presentation.

Diagnosis during labour

Abdominal palpation

- The findings are as above but when the membranes have ruptured the irregular outline of the uterus is more marked.
- If the uterus is contracting strongly and becomes moulded around the fetus, palpation is very difficult.
- The pelvis is no longer empty, the shoulder being wedged into it.

Vaginal examination

- *This should not be performed without first excluding placenta praevia.*
- In early labour the presenting part may not be felt.
- The membranes usually rupture early.
- If the labour has been in progress for some time, the shoulder may be felt as a soft irregular mass.

- It is sometimes possible to palpate the ribs, their characteristic grid-iron pattern being diagnostic.
- When the shoulder enters the pelvic brim an arm may prolapse; this should be differentiated from a leg.

Possible outcomes of labour

If shoulder presentation persists in labour, delivery must be by caesarean section to avoid obstructed labour and subsequent uterine rupture.

Management

Antenatal

A cause must be sought before deciding on a course of management. Once placenta praevia or uterine abnormalities have been excluded, ECV may be attempted. If this fails, or if the lie is again transverse at the next antenatal visit, the woman is admitted to hospital while further investigations into the cause are made. She frequently remains there until delivery because of the risk of cord prolapse if the membranes rupture.

Intrapartum

If a transverse lie is detected in early labour while the membranes are still intact, the obstetrician or competent health professional may attempt an ECV, followed, if this is successful, by a controlled rupture of the membranes. If the membranes have already ruptured spontaneously, a vaginal examination must be performed immediately to exclude cord prolapse.

Immediate caesarean section must be performed:

- if the cord prolapses
- when the membranes are already ruptured
- when ECV is unsuccessful
- when labour has already been in progress for some hours.

Complications

- Prolapsed cord.
- Prolapsed arm.
- Impacted shoulder presentation leading to obstructed labour, ruptured uterus and stillbirth.

Unstable Lie

The lie is defined as unstable when, after 36 weeks' gestation, instead of remaining longitudinal, it varies from one examination to another between longitudinal and oblique or transverse.

Causes

Any condition in late pregnancy that increases the mobility of the fetus or prevents the head from entering the pelvic brim can cause an unstable lie.

Maternal causes include:

- lax uterine muscles in multigravidae
- contracted pelvis.

Fetal causes include:

- polyhydramnios
- placenta praevia.

Management

Antenatal

- Advise the woman to go to the labour ward as soon as labour commences or membranes rupture.
- Exclude placenta praevia.

■ Attempts to correct the abnormal presentation by ECV may be made. If unsuccessful, caesarean section is considered.

Intrapartum

Many obstetricians induce labour after 38 weeks' gestation, having first ensured that the lie is longitudinal; the induction may be performed by commencing an intravenous infusion of oxytocin to stimulate contractions. A controlled rupture of the membranes is performed so that the head enters the pelvis.

The midwife should ensure that the woman has an empty rectum and bladder before the procedure. The abdomen should be palpated at frequent intervals to ensure that the lie remains longitudinal and to assess the descent of the head. Labour is regarded as a trial.

Complications

If labour commences with the lie other than longitudinal, the complications are the same as for a transverse lie.

Compound Presentation

A compound presentation is when a hand, or occasionally a foot, lies alongside the head. If diagnosed during the first stage of labour, medical aid must be sought. If, during the second stage, the midwife sees a hand presenting alongside the vertex, she could try to hold the hand back.

Chapter 22

Operative Deliveries

Birth by Forceps

Forceps are most commonly employed to expedite delivery of the fetal head or to protect the fetus or the mother, or both, from trauma and exhaustion. They are also used to assist the delivery of the after-coming head of the breech or to draw the head of the baby up and out of the pelvis at caesarean section birth.

The three main indications for the use of forceps are:

- delay in the second stage of labour
- fetal compromise
- maternal distress.

Types of obstetric forceps

- *Wrigley's forceps.* These are designed for use when the head is on the perineum. They are also used for the after-coming head of a breech delivery, or at caesarean section.
- *Neville-Barnes or Simpson's forceps.* These are generally used for a low or mid-cavity forceps delivery when the sagittal suture is in the anteroposterior diameter of the cavity/outlet of the pelvis.

> **Box 22.1** The 'forceps' mnemonic
>
> - **F**ull dilatation of the cervix
> - **O**-fifths of the head palpable abdominally
> - **R**oom in pelvis and **r**uptured membranes
> - **C**ephalic presentation
> - **E**mpty bladder
> - **P**osition recognised
> - **S**uitable pain relief — epidural or pudendal block plus perineal infiltration of local anaesthetic

■ *Kielland's forceps.* These are generally used for the rotation and extraction of the head that is arrested in the deep transverse or the occipitoposterior position.

Prerequisites for forceps delivery

'Forceps' is a useful mnemonic (Box 22.1).

The paediatrician may not be required at birth, but should be kept informed of circumstances. Neonatal resuscitation equipment must be checked and prepared in case it is needed.

Complications

These are listed in Box 22.2.

Birth by the Ventouse Method

The ventouse vacuum extractor is an instrument that applies traction. It can be used as an alternative to forceps. The cup cleaves to the fetal scalp by suction and is used to assist maternal effort. It may be employed when there is a delay in labour, when the cervix is no

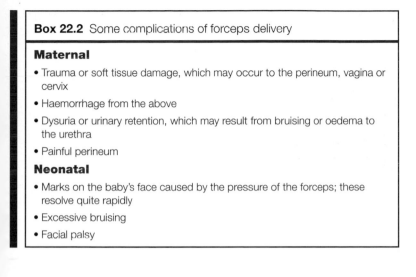

> **Box 22.2** Some complications of forceps delivery
>
> ### Maternal
>
> - Trauma or soft tissue damage, which may occur to the perineum, vagina or cervix
> - Haemorrhage from the above
> - Dysuria or urinary retention, which may result from bruising or oedema to the urethra
> - Painful perineum
>
> ### Neonatal
>
> - Marks on the baby's face caused by the pressure of the forceps; these resolve quite rapidly
> - Excessive bruising
> - Facial palsy

quite fully dilated. It may also be useful in the case of a second twin, when the head remains relatively high.

Procedure

- The woman is usually in the lithotomy position and the same precautions are observed as for a forceps birth.

- The cup of the ventouse is placed as near as possible to, or on, the flexing point of the fetal head.

- The vacuum in the cup is increased gradually so as to achieve a close application to the fetal head. Usually a vacuum of $0.8\,\text{kg/cm}^2$ is reached, by an increase of $0.2\,\text{kg/cm}^2$ in stages, or an increase from 0.2 to $0.8\,\text{kg/cm}^2$ is achieved directly.

- When the vacuum is achieved, traction is applied with a contraction and with maternal effort. This traction is applied in a downwards and backwards direction, then forwards and upwards, thus following the natural curve of the pelvis.

- The vacuum is released and the cup is removed at the crowning of the fetal head.
- The mother can then push the baby for the final part of the birth.

Complications

Prolonged traction will increase the likelihood of:

- scalp abrasions
- cephalhaematoma
- subaponeurotic bleeding.

Caesarean Section

Caesarean section is an operative procedure that is carried out under anaesthesia, whereby the fetus, placenta and membranes are delivered through an incision in the abdominal wall and the uterus. This is usually carried out after viability has been reached (i.e. 24 weeks of gestation onwards).

Preparation

Women expect to be actively involved in their care and the midwife must ensure that recent, valid and relevant information is provided.

The usual preoperative preparation is observed, including:

- an anaesthetic chart/preoperative assessment
- measurement of weight
- baseline observations of blood pressure, pulse and temperature
- gowning and removal of make-up and jewellery.

Results are obtained of any blood tests that have been requested and a full blood count is carried out. Blood is grouped and saved. In the case of pre-eclampsia, urea and electrolyte levels will be examined and clotting factors assessed. The woman will have fasted and taken the prescribed antacid therapy. Attitudes and practices vary regarding pubic shaving.

The woman may choose to be catheterised in theatre under epidural or general anaesthetic, or in her room where it may be more private.

Positioning of the woman

As the woman will need to lie flat it is essential that a wedge or cushion is used, or the table is tilted, to direct the weight of the gravid uterus away from the inferior vena cava and so avoid supine hypotensive syndrome.

Elective caesarean section

This implies that the decision to carry out the procedure has been taken during the pregnancy; therefore before labour has commenced.

Indications for elective caesarean section are shown in Box 22.3.

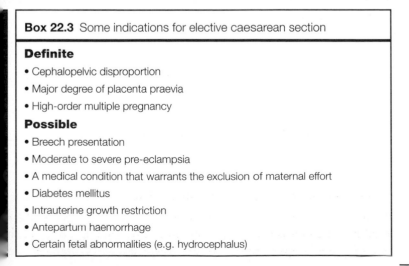

Box 22.3 Some indications for elective caesarean section

Definite
- Cephalopelvic disproportion
- Major degree of placenta praevia
- High-order multiple pregnancy

Possible
- Breech presentation
- Moderate to severe pre-eclampsia
- A medical condition that warrants the exclusion of maternal effort
- Diabetes mellitus
- Intrauterine growth restriction
- Antepartum haemorrhage
- Certain fetal abnormalities (e.g. hydrocephalus)

> **Box 22.4** Some indications for emergency caesarean section
>
> - Antepartum haemorrhage
> - Cord prolapse
> - Uterine rupture (dramatic/scar dehiscence)
> - Cephalopelvic disproportion diagnosed in labour
> - Fulminating pre-eclampsia
> - Eclampsia
> - Failure to progress in the first or second stage of labour and fetal compromise if birth is not imminent

Emergency caesarean section

This is carried out when adverse conditions develop during pregnancy or labour. Some examples of urgent/emergency reasons for caesarean birth are given in Box 22.4.

Vaginal birth after caesarean section (VBAC)

If the indication for caesarean section has been a non-recurring one — for example, placenta praevia — VBAC may be attempted. Repeat caesarean section may be indicated in, for example, cephalopelvic disproportion, or on a uterus that has been scarred twice.

Trial of labour

A trial of labour is carried out whenever there is doubt about the outcome of the labour because of a previous caesarean section. Criteria include the following:

- It is established that the presenting part is capable of flexing adequately to pass through the brim of the pelvis.
- All the facilities for assisted birth are readily available.
- Progress of the labour is sufficient, observed both in the descent of the presenting part and by the dilatation of the cervix.
- Time limits as to the duration of the trial are set.

Anaesthesia

Regional anaesthesia normally remains the safer option for caesarean birth; however, general anaesthesia is sometimes required.

- Regional anaesthesia is incompatible with any maternal coagulation disorder.

- General anaesthesia can be more rapidly administered.

- Some women choose general rather than regional anaesthesia.

Mendelson's syndrome

This is caused if acid gastric contents are inhaled and result in a chemical pneumonitis. This regurgitation may occur during the induction of a general anaesthetic. The acidic gastric contents damage the alveoli, impairing gaseous exchange, and death may result.

Prevention of Mendelson's syndrome

- *Antacid therapy.* A usual regimen is for women having an elective operation to be given two doses of oral ranitidine 150 mg approximately 8 hours apart, plus 30 ml sodium citrate immediately before transfer to theatre. Women in labour who are thought to have a high risk of caesarean section should have ranitidine 150 mg every 8 hours.

- *Cricoid pressure.* This is applied during intubation.

Complications associated with caesarean section

- Infection, e.g. wound, intrauterine, urinary tract and pelvic infections, thrombophlebitis.

- Thromboembolic disorders.

Postoperative care

Immediate care

If the mother intends to breastfeed, the baby should be put to the breast as soon as possible. This can usually be achieved with minimal disturbance to the mother. Ideally, the baby should remain with the mother and they should be transferred to the postnatal ward together as soon as possible.

Observations

- Blood pressure and pulse should be recorded every quarter-hour in the immediate recovery period.
- Temperature should be recorded every 2 hours.
- Lochia and the wound should be inspected every half-hour.
- Following general anaesthesia, level of consciousness and respirations should be monitored.

Analgesia and antiemetics

Analgesia is prescribed and given as required — for example:

- an epidural opioid
- rectal analgesia (e.g. diclofenac)
- intramuscular analgesia
- oral medications (e.g. dihydrocodeine, paracetamol).

Antiemetics (e.g. cyclizine, prochlorperazine) are usually prescribed.

Care following regional block

- Following epidural or spinal anaesthesia the woman may sit up as soon as she wishes, provided her blood pressure is not low.
- Fluids are introduced gradually, followed by a light diet.
- The intravenous infusion remains in progress for about 12 hours
- Care must be taken to avoid any damage to the legs, which will gradually regain sensation and movement.

- As it is possible that an opiate administered via the epidural route may cause some respiratory depression, the woman's respiratory rate must be recorded. This means of pain relief offers the advantage of excellent analgesia without motor block and also seems to give a feeling of well-being. Women are usually able to become mobile very quickly, which reduces the risk of deep venous thrombosis.

Care in the postnatal ward

- Blood pressure, temperature and pulse are usually checked every 4 hours.
- The urinary catheter may remain in situ until the woman is able to get up to the toilet. Urinary output should be monitored after removal of the catheter. Any haematuria must be reported to the doctor.
- The wound and lochia must initially be observed at least hourly.
- Leg and breathing exercises are encouraged.
- Prophylactic low-dose heparin and TED antiembolism stockings are often prescribed.
- Appropriate analgesia must be given as frequently, as necessary.
- Help may be needed with care for the baby.
- The woman may value an opportunity to talk with the midwife about her feelings about having had a caesarean section.

Symphysiotomy

This is an incision of the fibrocartilage partly through the symphysis pubis and is performed in labour to enlarge the transverse diameter of the pelvis. It is rarely seen in the UK, but is carried out in countries where the risk of caesarean section is particularly high for the management of cephalopelvic disproportion.

Chapter 23

Obstetric Emergencies

Vasa Praevia

The term vasa praevia is used when a fetal blood vessel lies over the os, in front of the presenting part. This occurs when fetal vessels from a velamentous insertion of the cord cross the area of the internal os to the placenta. Vasa praevia may sometimes be palpated on vaginal examination when the membranes are still intact. It may also be visualised on ultrasound. If it is suspected, a speculum examination should be made.

Ruptured vasa praevia

When the membranes rupture in a case of vasa praevia, a fetal vessel may also rupture. This leads to exsanguination of the fetus unless birth occurs within minutes.

Diagnosis
- Slight fresh vaginal bleeding, particularly if it commences at the same time as rupture of the membranes.
- Fetal distress disproportionate to blood loss.

Management
See Box 23.1.

> **Box 23.1** Management of vasa praevia
>
> - Request urgent medical aid
> - Monitor the fetal heart rate
> - If the mother is in the first stage of labour and the fetus is still alive, an emergency caesarean section is carried out
> - If in the second stage of labour, delivery should be expedited and a vaginal birth may be achieved
> - A paediatrician should be present at delivery. If the baby is alive, Hb estimation will be necessary after resuscitation

---

Presentation and Prolapse of the Umbilical Cord

See Box 23.2 for definitions.

Predisposing factors

Any situation where the presenting part is neither well applied to the lower uterine segment nor well down in the pelvis may make it possible for a loop of cord to slip down in front of the presenting part. Such situations include:

- high or ill-fitting presenting part
- high parity
- prematurity
- malpresentation
- multiple pregnancy
- polyhydramnios.

Cord presentation

This is diagnosed on vaginal examination when the cord is felt behind intact membranes. It is, however, rarely detected but may be associated

---

Box 23.2 Definitions

Cord presentation

• The umbilical cord lies in front of the presenting part, with the fetal membranes still intact

Cord prolapse

• The cord lies in front of the presenting part and the fetal membranes are ruptured

Occult cord prolapse

• The cord lies alongside, but not in front of, the presenting part

---

Box 23.3 Management of cord presentation

• Under no circumstances should the membranes be ruptured

• Summon medical aid

• Assess fetal well-being, using continuous electronic fetal monitoring, if available

• Help the mother into a position that will reduce the likelihood of cord compression

• Caesarean section is the most likely outcome

---

with aberrations in fetal heart monitoring such as decelerations, which occur if the cord becomes compressed.

Management

See Box 23.3.

Cord prolapse

Diagnosis

■ Diagnosis is made when the cord is felt below or beside the presenting part on vaginal examination.

- A loop of cord may be visible at the vulva.
- Whenever there are factors present that predispose to cord prolapse, a vaginal examination should be performed immediately on spontaneous rupture of membranes.
- Variable decelerations and prolonged decelerations of the fetal heart are associated with cord compression, which may be caused by cord prolapse.

Immediate action and management

See Box 23.4.

Shoulder Dystocia

Definition

The term 'shoulder dystocia' is used to describe failure of the shoulders to traverse the pelvis spontaneously after delivery of the head. The anterior shoulder becomes trapped behind or on the symphysis pubis, whilst the posterior shoulder may be in the hollow of the sacrum or high above the sacral promontory. This is, therefore, a bony dystocia, and traction at this point will further impact the anterior shoulder, impeding attempts at delivery.

Risk factors

These can only give a high index of suspicion:

- post-term pregnancy
- high parity
- maternal obesity (weight over 90 kg)
- fetal macrosomia (birth weight over 4000 g)
- maternal diabetes and gestational diabetes
- prolonged labour (first and second stages)
- operative delivery.

Box 23.4 Management of cord prolapse

Immediate action

- Call for urgent assistance

- If an oxytocin infusion is in progress, this should be stopped

- A vaginal examination is performed to assess the degree of cervical dilatation and identify the presenting part and station. If the cord can be felt pulsating, it should be handled as little as possible

- If the cord lies outside the vagina, replace it gently to try to maintain temperature

- Auscultate the fetal heart rate

- Relieve pressure on the cord.

  Keep your fingers in the woman's vagina and, especially during a contraction, hold the presenting part off the umbilical cord

  Help the mother to change position so that her pelvis and buttocks are raised. The knee–chest position causes the fetus to gravitate towards the diaphragm, relieving the compression on the cord

  Alternatively, help the mother to lie on her left side, with a wedge or pillow elevating her hips (exaggerated Sims' position)

  The foot of the bed may be raised

  These measures need to be maintained until the delivery of the baby, either vaginally or by caesarean section

- Consider inserting 500 ml of warm saline into the bladder to relieve the pressure if transfer to an obstetric unit is required

Treatment

- Delivery must be expedited with the greatest possible speed

- Caesarean section is the treatment of choice if the fetus is still alive and delivery is not imminent, or vaginal birth cannot be indicated

- In the second stage of labour the mother may be able to push and you may perform an episiotomy to expedite the birth

- Where the presentation is cephalic, assisted birth may be achieved through ventouse or forceps

Warning signs and diagnosis

The birth may have been uncomplicated initially, but the head may have advanced slowly and the chin may have had difficulty in sweeping over the perineum. Once the head is born, it may look as if it is trying to return into the vagina.

Shoulder dystocia is diagnosed when manœuvres normally used by the midwife fail to accomplish birth.

Management

See Box 23.6.

The mnemonic HELPERR is widely used in obstetric drills (Box 23.5). An algorithm (Fig. 23.4) can also be helpful.

Complications associated with shoulder dystocia

- Postpartum haemorrhage.
- Uterine rupture.
- Neonatal asphyxia.
- Erb's palsy.
- Intrauterine death.

Box 23.5 The 'HELPERR' mnemonic

- **H**elp
- **E**pisiotomy need assessed
- **L**egs in McRoberts position
- **P**ressure suprapubically
- **E**nter vagina (internal rotation)
- **R**emove posterior arm
- **R**oll over and try again

Box 23.6 Management of shoulder dystocia

- Summon help — an obstetrician, an anaesthetist and a person proficient in neonatal resuscitation
- Attempt to disimpact the shoulders and accomplish delivery. An accurate and detailed record of the type of manoeuvre(s) used, the time taken, the amount of force used and the outcome of each attempted manoeuvre should be made
- Try the procedures for 30–60 seconds; if the baby is not born, move on to the next procedure

Non-invasive procedures

- *Change in maternal position*
- *McRoberts manoeuvre.* Involves helping the woman to lie flat and to bring her knees up to her chest as far as possible to rotate the angle of the symphysis pubis superiorly and use the weight of her legs to create gentle pressure on her abdomen, releasing the impaction of the anterior shoulder
- *Suprapubic pressure* (Fig. 23.1). Pressure is exerted on the side of the fetal back and towards the fetal chest to adduct the shoulders and push the anterior shoulder away from the symphysis pubis. Can be used with the McRoberts manoeuvre.

Manipulative procedures

Where non-invasive procedures have not been successful, direct manipulation of the fetus must now be attempted:

- *Positioning of the mother.* McRoberts or the all-fours position may be used
- *Episiotomy.* May be necessary to gain access to the fetus and reduce maternal trauma
- *Rubin's manoeuvre.* The posterior shoulder is pushed in the direction of the fetal chest, thus rotating the anterior shoulder away from the symphysis pubis into the oblique diameter
- *Wood's manoeuvre* (Fig. 23.2). A hand is inserted into the vagina, pressure is exerted on the posterior fetal shoulder, and rotation is achieved
- *Reverse Wood's manoeuvre.* Fingers on the back of the posterior shoulder apply pressure to rotate in opposite direction

- *Delivery of the posterior arm* (Fig. 23.3). A hand is inserted into the vagina, and two fingers splint the humerus of the posterior arm, flex the elbow, and sweep the forearm over the chest to deliver the hand. If the rest of the delivery is not then accomplished, the second arm can be delivered following rotation of the shoulder using either Wood's or Rubin's manoeuvre or by reversing the Løvset manoeuvre. Has a high complication rate

- *Zavanelli manoeuvre*. If the manoeuvres described above have been unsuccessful, the obstetrician may consider the Zavanelli manoeuvre. Requires the reversal of the mechanisms of delivery so far and success rates vary

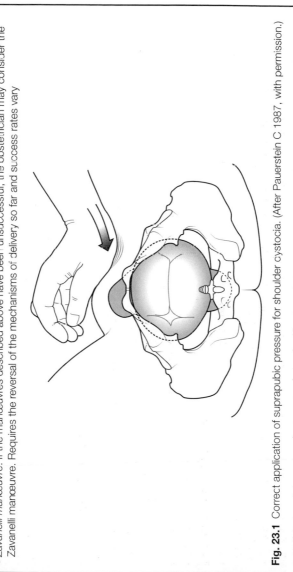

Fig. 23.1 Correct application of suprapubic pressure for shoulder cystocia. (After Pauerstein C 1987, with permission.)

(Continued)

Box 23.6 (Continued)

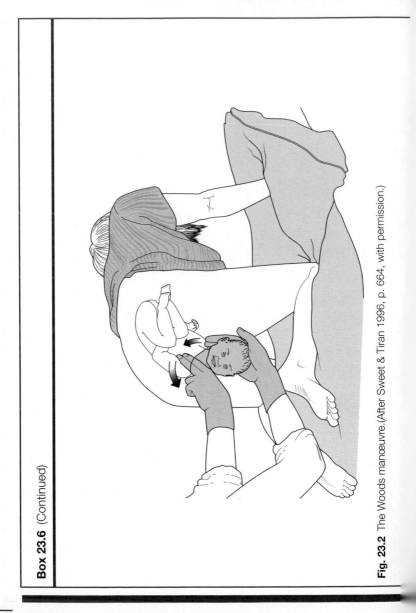

Fig. 23.2 The Woods manoeuvre.(After Sweet & Tiran 1996, p. 664, with permission.)

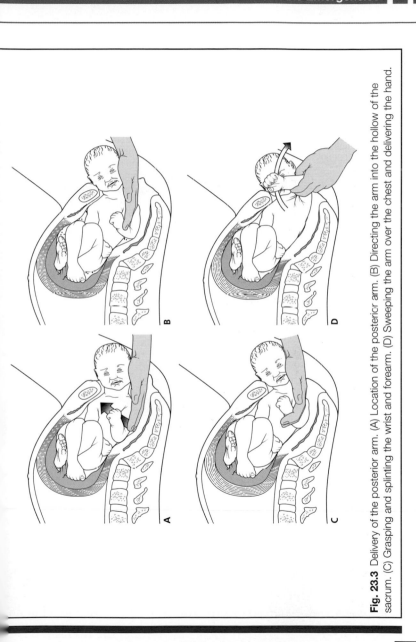

Fig. 23.3 Delivery of the posterior arm. (A) Location of the posterior arm. (B) Directing the arm into the hollow of the sacrum. (C) Grasping and splinting the wrist and forearm. (D) Sweeping the arm over the chest and delivering the hand.

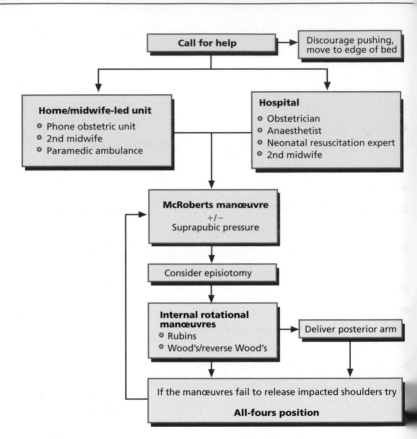

Fig. 23.4 Algorithm for the management of shoulder dystocia.

Rupture of the Uterus

Rupture of the uterus is defined as:

- *complete rupture* — involves a tear in the wall of the uterus with or without expulsion of the fetus.
- *incomplete rupture* — involves tearing of the uterine wall but no the perimetrium.

The life of both mother and fetus may be endangered in either situation.

Dehiscence of an existing uterine scar may also occur.

Causes

- High parity.
- Injudicious use of oxytocin, particularly where the mother is of high parity.
- Obstructed labour.
- Neglected labour, where there is previous history of caesarean section.
- Extension of severe cervical laceration upwards into the lower uterine segment.
- Trauma, as a result of a blast injury or an accident.
- Antenatal rupture of the uterus, where there has been a history of previous classical caesarean section.

Signs of rupture of the uterus

- Maternal tachycardia.
- Scar pain and tenderness (where there has been previous caesarean section).
- Abnormalities of the fetal heart rate and pattern.
- Poor progress in labour.
- Vaginal bleeding.

Management

- immediate caesarean section
- repair of the rupture or a hysterectomy, depending on the extent of the trauma and the mother's condition.

Amniotic Fluid Embolism/Anaphylactoid Syndrome of Pregnancy

This rare but potentially catastrophic condition occurs when amniotic fluid enters the maternal circulation via the uterus or placental site. The presence of amniotic fluid in the maternal circulation triggers an anaphylactoid response and the term 'embolus' is a misnomer.

The body responds in two phases:

- The initial phase is one of pulmonary vasospasm causing hypoxia, hypotension, pulmonary oedema and cardiovascular collapse.

- The second phase sees the development of left ventricular failure, with haemorrhage and coagulation disorder and further uncontrollable haemorrhage.

Amniotic fluid embolism can occur at any time, but during labour and its immediate aftermath is most common. It should be suspected in cases of sudden collapse or uncontrollable bleeding. Maternal and fetal/neonatal mortality and morbidity are high.

Acute Inversion of the Uterus

This is a rare but potentially life-threatening complication of the third stage of labour.

Classification of inversion

Inversion can be classified according to severity as follows:

- *First-degree*. The fundus reaches the internal os.
- *Second-degree*. The body or corpus of the uterus is inverted to the internal os.
- *Third-degree*. The uterus, cervix and vagina are inverted and are visible.

Causes

Causes of acute inversion are associated with uterine atony and cervical dilatation, and include:

- mismanagement in the third stage of labour, involving excessive cord traction to manage the delivery of the placenta actively
- combining fundal pressure and cord traction to deliver the placenta
- use of fundal pressure while the uterus is atonic, to deliver the placenta
- pathologically adherent placenta
- spontaneous occurrence of unknown cause
- short umbilical cord
- sudden emptying of a distended uterus.

Warning signs and diagnosis

- There is haemorrhage, the amount of which will depend on the degree of placental adherence to the uterine wall.
- There is shock and sudden onset of pain.
- The fundus will not be palpable on abdominal examination.
- A mass may be felt on vaginal examination.
- The fundus may be visible at the introitus.

Management

See Box 23.7.

Basic Life-support Measures

Before starting any resuscitation, assessment of any risk to the carer and the patient is needed. The basic principles of life support are:

A — airway

B — breathing

C — circulation.

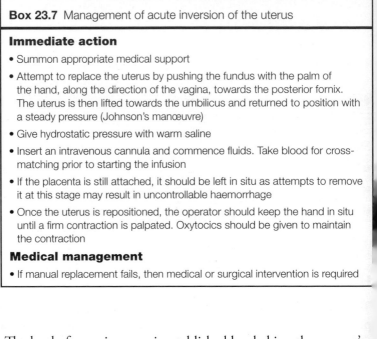

Box 23.7 Management of acute inversion of the uterus

Immediate action

- Summon appropriate medical support
- Attempt to replace the uterus by pushing the fundus with the palm of the hand, along the direction of the vagina, towards the posterior fornix. The uterus is then lifted towards the umbilicus and returned to position with a steady pressure (Johnson's manœuvre)
- Give hydrostatic pressure with warm saline
- Insert an intravenous cannula and commence fluids. Take blood for cross-matching prior to starting the infusion
- If the placenta is still attached, it should be left in situ as attempts to remove it at this stage may result in uncontrollable haemorrhage
- Once the uterus is repositioned, the operator should keep the hand in situ until a firm contraction is palpated. Oxytocics should be given to maintain the contraction

Medical management

- If manual replacement fails, then medical or surgical intervention is required

- The level of consciousness is established by shaking the woman's shoulders and enquiring whether she can hear.
- Summon assistance.
- Lie the woman flat; if she is pregnant, position with a left lateral tilt to prevent aortocaval compression.
- Airway check — remove obstructions, tilt head back and lift chin upwards.
- Breathing — look, listen and feel for up to 10 seconds.
- Circulation — check carotid pulse; if no pulse felt, commence cardiopulmonary resuscitation (CPR).
- CPR

  Thirty chest compressions (rate of 100/min at a depth of 4–5 cm)

Two mouth-to-mouth ventilations (insert airway if one available, rate of 10 breaths/min)

Maintain ratio 30:2 (note — ratios may change in light of evidence; check resuscitation council guidelines).

Shock

Shock can be classified as follows:

- *hypovolaemic* — the result of a reduction in intravascular volume
- *cardiogenic* — impaired ability of the heart to pump blood
- *distributive* — an abnormality in the vascular system that produces a maldistribution of the circulatory system; this includes septic and anaphylactic shock.

Hypovolaemic shock

This is caused by any loss of circulating fluid volume that is not compensated for, as in haemorrhage, but may also occur when there is severe vomiting. The body reacts to the loss of circulating fluid in stages, as described below.

Initial stage

The reduction in fluid or blood decreases the venous return to the heart. The ventricles of the heart are inadequately filled, causing a reduction in stroke volume and cardiac output. As cardiac output and venous return fall, the blood pressure is reduced. The drop in blood pressure decreases the supply of oxygen to the tissues and cell function is affected.

Compensatory stage

The drop in cardiac output produces a response from the sympathetic nervous system through the activation of receptors in the aorta and carotid arteries. Blood is redistributed to the vital organs. Vessels in the gastrointestinal tract, kidneys, skin and lungs constrict. This response is seen as the skin becomes pale and cool. Peristalsis slows, urinary output is reduced and exchange of gas in the lungs is impaired as blood flow diminishes. The heart rate increases in an attempt to improve cardiac output and blood pressure. The pupils of the eyes dilate. The sweat glands are stimulated and the skin becomes moist and clammy. Adrenaline (epinephrine) is released from the adrenal medulla and aldosterone from the adrenal cortex. Antidiuretic hormone (ADH) is secreted from the posterior lobe of the pituitary. Their combined effect is to cause vasoconstriction, an increased cardiac output and a decrease in urinary output. Venous return to the heart will increase but, unless the fluid loss is replaced, will not be sustained.

Progressive stage

This stage leads to multisystem failure. Compensatory mechanisms begin to fail, with vital organs lacking adequate perfusion. Volume depletion causes a further fall in blood pressure and cardiac output. The coronary arteries suffer lack of supply. Peripheral circulation is poor, with weak or absent pulses.

Final, irreversible stage of shock

Multisystem failure and cell destruction are irreparable. Death ensues

Management

The priorities are listed in Box 23.8.

Septic shock

The most common form of sepsis in childbearing in the UK i reported to be that caused by beta-haemolytic *Streptococcus pyogene* (Lancefield group A). This is a Gram-positive organism, respondin to intravenous antibiotics, specifically those that are penicillin-base In the general population, infections from Gram-negative organism

---

Box 23.8 Priorities in the management of hypovolaemic shock

- *Call for help*

  Shock is a progressive condition and delay in correcting hypovolaemia can ultimately lead to maternal death

- *Maintain the airway*

  If the mother is severely collapsed, she should be turned on to her side and 40% oxygen administered at a rate of 4–6 L per minute

  If she is unconscious, an airway should be inserted

- *Replace fluids*

  Two wide-bore intravenous cannulae should be inserted to enable fluids and drugs to be administered swiftly

  Blood should be taken for cross-matching prior to commencing intravenous fluids

  A crystalloid solution such as Hartmann's or Ringer's lactate is given until the woman's condition has improved

  To maintain intravascular volume, colloids (e.g. Gelofusine, Haemaccel) are recommended

- *Ensure warmth*

  It is important to keep the woman warm, but not overwarmed or warmed too quickly, as this will cause peripheral vasodilatation and result in hypotension

- *Arrest haemorrhage*

  The source of the bleeding needs to be identified and stopped

- *Monitor vital signs*

---

uch as *E. coli, Proteus* or *Pseudomonas pyocyaneus* are predominant; hese are common pathogens in the female genital tract.

The placental site is the main point of entry for an infection ssociated with pregnancy and childbirth. This may occur following rolonged rupture of fetal membranes, obstetric trauma or septic bortion, or in the presence of retained placental tissue. Endotoxins resent in the organisms release components that trigger the body's mmune response, culminating in multiple organ failure.

Clinical presentation

The mother may present with a sudden onset of tachycardia, pyrexia, rigors and tachypnoea. She may also exhibit a change in her mental state. Signs of shock, including hypotension, develop as the condition takes hold. Haemorrhage may develop as a result of DIC.

Management

This is based on preventing further deterioration by restoring circulatory volume and eradication of the infection (Box 23.9).

Box 23.9 Management of septic shock

- Replacement of fluid volume will restore perfusion of the vital organs
- Satisfactory oxygenation is also needed
- Rigorous treatment with intravenous antibiotics, after blood cultures have been taken, is necessary to halt the illness
- Retained products of conception can be detected on ultrasound, and these can then be removed

---

Section 4

Puerperium

Chapter 24

Physiology and Care
in the Puerperium

Defining the Puerperium and
the Postnatal Period

Following the birth of the baby and expulsion of the placenta, the mother enters a period of physical and psychological recuperation. From a medical and physiological viewpoint this period, called the *puerperium*, starts immediately after delivery of the placenta and membranes and continues for 6 weeks.

Midwives and the Management of
Postpartum Care

The *postnatal period* means the period after the end of labour during which the attendance of a midwife upon the woman and baby is required, being not less than 10 days and for a longer period if the midwife considers it necessary (Nursing and Midwifery Council (NMC) Rule).

Physiological Observations

The uterus and vaginal fluid loss

After the birth, oxytocin is secreted from the posterior pituitary gland to act upon the uterine muscle and assist separation of the placenta. Following expulsion of the placenta, the uterine cavity collapses inwards; the now-opposed walls of the uterus compress the newly exposed placental site and effectively seal the exposed ends of the major blood vessels. The muscle layers of the myometrium are said to simulate the action of ligatures that compress the large sinuses of the blood vessels exposed by placental separation. These occlude the exposed ends of the large blood vessels and contribute further to reducing blood loss. In addition, vasoconstriction in the overall blood supply to the uterus results in the tissues being denied their previous blood supply; deoxygenation and a state of ischaemia arise. Through the process of autolysis, autodigestion of the ischaemic muscle fibres by proteolytic enzymes occurs, resulting in an overall reduction in their size. There is phagocytic action of polymorphs and macrophages in the blood and lymphatic systems upon the waste products of autolysis, which are then excreted via the renal system in the urine. Coagulation takes place through platelet aggregation and the release of thromboplastin and fibrin.

Renewal of the uterine lining and renewal of the placental site involve different physiological processes. What remains of the inner surface of the uterine lining, apart from the placental site, regenerates rapidly to produce a covering of epithelium. Partial coverage is said to have occurred within 7–10 days of the birth; total coverage is complete by the 21st day.

Once the placenta is expelled, the circulating levels of oestrogen, progesterone, human chorionic gonadotrophin and human placental lactogen are reduced. This leads to further physiological changes in muscle and connective tissues, as well as having a major influence on the secretion of prolactin from the anterior pituitary gland.

Once empty, the uterus can be likened to an empty sac, although it retains its muscular structure. It is therefore important to remember that the uterus, although at this point markedly reduced in size, still retains the potential to be a much larger cavity. This underpins the requirement to undertake immediate and then regular observations of fundal height and the degree of uterine contraction in the first few hours after the birth. Abdominal palpation of the uterus is usually performed soon after placental expulsion to ensure that the physiological processes described above are beginning to take place. On abdominal palpation, the fundus of the uterus should be located centrally, at the same level or slightly below the umbilicus, and should be in a state of contraction, feeling firm under the palpating hand. The woman may experience some uterine or abdominal discomfort, especially where uterotonic drugs have been administered to augment the physiological process.

The physiological process of the uterus returning to its non-pregnant state is known as *involution*. A well-contracted uterus will gradually reduce in size until it is no longer palpable above the symphysis pubis. The rate at which this occurs and the duration of time taken have been demonstrated to be highly individual. The uterus should not be tender during this process, although the woman may be experiencing afterpains.

The observations obtained by the midwife about the state of involution of the uterus should be placed into context alongside the colour, amount and duration of the woman's vaginal fluid loss and her general state of health at that time.

Postpartum vaginal fluid loss (lochia)

Blood products constitute the major part of the vaginal loss immediately after the birth of the baby and expulsion of the placenta. As involution progresses, the vaginal loss reflects this and changes from predominantly fresh blood loss to one that contains stale blood products, lanugo, vernix and other debris from the unwanted products of the conception. This loss varies from woman to woman, being lighter or darker in colour, but for any woman the shade and density tend to be consistent.

Assessment of vaginal blood loss

The mother should be asked about the current vaginal loss:

- whether this is more or less than previously
- whether it is lighter or darker than previously
- whether she herself has any concerns about it.

It is of particular importance to record any clots passed and when these occurred.

Perineal pain

Regardless of whether the birth resulted in actual perineal trauma, women are likely to feel bruised around the vaginal and perineal tissues for the first few days after the birth. Women who have undergone any degree of actual perineal injury will experience pain for several days until healing takes place.

All women should be asked about discomfort in the perineal area, regardless of whether there is a record of actual perineal trauma. Advice from the midwife may be welcomed, and clear information and reassurance are helpful where women have poor understanding of what happened and are anxious about urinary, bowel or sexual function in the future.

Where women appear to have no discomfort or anxieties about their perineum, it is not essential for the midwife to examine this area. For the majority of women, the perineal wound gradually becomes less painful and healing should occur by 7–10 days after the birth.

Advice on what might help perineal pain

- Appropriate information and advice are important components in pain management and should take into account women's

individual experiences of their pain and their preferences for
its relief.

- Women may find soaking in a bath of great comfort to them
  regardless of any additive, and relief may be derived from the use
  of a bidet or cool water poured over the area that is tender.

- There is increasing interest in complementary therapeutic
  preparations and more and more research is being undertaken into
  their use. Essential oils such as lavender and tea tree have been
  found to be beneficial when used as bath additives or topical
  compresses. Homeopathic remedies such as arnica, calendula and
  Bellis perennis can be applied topically or taken orally.

Vital signs and general health

Observations of pulse, temperature, respiration and blood pressure

Making a note of the pulse rate is probably one of the least invasive
and most cost-effective observations a midwife can undertake. While
monitoring the pulse rate, particularly if this is done for a full
minute, the midwife can also observe a number of related signs of
well-being, as well as just listening to what the woman is saying:

- respiratory rate
- overall body temperature
- any untoward body odour
- skin condition
- overall colour and complexion.

It is not necessary to undertake observations of temperature routinely
for women who appear to be physically well and who do not complain of any symptoms that could be associated with an infection.
However, where the woman complains of feeling unwell with flu-like
symptoms, or there are signs of possible infection or information

that might be associated with a potential environment for infection, the midwife should undertake and record the temperature.

Blood pressure

Following the birth of the baby, a baseline recording of the woman's blood pressure will be made. In the absence of any previous history of morbidity associated with hypertension, it is usual for the blood pressure to return to a normal range within 24 hours of the birth. Routinely undertaking observations of blood pressure without a clinical reason is therefore not required.

Circulation

The body has to reabsorb a quantity of excess fluid following the birth. For the majority of women this results in passing large quantities of urine, particularly in the first day, as diuresis is increased. Women may also experience oedema of their ankles and feet and this swelling may be greater than that experienced in pregnancy. These are variations of normal physiological processes and should resolve within the puerperal time scale as the woman's activity levels also increase. Advice should be related to:

- taking reasonable exercise
- avoiding long periods of standing
- elevating the feet and legs when sitting, where possible.

Swollen ankles should be bilateral and not accompanied by pain; the midwife should note particularly if this is present in one calf only, as it could indicate pathology associated with a deep vein thrombosis.

Skin and nutrition

Women who have suffered from urticaria of pregnancy or cholestasis of the liver should experience relief once the pregnancy is over. The pace of life once the baby is born might lead to women having reduced fluid intake than formerly or to taking a different diet. This in turn might affect their skin and overall physiological state. Women should be encouraged to maintain a balanced fluid intake and to eat a diet that has a greater proportion of fresh food in it.

Urine and bowel function

Women need reassurance that, in the first few days after the birth, minor disorders of urinary and bowel function are common. These may be associated with retention or incontinence of urine or constipation, or both. The skill of midwifery care is to try to explore the possible cause of this and to decide whether it will resolve spontaneously or requires further investigation.

Exercise and healthy activity versus rest, relaxation and sleep

Within the current national policy for health promotion there is an emphasis on increasing the understanding in the general population about the value of different forms of exercise and health. Exploring each person's level of activity will encourage advice in relation to appropriate exercise and, by association, nutritional intake and rest or relaxation and sleep. Undertaking regular pelvic floor exercises is of benefit to women's long-term health.

Afterpains

Management of afterpains is by an appropriate analgesic; where possible, this should be taken prior to breastfeeding, as it is the production of oxytocin in relation to the let-down response that initiates the contraction in the uterus and causes pain. It is helpful to explain the cause of afterpains to women and to inform them that they might experience a heavier vaginal loss at this time, even to the extent of passing clots. Pain in the uterus that is constant or present on abdominal palpation is unlikely to be associated with afterpains and further enquiry should be made into this. Women might also confuse afterpains with flatus pain, especially after an operative birth or where they are constipated. Relief of the cause is likely to relieve the symptoms.

Future Health, Future Fertility

Midwives need to be aware of a range of different needs with regard to women's sexuality and should be able to offer sensitive and appropriate advice on contraception where this is needed.

Weighing up the 'evidence'

The midwife should have gained a considerable amount of information during her contact with mother and baby. The wide range of normality and the individuality within this spectrum can make it difficult to decide whether an observation is related to morbidity. It is more likely to be a relationship between several observations that causes concern; where these appear to be more strongly related to abnormality than to normality, the midwife has a responsibility to make an appropriate referral to a medical practitioner or other health care professional.

Chapter 25

Physical Problems and Complications in the Puerperium

The Need for Women-Centred and Women-Led Postpartum Care

The context of postpartum care within the woman's social and ethnic environment should take into account women's individual perceptions and experiences surrounding the pregnancy and the birth event. Where the birth involves obstetric or medical complications, a woman's postpartum care is likely to differ from that of women whose pregnancy and labour are considered straightforward; the role of the midwife in these cases is:

- to identify whether a potentially pathological condition exists
- if so, to refer the woman for appropriate investigations and care.

Immediate Untoward Events for the Mother Following the Birth of the Baby

Postpartum haemorrhage

- *Immediate (primary) postpartum haemorrhage (PPH)*. This is the most immediate and potentially life-threatening event occurring at the point, or within 24 hours, of delivery of the placenta and membranes. It presents as a sudden and excessive vaginal blood loss of 500 ml or more. (See ch. 19 for management.)

- *Secondary or delayed PPH*. This is where there is excessive or prolonged vaginal loss from 24 hours after delivery of the placenta and for up to 6 weeks postpartum. Unlike primary PPH, which includes a specified volume of blood loss as part of its definition, there is no such volume defined for secondary PPH.

Regardless of the timing of any haemorrhage, it is most frequently the placental site that is the source. Alternatively, a cervical or deep vaginal wall tear or trauma to the perineum might be the cause in women who have recently given birth. Retained placental fragments or other products of conception are likely to inhibit the process of involution, or reopen the placental wound. The diagnosis is likely to be determined by the woman's condition and pattern of events and is also often complicated by the presence of infection (see Box 25.1).

Maternal collapse within 24 hours of the birth without overt bleeding

Consider:

- inversion of the uterus
- amniotic fluid embolism
- cerebrovascular accident.

> **Box 25.1** Secondary PPH
>
> **Signs of secondary PPH**
> - Lochial loss is heavier than normal
> - Lochia returns to a bright red loss and may be offensive
> - Subinvolution of the uterus
> - Pyrexia and tachycardia
> - Haematoma formation
>
> **Treatment**
> - Call a doctor
> - Reassure the woman and her support person(s)
> - Rub up a contraction by massaging the uterus if it is still palpable
> - Express any clots
> - Encourage the mother to empty her bladder
> - Give an uterotonic drug, such as ergometrine maleate, by the intravenous or intramuscular route
> - Keep all pads and linen to assess the volume of blood lost
> - Antibiotics may be prescribed
> - If retained products of conception are seen on an ultrasound scan, it may be appropriate to transfer the woman to hospital and prepare her for theatre

Postpartum Complications and Identifying Deviations from the Normal

Following the birth of their baby, women recount feelings that are, at one level, elation that they have experienced the birth and survived and, at another, the reality of pain or discomfort from a number of unwelcome changes as their bodies recover from pregnancy and labour. The midwife needs to establish whether there are any signs of possible morbidity and determine whether these might indicate the need for referral. Figure 25.1 suggests a model for linking together key observations that suggest potential risk of, or actual, morbidity.

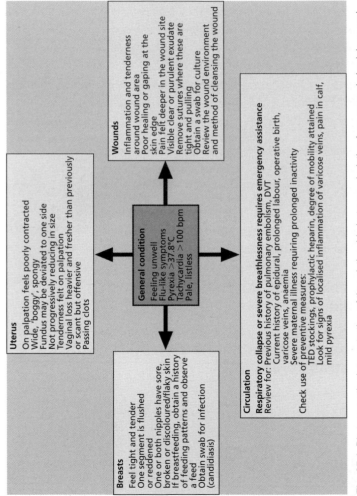

Uterus
On palpation feels poorly contracted
Wide, 'boggy', spongy
Fundus may be deviated to one side
Not progressively reducing in size
Tenderness felt on palpation
Vaginal loss heavier and fresher than previously
or scant but offensive
Passing clots

Wounds
Inflammation and tenderness
around wound area
Poor healing or gaping at the
skin edge
Pain felt deeper in the wound site
Visible clear or purulent exudate
Remove sutures where these are
tight and pulling
Obtain a swab for culture
Review the wound environment
and method of cleansing the wound

General condition
Feeling unwell
Flu-like symptoms
Pyrexia >37.8°C
Tachycardia >100 bpm
Pale, listless

Breasts
Feel tight and tender
One segment is flushed
or reddened
One or both nipples have sore,
broken or discoloured/flaky skin
If breastfeeding, obtain a history
of feeding patterns and observe
a feed
Obtain swab for infection
(candidiasis)

Circulation
Respiratory collapse or severe breathlessness requires emergency assistance
Review for: Previous history of pulmonary embolism, DVT
Current history of epidural, prolonged labour, operative birth,
varicose veins, anaemia
Severe maternal illness requiring prolonged inactivity
Check use of preventive measures:
TED stockings, prophylactic heparin, degree of mobility attained
Look for signs of localised inflammation of varicose veins, pain in calf,
mild pyrexia

Fig. 25.1 Diagrammatic demonstration of the relationship between deviation from normal physiology and potential morbidity.

The central point, as with any personal contact, is the midwife's initial review of the woman's appearance, psychological state and vital signs:

■ A rise in temperature above 37.8°C is usually considered to be of clinical significance. A mildly raised temperature may be related to normal physiological hormonal responses: for example, the increasing production of breast milk.

■ A weak and rapid pulse rate in a woman who is in a state of collapse with signs of shock and a low blood pressure, but no evidence of vaginal haemorrhage, may indicate the formation of a haematoma. A rapid pulse rate in an otherwise well woman might suggest that she is anaemic but could also indicate increased thyroid or other dysfunctional hormonal activity.

■ The midwife needs to be alert to any possible relationship between the observations overall and their potential cause, keeping common illnesses in mind — for example, the woman may have a common cold.

The uterus and vaginal loss following vaginal birth

The midwife will undertake assessment of uterine involution where the woman:

◀ is feeling generally unwell

◀ has abdominal pain

◀ has a vaginal loss that is markedly brighter red or heavier than previously

◀ is passing clots

◀ reports her vaginal loss to be offensive.

Where palpation of the uterus identifies deviation to one side, this might be the result of a full bladder. Where the woman had emptied her bladder prior to palpation, the presence of urinary retention must be considered. Catheterisation of the bladder in these circumstances is indicated for two reasons: to remove any obstacle that is preventing the process of involution taking place and to provide relief to the bladder itself. If deviation is not the result of a full bladder, further investigations need to be undertaken to determine the cause.

Morbidity might be suspected where the uterus:

- fails to follow the expected progressive reduction in size
- feels wide or 'boggy' on palpation
- is less well contracted than expected.

This might be described as subinvolution of the uterus, which can indicate postpartum infection, or the presence of retained products of the placenta or membranes, or both.

Treatment involves:

- antibiotics
- oxytocic drugs
- hormonal preparations

  or

- evacuation of the uterus (ERPC).

Vulnerability to infection: potential causes and prevention

Causes include:

- poor immunity
- pre-existing resistance to the invading organism
- virulence of the organism
- presence of hospital 'superbugs'.

The bacteria responsible for the majority of puerperal infection belong to the streptococcal or staphylococcal species.

- The *Streptococcus* bacterium may be haemolytic or non-haemolytic, aerobic or anaerobic; the most common species associated with puerperal sepsis is the beta-haemolytic *S. pyogenes* (Lancefield group A).

■ The *Staphylococcus* bacterium has a grape-like structure; the most important species are *Staph. aureus* or *pyogenes*. Staphylococci are the most frequent cause of wound infections; where these bacteria are coagulase-positive they form clots on the plasma, which can lead to more widespread systemic morbidity. There is additional concern about their resistance to antibiotics and about subsequent management to control spread of the infection.

The uterus and vaginal loss following operative delivery

It may be some hours after the operation before the woman sits up or moves about. Blood and debris will have been slowly released from the uterus during this time and, when the woman begins to move, this will be expelled though the vagina and may appear as a substantial fresh-looking red loss. Following this initial event, it is usual for the amount of vaginal loss to lessen and for further fresh loss to be minimal. All this can be observed without actually palpating the uterus, which is likely to be very painful in the first few days after the operation. For women who have undergone an operative delivery, abdominal palpation to assess uterine involution can be undertaken by the midwife once 3 or 4 days have elapsed, where this appears to be clinically appropriate. By this time the uterus and the area around it should no longer be painful on palpation.

Where clinically indicated — for example, where vaginal bleeding is heavier than expected — the uterine fundus can be gently palpated. If the uterus is not well contracted, then medical intervention is needed. The following may be required:

■ uterotonics (e.g. intravenous infusion of oxytocin, intravenous ergometrine, intramuscular syntometrine)

■ blood tests for clotting factors

■ exploration of the uterine cavity.

Wound problems

Perineal problems

Severe perineal pain might be the result of:

- the analgesia no longer being effective
- increased oedema in the surrounding tissues
- haematoma formation.

The blood contained within a haematoma can exceed 1000 ml and may significantly affect the overall state of the woman, who can present with signs of acute shock. Treatment is by evacuation of the haematoma and resuturing of the perineal wound, usually under a general anaesthetic.

Oedema can cause the stitches to feel excessively tight. Local application of cold packs can bring relief, as these reduce the immediate oedema. The use of oral analgesia, as well as complementary medicines such as arnica and witch hazel, is said to have a beneficial effect.

Pain in the perineal area that occurs at a later stage or pain that reoccurs might be associated with an infection. The skin edges are likely to have a moist, puffy and dull appearance; there may also be an offensive odour and evidence of pus in the wound.

- A swab should be obtained for microorganism culture and referral should be made to a GP.

- Antibiotics might be commenced immediately when there is specific information about any infective agent

- Advice should be given about cleaning the area, using cotton underwear, avoiding tights and trousers and changing sanitary pads frequently.

- Women should also be advised to avoid using perfumed bath additives or talcum powder.

If the perineal area fails to heal or continues to cause pain by the time the initial healing process should have begun, resuturing or refashioning might be advised. Women should be pain-free and able to resume sexual intercourse without pain by 6 weeks after the birth; some discomfort might still be present, however, depending on the degree of trauma experienced.

Caesarean section wounds

It is now common practice for women undergoing an operative birth to be given prophylactic antibiotics at the time of the surgery. This has been demonstrated to reduce the incidence of subsequent wound infection and endometritis significantly. It is usual for the wound dressing to be removed after the first 24 hours, as this also aids healing and reduces infection.

A wound that is hot, tender and inflamed and is accompanied by a pyrexia is highly suggestive of an infection. Where this is observed:

- a swab should be obtained for microorganism culture
- medical advice should be sought.

Haematoma and abscesses can also form underneath the wound, and women may identify increased pain around the wound where these are present. Rarely, a wound may need to be probed to reduce the pressure and to allow infected material to drain, reducing the likelihood of the formation of an abscess.

Circulation problems

Pulmonary embolism remains a major cause of maternal deaths in the UK. Women at higher risk include those with the factors listed in Box 25.2.

Women who undergo surgery and have these pre-existing factors should be:

- provided with TED stockings during, or as soon as possible after, the birth
- prescribed prophylactic heparin until they attain normal mobility.

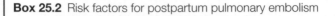

> **Box 25.2** Risk factors for postpartum pulmonary embolism
>
> - *Previous* history of pulmonary embolism
> - Deep vein thrombosis
> - Varicose veins
> - Epidural anaesthetic
> - Anaemia
> - Prolonged labour
> - Operative birth

Clinical signs that women might report include the conditions listed below (the most common given first, progressing to the most serious):

■ Signs of circulatory problems related to varicose veins usually include localised inflammation or tenderness around the varicose vein, sometimes accompanied by a mild pyrexia. This is superficial thrombophlebitis, which is usually resolved by applying support to the affected area and administering anti-inflammatory drugs, where these do not conflict with other medication being taken or with breastfeeding.

■ Unilateral oedema of an ankle or calf, accompanied by stiffness or pain and a positive Homan's sign, might indicate a deep vein thrombosis that has the potential to cause a pulmonary embolism. Urgent medical referral must be made to confirm the diagnosis and commence anticoagulant or other appropriate therapy.

■ The most serious outcome is the development of a pulmonary embolism. The first sign might be the sudden onset of breathlessness, which may not be associated with any obvious clinical sign of a blood clot. Women with this condition are likely to become seriously ill and could suffer respiratory collapse with very little prior warning.

Some degree of oedema of the lower legs, ankles and feet can be viewed as being within normal limits where it is not accompanied by calf pain (especially unilaterally), pyrexia or raised blood pressure.

Hypertension

Women who have had previous episodes of hypertension in pregnancy may continue to demonstrate this postpartum. Mothers with clinical signs of pregnancy-induced hypertension still run the risk of developing eclampsia in the hours and days following the birth, although this is a relatively rare outcome in the normal population. Some degree of blood pressure monitoring should be continued for women who suffered hypertension antenatally, and postpartum management should proceed on an individual basis. For these women the medical advice should cover:

■ optimal systolic and diastolic levels
■ instructions for treatment with antihypertensive drugs if the blood pressure exceeds these levels.

Occasionally, women can develop postnatal pre-eclampsia without associated antenatal problems. Therefore, if a postpartum woman presents with signs associated with pre-eclampsia, the midwife should:

■ undertake observations of the blood pressure and urine
■ obtain medical advice.

For women with essential hypertension, management of their overall medical condition will be reviewed postpartum by their usual caregivers. Clinical observation of blood pressure for a period after the birth is advisable so that information is available upon which to base future management.

Headache

Concern about postpartum morbidity should centre around the history of:

■ the severity, duration and frequency of the headaches
■ the medication being taken to alleviate them
  how effective this is.

If an epidural anaesthetic was administered for the birth (or at any time postpartum), medical advice should be sought and the anaesthetist who sited the epidural might need to be contacted. Headaches from a dural tap typically arise once the woman has become mobile after the birth; these headaches are at their most severe when the woman is standing, lessening when she lies down. They are often accompanied by:

■ neck stiffness

■ vomiting

■ visual disturbances.

These headaches are very debilitating and are best managed by stopping the leakage of cerebrospinal fluid (CSF) by the insertion of 10–20 ml of blood into the epidural space; this should resolve the clinical symptoms. If women have returned home after the birth, they would need to return to the hospital to have this procedure carried out.

Headaches might also be precursors of psychological distress and it is important for other issues related to the birth event to be explored.

Backache

Many women experience pain or discomfort from backache in pregnancy as a result of separation or diastasis of the abdominal muscle (rectus abdominis diastasis, RAD). It might be sufficient to:

■ give advice on skeletal support to attain a good posture when feeding and lifting

■ suggest a feasible personal exercise plan and how to achieve this

■ discuss a range of relaxation techniques.

Where backache is causing pain that affects the woman's activities of daily living, referral can be made to local physiotherapy services. If the symphysis pubis has been affected in pregnancy, this should resolve in the weeks after the baby is born, with relief being gained from no longer having to carry the weight of the fetus and gradual resolution of the problem as hormonal levels return to the non-pregnant state.

Urinary problems

Although acute retention of urine following the birth is not common, it is important to monitor urinary function and to ask women about this and the sensations associated with normal bladder control. A short period of poor bladder control may be present for a few days after the birth, but this should resolve within a week. Epidural or spinal anaesthetic can have an effect on the neurological sensors that control urine release and flow; this might cause acute retention. Women with perineal trauma may have difficulty in deciding whether they have normal urinary control; retention of urine might be detected by the midwife as a result of abdominal palpation of the uterus. Abdominal tenderness in association with other urinary symptoms — for example, poor output, dysuria or offensive urine, and a pyrexia or general flu-like symptoms — might indicate a urinary tract infection. Very rarely, urinary incontinence might be a result of a urethral fistula following complications from the labour or birth.

The main complication of any form of urine retention is that the uterus might be prevented from effective contraction, which leads to increased vaginal blood loss. There is also increased potential for the development of a urine infection.

It is not uncommon for some women to have a small degree of leakage or retention of urine within the first 2 or 3 days after the birth while the tissues are recovering, but this should resolve with the practice of postnatal exercise and healing of any localised trauma. Referral to a physiotherapist might be appropriate. Specific enquiry about these issues should be made when women attend for their 6-week postnatal examination.

Bowels and constipation

Any disruption to a woman's normal bowel pattern that occurred during pregnancy should resolve within days of the birth, taking into consideration the recovery time required if perineal trauma is present.

Women who have haemorrhoids or difficulty with constipation should be given:

■ advice on following a diet high in fibre and fluids, preferably water

■ instructions on the use of appropriate laxatives to soften the stools

■ topical applications to reduce the oedema and pain.

It is also a matter of concern if women experience a loss of bowel control or faecal incontinence. It is important to determine the nature of the incontinence and distinguish it from an episode of diarrhoea. Women who identify any change to their pre-pregnant bowel pattern by the end of the puerperal period should have this reviewed.

Anaemia

The impact of the events of the labour and birth may leave many women looking pale and tired for a day or so afterwards.

■ Where it is evident that a larger than normal blood loss has occurred, red blood cell volume and Hb can be assessed and appropriate treatment provided to reduce the effects of anaemia.

■ Where the Hb level is less than 9.0 g/dl, a blood transfusion might be appropriate; oral iron and appropriate dietary advice are advocated when women decline a blood transfusion or when the Hb level is less than 11.0 g/dl.

■ If Hb values have not been assessed, clinical symptoms such as lethargy, tachycardia, breathlessness or pale mucous membranes may suggest anaemia; a blood profile should then be considered.

Breast problems

Regardless of whether women are breastfeeding, they may experience tightening and enlargement of their breasts towards the 3rd or 4th day, as hormonal influences encourage the breasts to produce milk.

■ For women who are breastfeeding, the general advice is to feed the baby and avoid excessive handling of the breasts. Simple analgesics may be required to reduce discomfort.

- For women who are not breastfeeding, the advice is to ensure that the breasts are well supported but that the support is not too constrictive; again, taking regular analgesia for 24–48 hours should reduce any discomfort. Heat and cold applied to the breasts via a shower or a soaking in the bath may temporarily relieve acute discomfort.

It is important to gauge whether the duration of the engorgement is excessive and whether there are any other signs of a possible infection, such as overt tenderness or inflammation, pyrexia or flu-like symptoms. If infective mastitis is suspected, then antibiotics should be prescribed. If a woman is breastfeeding, it is important that this continues or that the breast milk is expressed.

Chapter 26

The Psychology and Psychopathology of Pregnancy and Childbirth

The Transition to Motherhood

Postnatally, parents may find coping with the demands of a new baby — infant feeding, financial constraints and adjusting to changes in roles and relationships — particularly testing emotionally. Disturbed sleep is inevitable with a new baby. Soreness and pain from perineal trauma will affect libido; so too will the feelings of exhaustion, despair and unhappiness that may be associated with the round-the-clock demands of caring for a new baby. Postnatal care from midwives plays a significant role in the positive adjustment to motherhood, as it assists in the acquisition of confident and well-informed parenting skills.

Normal Emotional Changes During Pregnancy, Labour and the Puerperium

It is perfectly normal for women to have periods of self-doubt and crises of confidence. The fluctuations between positive and negative emotions may include the emotions described below.

First trimester

- Pleasure, excitement, elation.
- Dismay, disappointment.
- Ambivalence.
- Emotional lability.
- Increased femininity.

Second trimester

- A feeling of well-being.
- A sense of increased attachment to the fetus.
- Stress and anxiety about antenatal screening and diagnostic tests.
- Increased demand for knowledge and information.
- Feelings relating to the need for increasing detachment from work commitments.

Third trimester

- Loss of or increased libido.
- Altered body image.
- Psychological effects from physiological discomforts such as backache and heartburn.
- Anxiety about labour (e.g. pain).
- Anxiety about fetal abnormality.
- Increased vulnerability to major life events, such as a precarious financial status, moving house or lack of a supportive partner.

Antenatal depression

Midwives must be knowledgeable and confident enough in their skills to differentiate between distress and depression. It is crucial to recognise that the majority of cases of emotional distress in the first

> **Box 26.1** Key points for practice
>
> - Prevalence of mental illness at conception is the same as the general population
> - Antenatal depression will improve over the course of the pregnancy
> - Prevalence of antenatal depression has not been accurately determined
> - Incidence of mild morbidity in the first trimester increases, but then decreases in the second and third trimesters
> - An elevated anxiety state is often a reaction to events and is therefore understandable, but the woman will need careful assessment and support

trimester of pregnancy are normal and do not pose a risk to a woman's mental health following birth. However, the midwife should be alert to the importance of social support. Box 26.1 lists key points for practice relating to antenatal emotional changes.

Emotional changes during labour

For many women, labour will be greeted with varied emotional responses ranging from:

- great excitement and anticipation to utter dread
- fear of the unknown
- fear of technology, intervention and hospitalisation
- tension, fear and anxiety about pain and the ability to exercise control during labour
- concerns about the well-being of the baby and ability of the partner to cope
- a fear of lack of privacy or utter embarrassment.

Having choice in pregnancy and childbirth, along with a sense of being in control, may lead to a more satisfying birth experience. Midwives should be aware that:

- Women's perception of labour and childbirth are crucial to their emotional adjustment.

- Interventions per se do not equate to postnatal psychological sequelae, provided that the woman feels that the right decision was made.

- Adequate information decreases the likelihood of psychological morbidity.

- Being involved in the discussion of what happened is not enough for women, but having some say in the outcome may be viewed more positively.

- Being unable to be assertive in interactions with health care professionals is more likely to result in lowering of women's mood.

- Emergency caesarean section is linked with more negative feelings about the baby.

- A woman's view of her baby is linked with her prior sense of control.

During labour, midwives must consider the factors that induce stress, and these should be prevented, or at least minimised, as the woman's long-term emotional health may be severely compromised by an adverse birth experience.

The puerperium

Normal emotional changes in the puerperium are eclectic and complex and may encompass the following:

- Contradictory and conflicting feelings may range from satisfaction, joy and elation to exhaustion, helplessness, discontentment and disappointment as the early weeks seem to be dominated by the novelty and unpredictability of the new baby.

- Relief — 'thank goodness that's over' — may be experienced by many women immediately following birth; sometimes the woman conveys a cool detachment from events, especially if labour was protracted, complicated and difficult.

- Some may experience a closeness to partner or baby and those who intend to breastfeed may want to initiate skin-to-skin contact and feed straight away. They may be very attentive towards the baby.

- Equally, women may feel disinterested in their baby.

- There may be fear of the unknown and a sudden realisation of overwhelming responsibility.

- Exhaustion and increased emotionality are normal.

- Some women may still have pain (e.g. perineal, in nipples).

- Increased vulnerability and indecisiveness (e.g. in feeding) are not unusual; neither is loss of libido, disturbed sleep or anxiety.

Postnatal 'blues'

This normal and transient phase is experienced by 50–80%, of women depending on parity. The onset typically occurs between 3 and 4 days postpartum, but may last up to a week or more, though rarely persisting for longer than a few days. The features of this state are mild and transitory and may include a state in which women usually experience labile emotions. The actual aetiology is unclear but hormonal influences seem to be implicated, as the period of increased emotionality appears to coincide with the production of milk in the breasts. Although the condition is self-limiting, occurrence of the postnatal 'blues' illuminates the need for psychosocial support.

Emotional distress associated with traumatic birth events

Over recent years the label 'post-traumatic stress disorder' (PTSD) has emerged in midwifery practice. Many women will eventually overcome the pain, fear and crippling anxiety of labour and childbirth. However, for others, the traumatic events surrounding the

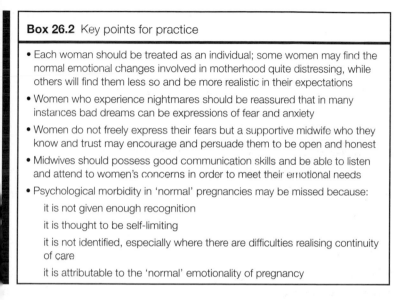

Box 26.2 Key points for practice

- Each woman should be treated as an individual; some women may find the normal emotional changes involved in motherhood quite distressing, while others will find them less so and be more realistic in their expectations

- Women who experience nightmares should be reassured that in many instances bad dreams can be expressions of fear and anxiety

- Women do not freely express their fears but a supportive midwife who they know and trust may encourage and persuade them to be open and honest

- Midwives should possess good communication skills and be able to listen and attend to women's concerns in order to meet their emotional needs

- Psychological morbidity in 'normal' pregnancies may be missed because:

    it is not given enough recognition

    it is thought to be self-limiting

    it is not identified, especially where there are difficulties realising continuity of care

    it is attributable to the 'normal' emotionality of pregnancy

birth experience will remain ingrained in their psyche, and may blight their lives and affect their relationship with their partner and baby. PTSD following childbirth may result in nightmares and 'flashbacks', which could be very distressing and frightening when women are again confronted with real images of labour. Key points for practice relating to emotional distress linked to giving birth are listed in Box 26.2.

Perinatal Psychiatric Disorders

There is a steep rise in the prevalence of psychotic illness and, to a lesser extent, mild to moderate 'postnatal depression' (PND) associated with having children. For women with pre-existing mental health problems, childbirth increases the risk of recurrence. For those with chronic illness such as schizophrenia, pregnancy and childbirth

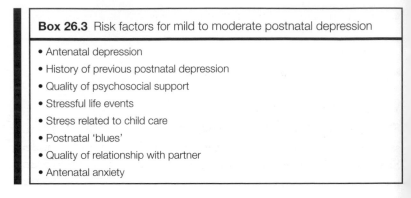

Box 26.3 Risk factors for mild to moderate postnatal depression

- Antenatal depression
- History of previous postnatal depression
- Quality of psychosocial support
- Stressful life events
- Stress related to child care
- Postnatal 'blues'
- Quality of relationship with partner
- Antenatal anxiety

cause even greater concern about their risk of relapse and their ability to care for the baby. Although the risk of a serious depressive illness increases significantly postpartum, difficulties may also emerge during pregnancy.

Mild to moderate postnatal depression

Over 10% of mothers will suffer from a mild to moderate depressive illness for the first time after the birth. Postnatal depression begins within 3 months of the birth but has a later onset than the postnatal 'blues'. The majority of women with identified risk factors (Box 26.3) will not subsequently suffer from postnatal depression. The non-specificity of these risk factors means that they are widely found in the population, but they are helpful for targeting vulnerable groups of women who may need special resources.

Recognition and aetiology

Early signs of postnatal depression may include:

- anxiety and worries about the baby
- inability to cope
- sleep disturbance

- feelings of sadness, inadequacy, worthlessness, loss of appetite, low self-esteem, lowered mood, loss of enjoyment and spontaneity
- feelings of guilt, isolation and failure.

Value of screening tools

The Edinburgh postnatal depression score (EPDS) is a simple 10-item self-completion questionnaire that takes only minutes to complete. Scores for each item range from 0 to 3, according to the woman's mood and responses. The value and limitations of the EPDS are summarised in Box 26.4.

Box 26.4 Value and limitations of the Edinburgh postnatal depression scale

Value

- Useful screening tool
- Acceptable to women
- Takes minutes to complete and score
- Results can be discussed immediately, leading to early identification of problems
- A score of 12+ indicates the likelihood of depression
- Provides women with tangible 'permission' to talk, be listened to and have feelings validated

Limitations

- May lead to misdiagnosis, i.e. false positives and medicalisation of low moods and situational distress
- Depression about depression
- Only predictive not diagnostic
- Is not a magic wand
- Does not and should not replace clinical judgement
- Does not give women opportunity to describe symptoms fully

Care and management and the role of the midwife

Mild to moderate PND is usually self-limiting, and many mothers will recover by about 6 months postpartum. However, 30% of women will remain ill at 1 year and over 10% at 2 years postpartum, with consequences for the cognitive development of the infant. How the mother interacts with her child should be assessed, taking into account cultural influences. Any untoward problems with infant feeding, sleeping and general temperament should alert the midwife and health professionals to the need for psychosocial support. The partner should also be involved in these interactions to help address and alleviate any tensions that may exist within the couple's relationship.

Antidepressants may be used in the treatment of PND but specific psychological treatments are as effective. Psychological and social support may suffice for mild cases. Collaboration with voluntary support agencies (e.g. postnatal support groups) is also valuable.

Motherhood and Serious Mental Illness

Severe depressive illness

Approximately 3–5% of mothers will be affected by a more severe form of depressive illness. It develops in the early postpartum period but later presentations (8–12 weeks) may be missed. Women who are severely depressed may look mentally anguished and ill.

Recognition and aetiology

The actual aetiology is unclear; however, the most powerful predicto appears to be a previous history of depressive illness, either post partum or at other times. It is thought that neuroendocrine factor play a part; particularly precipitous is the role of oestradiol. The onse is insidious and is often in the first 2–6 weeks postpartum. The main characteristics are:

- 'biological syndrome' of sleep disturbance — waking early in the morning; the woman will feel most depressed and her symptoms will be worst at the start of the day
- impaired concentration, disturbed thought processes, indecisiveness and an inability to cope with everyday life
- emotional detachment and profound lowering of mood
- loss of ability to feel pleasure (anhedonia)
- feelings of guilt, incompetence and of being a 'bad' mother
- in approximately one-third of women, distressing intrusive obsessional thoughts and ruminations
- commonly, extreme anxiety and even panic attacks
- impaired appetite and weight loss
- in a small number, a depressive psychosis and morbid, delusional thoughts and hallucinations.

Variations

Phobic anxiety, panic disorders and obsessive compulsive disorders (OCD) might be variations on the theme. OCD may present with unpleasant, intrusive and distressing thoughts. The thoughts often relate to obscenities, dirt or disease, which are incongruent with the woman's true nature. Thoughts may also include harm coming to the baby or a member of the family, excessive cleanliness, disproportionate anxiety about the baby and obsession with personal health and hygiene.

Puerperal psychosis

Puerperal psychosis is regarded as the most severe and dramatic of the psychiatric disturbances to occur in the postpartum period.

Recognition and aetiology

Symptoms are florid, presenting dramatically and very early and tending to change rapidly, altering from day to day during the acute phase of the illness. These typically include changes of mood state, irrational behaviour and disturbed agitation, fear and perplexity as the woman quickly loses touch with reality. The onset is very sudden, commonly occurring within the 1st postnatal week but rarely before the 3rd postpartum day, with the majority presenting before the 16th postnatal day.

Features may include:

- restlessness and agitation
- confusion and perplexity
- suspicion and fear, even terror
- insomnia
- episodes of mania, making the woman hyperactive (e.g. talking rapidly and incessantly, and being very overactive and elated)
- neglect of basic needs (e.g. nutrition and hydration)
- hallucinations and morbid delusional thoughts involving self and baby
- major behavioural disturbance
- profound depressive mood.

Puerperal psychosis appears to be much less related to stress factors than to biochemical changes. Most mothers with puerperal psychosis will be experiencing mental illness for the first time. The strong association between a family history of bipolar illness/manic depressive disorder (mother or father) and puerperal psychosis suggests a genetic link.

Care and management and the role of the midwife

Documentation of any past history of psychiatric disturbances should clearly spell out the precise onset, duration, diagnosis and treatment regimen. In the case of psychosis, where delusional thoughts and hallucinations are implicated, the woman must be referred urgently to the mental health team, as it is likely that she will need admission. This should be to a specialist mother and baby unit, with an out-of-area referral if necessary.

Ideally, care and management should be based primarily on preventative measures and begin preconception, or at least during the antenatal period, for women with a past history and known risk factors. Tremendous cooperation and interprofessional collaboration are required during the acute phase of the illness. Skilled staff in a specialist mother and baby unit will be able to undertake an assessment of the mother's ability to care for her baby and her need for care to continue once she is back in the community.

It may be difficult for the woman or her partner and family to accept the symptoms and diagnosis of a psychotic illness.

Antipsychotic (neuroleptic) medication is often an essential initial part of treatment. Such medication will not only sedate the patient, but will also reduce perplexity, distress and fear; within 48 hours there should be some impact on hallucinations and delusions. Manic features are often managed effectively with medication such as lithium carbonate; however, this is contraindicated if the woman is breastfeeding. Although it is widely believed that electroconvulsive therapy (ECT) is the treatment of choice, modern management has resulted in much lower usage than in the past. However, it remains useful in states where there is a threat of suicide. Antidepressants could take up to 2 weeks to have any therapeutic effect so may not be appropriate for first-line management; however, they are useful to maintain recovery after ECT treatment has been terminated.

Risk of relapse is high and therefore medication will need to be continued for 6 months; by this time the majority of women will have recovered. If relapse occurs the psychiatrist may consider using lithium carbonate or other mood stabilisers for 6 months to 1 year postpartum, and up to 2 years prophylactically if the woman presents with a non-postpartum bipolar illness/manic depressive disorder. Note: psychotropic medication is constantly changing).

Suicide

Suicide is a leading cause of maternal mortality in the UK. The majority of postpartum maternal suicides are the sequelae of a serious illness, such as puerperal psychosis or severe depressive illness. The most important factors in the reduction of risk posed by mental illness to both mother and baby are:

- prompt detection
- appropriate referral
- early intervention
- effective and vigorous management.

Psychotropic Medication During Pregnancy and Implications for Breastfeeding

Given that there is a paucity of systematic research into the efficacy and risks of pharmacological intervention in the management of postnatal depression, balancing risk to the fetus against the risk of not treating the mother is a challenge. Women should be actively supported to breastfeed their baby, if this is their wish.

General principles

- Whenever possible, conception and birth should be medication-free.
- Most new episodes of mental illness in pregnancy are early and improve as pregnancy progresses with appropriate psychosocial interventions.
- Liaison between the midwife, GP, obstetrician, psychiatrist, community psychiatric nurse, health visitor and, where necessary, social worker is of great importance.
- No medication is of proven safety.

- Medications that carry a significant risk of teratogenesis have been shown to affect 1–2% of exposed pregnancies, so may be considered of low risk. Nevertheless they may contribute to fetal demise, intrauterine growth restriction, organ dysgenesis and adverse effects on the neonate, such as withdrawal.

- Babies more than 12 weeks old are at low risk of exposure to antidepressants in breast milk.

- Breast milk levels will reflect the serum levels of the medication. Therefore women should be advised to avoid feeding at times of peak plasma level, and preferably should time their medication after a feed and before the baby's longest sleep.

- The baby should be monitored for any deleterious effects, particularly weight gain and drowsiness.

A summary of key recommendations for best practice is given in Box 26.5.

Box 26.5 Summary of key recommendations for best practice

Prevention of perinatal psychiatric disorders

- Prepare couples realistically to aim for achievable birth expectations and to deal ably with the demands and challenges of parenthood
- Recognise the value of interagency networking to afford more responsive helplines and points of contact for parents in crisis
- Develop an evidence base of effective mental health promotion strategies
- Be aware that the risk of recurrence of a severe mental illness is at its greatest in the first 30 days postpartum
- Antenatally, screen for risk factors that may culminate in antenatal or postnatal depression: person or family history of mental illness, history of substance (drug or alcohol) abuse, domestic violence, and self-harm and suicidal traits
- Be vigilant with record keeping to ensure good communication and continuity of care. Promote good liaison between members of the interprofessional team

(Continued)

Box 26.5 (Continued)

• Avoid misdiagnosis and prevent errors and missed opportunities in care by employing the correct terminology. Use of the umbrella term, 'PND', to describe all types of postpartum mental health problems must cease; use it only when referring to non-psychotic depressive illness of mild to moderate severity that has an onset following childbirth

Standards and targets

• Set national targets for perinatal mental health services

• Develop clear care pathways for women with a history of mental health problems, substance abuse and abusive relationships

• Set targets to establish the incidence of antenatal depression and reduce the prevalence of postnatal depression; one way of achieving this is to standardise the criteria used for screening

Services

• Improve access to perinatal mental health services

• Increase consultants specialising in perinatal mental health problems

• Increase specialist activities to avoid risk of mother and baby being admitted to a general psychiatric ward

• Form a strategy group reflective of all key members of the multiprofessional team to review services for the childbearing woman with perinatal mental health problems

• Ensure interprofessional and interagency collaboration, especially within the primary and secondary care sectors

Research, education and training

• Evaluate perinatal mental health services

• Develop interprofessional or interagency education programmes to aid learning and to improve and understand lines of communication or delineate professional boundaries

• Distinguish between psychology and pathology in order to avoid or reduce inappropriate referrals

Section 5

The Newborn Baby

Chapter 27

The Baby at Birth

A newborn baby's survival is dependent on its ability to adapt to an extrauterine environment. This involves adaptations in cardiopulmonary circulation and other physiological adjustments to replace placental function and maintain homeostasis. Birth is also the commencement of the early parent/baby relationship and, once the health of both mother and baby has been confirmed, privacy for the parents to talk to, touch and be alone with their baby is important.

Adaptation to Extrauterine Life

Subjected to intermittent diminution of the oxygen supply during uterine contractions, compression followed by decompression of the head and chest, and extension of the limbs, hips and spine during birth, the baby emerges from the mother to encounter light, noises, cool air, gravity and tactile stimuli for the first time. Simultaneously, the baby has to make major adjustments in the respiratory and circulatory systems, as well as controlling body temperature.

Respiratory and cardiovascular changes are interdependent and concurrent.

Pulmonary adaptation

Prior to birth, the fetus makes breathing movements and the lungs will be mature enough, both biochemically and anatomically, to produce surfactant and will have adequate numbers of alveoli for gas exchange. The fetal lung is full of fluid, which is excreted by the lung itself.

- During birth, this fluid leaves the alveoli, either by being squeezed up the airway and out of the mouth and nose, or by moving across the alveolar walls into the pulmonary lymphatic vessels and into the thoracic duct, or to the lung capillaries.

- Stimuli to respiration include the mild hypercapnia, hypoxia and acidosis that result from normal labour, due partially to the intermittent cessation of maternal–placental perfusion with contractions. The rhythm of respiration changes from episodic shallow fetal respiration to regular deeper breathing, as a result of a combination of chemical and neural stimuli: notably, a fall in pH and PaO_2 and a rise in $PaCO_2$. Other stimuli include cold, light, noise, touch and pain.

- Considerable negative intrathoracic pressure of up to 9.8 kPa (100 cm water) is exerted as the first breath is taken. Pressure exerted to effect inhalation diminishes with each breath taken until only 5 cm water pressure is required to inflate the lungs. This is an effect of surfactant, which lines the alveoli, lowering surface tension thus permitting residual air to remain in the alveoli between breaths. Surfactant is a complex of lipoproteins and proteins produced by the alveolar type 2 cells in the lungs; it is primarily concerned with the reduction in surface tension at the alveolar surface, thus reducing the work of breathing.

Cardiovascular adaptation

The baby's circulatory system must make major adjustments in order to divert deoxygenated blood to the lungs for reoxygenation.

- With the expansion of the lungs and lowered pulmonary vascular resistance, virtually all of the cardiac output is sent to the lungs.

- Oxygenated blood returning to the heart from the lungs increases the pressure within the left atrium.

- Pressure in the right atrium is lowered because blood ceases to flow through the cord.

- A functional closure of the foramen ovale takes place. During the first days of life this closure is reversible and reopening may occur if pulmonary vascular resistance is high — for example, when crying — resulting in transient cyanotic episodes in the baby.

- The septa usually fuse within the first year of life to form the interatrial septum, though in some individuals perfect anatomical closure may never be achieved.

- Contraction of the muscular walls of the ductus arteriosus takes place; this is thought to occur because of sensitivity of the muscle of the ductus arteriosus to increased oxygen tension and reduction in circulating prostaglandin. As a result of altered pressure gradients between the aorta and pulmonary artery, a temporary reverse left-to-right shunt through the ductus may persist for a few hours, though there is usually functional closure of the ductus within 8–10 hours of birth.

- The remaining temporary structures of the fetal circulation — the umbilical vein, ductus venosus and hypogastric arteries — close functionally within a few minutes after birth and constriction of the cord. Anatomical closure by fibrous tissue occurs within 2–3 months, resulting in the formation of the ligamentum teres, ligamentum venosum and the obliterated hypogastric arteries. The proximal portions of the hypogastric arteries persist as the superior vesical arteries.

Thermal adaptation

The baby enters a much cooler atmosphere, the birthing room temperature of 21°C contrasting sharply with an intrauterine temperature

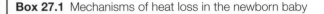

> **Box 27.1** Mechanisms of heat loss in the newborn baby
>
> **Evaporation**
> - Amniotic fluid evaporates from the skin. Each millilitre that evaporates removes 560 calories of heat. The baby's large surface area:body mass ratio potentiates heat loss, especially from the head, which comprises 25% of body mass
>
> **Poor insulation**
> - The subcutaneous fat layer is thin, allowing rapid transfer of core heat to the skin and the environment
>
> **Conduction**
> - Conduction takes place when the baby is in contact with cold surfaces
>
> **Radiation**
> - Heat radiates to cold objects in the environment that are not in contact with the baby
>
> **Convection**
> - This is caused by currents of cool air passing over the surface of the body

of 37.7°C. Heat loss can be rapid, and takes place through the mechanisms listed in Box 27.1.

The heat-regulating centre in the baby's brain has the capacity to promote heat production in response to stimuli received from thermoreceptors. However, this is dependent on increased metabolic activity, compromising the baby's ability to control body temperature especially in adverse environmental conditions. The baby has a limited ability to shiver and is unable to increase muscle activity voluntarily in order to generate heat. Therefore the baby must depend on his or her ability to produce heat by metabolism.

The neonate has brown adipose tissue, which assists in the rapid mobilisation of heat resources (namely, free fatty acids and glycerol) in times of cold stress. This mechanism is called non-shivering thermogenesis. Babies derive most of their heat production from the metabolism of brown fat. The term baby has sufficient brown fat to meet minimum heat needs for 2–4 days after birth, but cold stress results in increased oxygen consumption as the baby strives to maintain sufficient heat for survival. Brown fat uses up to three times as much oxygen as other tissue, with the undesired effect of diverting oxygen and glucose from vital centres such as the brain and cardiac muscle. In addition, cold stress causes vasoconstriction, thus reducing pulmonary perfusion, and respiratory acidosis develops as the pH and PaO_2 of the blood decrease and the $PaCO_2$ increases, leading to respiratory distress, exhibited by tachypnoea, and grunting respirations. This, together with the reduction in pulmonary perfusion, may result in the reopening or maintenance of the right-to-left shunt across the ductus arteriosus. Anaerobic glycolysis (i.e. the metabolism of glucose in the absence of oxygen) results in the production of acid, compounding the situation by adding a metabolic acidosis. Protraction of cold stress, therefore, should be avoided. The peripheral vasoconstrictor mechanisms of the baby are unable to prevent the fall in core body temperature that occurs within the first few hours after birth. It is important, therefore, to minimise heat loss at birth.

Immediate Care of the Baby at Birth

Prevention of heat loss

It is important to provide an ambient temperature in the range 21–25°C. The baby's temperature can drop by as much as 3–4.5°C within the first minute. Measures to conserve heat include:

- drying the baby at birth
- removing wet towels
- encouraging skin-to-skin contact with the mother
- wrapping the baby in dry, prewarmed towels.

Clearing the airway

As the baby's head is born, excess mucus may be wiped gently from the mouth. Care must be taken to avoid touching the nares, as such action may stimulate reflex inhalation of debris in the trachea. Although fetal pulmonary fluid is present in the mouth, most babies will achieve a clear airway unaided. Only rarely will it be necessary to clear the airway with the aid of a soft suction catheter attached to low-pressure (10 cm water) mechanical suction. It is important to aspirate the oropharynx prior to the nasopharynx so that, if the baby gasps as the nasal passages are aspirated, mucus or other material is not drawn down into the respiratory tract. Suction at the back of the pharynx can result in vagal stimulation, with laryngospasm and bradycardia.

Cutting the cord

The optimal time for umbilical cord clamping after birth remains unknown. Some centres advocate delay until respirations are established and cord pulsation has ceased. What is agreed is that a term baby at birth can be drawn up on to the mother's abdomen but raised no higher, and a preterm baby should be kept at the level of the placenta. This is because:

- if a preterm baby is held above the placenta, blood can drain from the baby to the placenta, resulting in anaemia
- if the baby is held below the placenta, it can cause him or her to receive a blood transfusion.

Early clamping and cutting of the cord is advocated in preterm babies.

Identification

The time of birth and sex of the baby are noted and recorded once the baby has been completely expelled from the mother.

When babies are born in hospital, it is essential that they are readily identifiable from one another. Various methods of indicating identity can be employed: for example, name bands or identity tags. In the UK each baby is issued with a National Unique Reference Number for receipt of Health and Social Care services.

Assessment of the baby's condition

At 1 minute and 5 minutes after the birth, an assessment is made of the baby's general condition using the Apgar score (Table 27.1).

■ The assessment at 1 minute is important for the further management of resuscitation.

■ An assessment at 5 minutes provides a record of response to resuscitation and immediate care needs.

The higher the score, the better the outcome for the baby.

A mnemonic — APGAR — for the Apgar score is given in Box 27.2.

Table 27.1 The Apgar score

Sign	Score		
	0	**1**	**2**
Heart rate	Absent	<100 bpm	>100 bpm
Respiratory effort	Absent	Slow, irregular	Good or crying
Muscle tone	Limp	Some flexion of limbs	Active
Reflex response to stimulus	None	Minimal grimace	Cough or sneeze
Colour	Blue, pale	Body pink, extremities blue	Completely pink

The score is assessed at 1 minute and 5 minutes after birth. Medical aid should be sought if the score is less than 7.

'Apgar minus colour' score omits the fifth sign. Medical aid should be sought if the score is less than 6.

Box 27.2 A mnemonic for the Apgar score

- **A** Appearance, i.e. colour
- **P** Pulse, i.e. heart rate
- **G** Grimace, i.e. response to stimuli
- **A** Active, i.e. tone
- **R** Respirations

Continued early care

Prior to leaving the mother's home or transferring the baby to the ward, the midwife undertakes a detailed examination of the baby, checking for obvious abnormalities such as:

- spina bifida
- imperforate anus
- cleft lip or palate
- abrasions
- fractures
- haemorrhage due to trauma.

The initial cord clamp is replaced with another method of securing haemostasis — the application of a disposable plastic clamp (or rubber band or three cord ligatures) approximately 2–3 cm from the umbilicus and the cutting off of the redundant cord. The baby's temperature is now recorded. The first bath and other non-urgent procedures may be deferred in order to minimise thermal stress.

Vitamin K

Depending on local policy and the mother's informed choice, vitamin K may be given intramuscularly or orally, as prophylaxis against bleeding disorders. Vitamin K is fat soluble and can only be absorbed from the intestine in the presence of bile salts. The body's capacity to store vitamin K is very low and the half-life of the vitamin K-dependent coagulation factors is short. A single dose (1.0 mg) of intramuscular vitamin K after birth has been found to be effective in the prevention of classic haemorrhagic disease of the newborn. Either intramuscular or oral (1.0 mg) vitamin K prophylaxis improves biochemical indices of coagulation status at 1–7 days. When three doses of oral vitamin K are compared to a single dose of intramuscular vitamin K, the plasma vitamin K levels are higher in the oral group at 2 weeks and 2 months, but again there is no evidence of a difference in coagulation studies.

Failure to Establish Respiration at Birth

Although the majority of babies gasp and establish respirations within 60 seconds of birth, some do not, mainly as a consequence of intrauterine hypoxia.

Intrauterine hypoxia

Possible causes include:

- maternal cardiac or respiratory disease
- eclamptic fit
- delayed intubation for induction of general anaesthesia
- hypertension
- hypotension due to haemorrhage or shock
- hypertonic uterine action
- prolapsed or compressed umbilical cord
- abnormal fetal cardiac function
- reduced fetal haemoglobin, e.g. Rhesus incompatibility, ruptured vasa praevia.

The fetus responds to hypoxia by accelerating the heart rate in an effort to maintain supplies of oxygen to the brain. If hypoxia persists, glucose depletion will stimulate anaerobic glycolysis, resulting in a metabolic acidosis. Cerebral vessels will dilate and some brain swelling may occur. Peripheral circulation will be reduced. As the fetus becomes acidotic and cardiac glycogen reserves are depleted, bradycardia develops, the anal sphincter relaxes and the fetus may pass meconium into the liquor. Gasping breathing movements triggered by hypoxia may result in the aspiration of meconium-stained liquor into the lungs, which presents an additional problem after birth.

The length of time during which the fetus or neonate is subjected to hypoxia determines the outcome.

- The initial response of gasping respirations is followed by a period of apnoea lasting $1\frac{1}{2}$ minutes — *primary apnoea*.

- If this is not resolved by means of intervention techniques, it is followed by a further episode of gasping respirations. These accelerate while diminishing in depth until, approximately 8 minutes after birth, respirations cease completely — *secondary apnoea*.

The essential difference between primary and secondary apnoea is the baby's circulatory status:

- During primary apnoea, the circulation and heart rate are maintained and such babies respond quickly to simple resuscitation measures.

- In secondary apnoea, the circulation is impaired, the heart rate is slow and the baby looks shocked (Table 27.2).

Table 27.2 Degrees of respiratory depression

Mildly depressed	**Severely depressed**
Heart rate not severely depressed (60–80 bpm)	Slow feeble heart rate (<40 bpm)
Short delay in onset of respiration	No attempt to breathe
Good muscle tone	Poor muscle tone
Responsive to stimuli	Limp, unresponsive to stimuli
Deeply cyanosed	Pale, grey
Apgar score 5–7	Apgar score <5
No significant deprivation of oxygen during labour (primary apnoea)	Oxygen lack has been prolonged before or after delivery, circulatory failure is present, baby is shocked (secondary apnoea)

Respiratory depression

Obstruction of the baby's airway by mucus, blood, liquor or meconium is one of the most common reasons for a baby failing to establish respirations. Depression of the respiratory centre may be due to:

- the effects of drugs administered to the mother, e.g. narcotics or diazepam
- cerebral hypoxia during labour or traumatic delivery
- immaturity of the baby, which causes mechanical dysfunction because of underdeveloped lungs, lack of surfactant and a soft pliable thoracic cage
- intranatal pneumonia, which can inhibit successful establishment of respirations and should be considered, especially if the membranes have been ruptured for some time
- severe anaemia, caused by fetomaternal haemorrhage or Rhesus incompatibility, which diminishes the oxygen-carrying capacity of the blood
- respiratory function, which may be compromised by major congenital abnormalities, particularly by abnormalities of the central nervous system or within the respiratory tract
- a congenital abnormality such as choanal or tracheal atresia which may be present. (Choanal atresia should be suspected when a baby is pink when crying but becomes cyanosed at rest.)

Resuscitation of the Newborn

The aims of resuscitation are:

- to establish and maintain a clear airway, by ventilation and oxygenation
- to ensure effective circulation
- to correct acidosis
- to prevent hypothermia, hypoglycaemia and haemorrhage.

As soon as the baby is born, the clock timer should be started. The Apgar score is assessed in the normal manner at 1 minute. In the absence of any respiratory effort, resuscitation measures are commenced. The baby's upper airways may be cleared by gentle suction of the oropharynx and nasopharynx and the presence of a heart beat verified. The baby is dried quickly, transferred to a well-lit resuscitaire and placed on a flat, firm surface at a comfortable working height and under a radiant heat source to prevent hypothermia. The baby's shoulders may be elevated on a small towel, which causes slight extension of the head and straightens the trachea. Hyperextension may cause airway obstruction owing to the short neck of the neonate and large, ill-supported tongue.

Stimulation

Rough handling of the baby merely serves to increase shock and is unnecessary. Gentle stimulation by drying the baby may initiate breathing.

Warmth

Hypothermia exacerbates hypoxia, as essential oxygen and glucose are diverted from the vital centres in order to create heat for survival. As stated above, wet towels should be removed and the baby's body and head should be covered with a prewarmed blanket, leaving only the chest exposed. *Note that it is hazardous to use a silver swaddle under a radiant heater because it could cause burning.*

Clearing the airway

Most babies require no airway clearance at birth; however, if there obvious respiratory difficulty a suction catheter may be used (size 10FG, or 8FG in preterm).

■ The catheter tip should not be inserted further than 5 cm and each suction attempt should not last longer than 5 seconds. Eve with a soft catheter, it is still possible to traumatise the delicate mucosa, especially in the preterm baby.

- If meconium is present in the airway, suction under direct vision should be performed by the passage of a laryngoscope blade and visualising the larynx. Care should be taken to avoid touching the vocal cords, as this may induce laryngospasm, apnoea and bradycardia. Thick meconium may need to be aspirated out of the trachea through an endotracheal tube.

Ventilation and oxygenation

If the baby fails to respond to these simple measures, assisted ventilation is necessary.

Facemask ventilation

- An appropriately sized mask (usually 00 or 0/1) is positioned on the face so that it covers the nose and mouth and ensures a good seal.
- A 500 ml bag is used, as a smaller 250 ml bag does not permit sustained inflation.
- Care should be taken not to apply pressure on the soft tissue under the jaw, as this may obstruct the airway.
- To aerate the lungs five sustained inflations are delivered, using oxygen or air or a combination of both, with a pressure of 30 cm H_2O applied for 2–3 seconds and repeated five times; then continue to ventilate at a rate of 40 respirations per minute.
- Insertion of a neonatal airway helps to prevent obstruction by the baby's tongue.

Note that over-extension of the baby's head causes airway obstruction. A longer inspiration phase improves oxygenation. Higher inflation pressures may be required to produce chest movement.

Endotracheal intubation

If the baby fails to respond to intermittent positive pressure ventilation (IPPV) by bag and mask, or if bradycardia is present, an endotracheal tube should be passed without delay. Intubating a baby requires special skill that, once acquired, must be practised if it is to be retained.

Technique for intubation

The equipment listed in Box 27.3 must be available and in working order.

- Position the baby on a flat surface, preferably a resuscitaire, and extend the neck into the 'neutral position'. A rolled-up towel placed under the shoulders will help maintain proper alignment.

- The blade of the laryngoscope is introduced over the baby's tongue into the pharynx until the epiglottis is seen.

- Elevation of the epiglottis with the tip of the laryngoscope reveals the vocal cords.

- Any mucus, blood or meconium which is obstructing the trachea should be cleared by careful suction prior to passing the endotracheal tube a distance of 1.5–2 cm into the trachea. (Pressure on the cricoid cartilage may facilitate visualisation of the larynx.)

- Intubation may be easier if a tracheal introducer made of plastic-covered soft metal wire is used. This will increase the stiffness and curvature of the tube.

- After the laryngoscope is removed, oxygen is administered by IPPV to the endotracheal tube via the Ambu bag. A maximum of 30 cm water pressure should be applied, as there is risk of rupture of alveoli or tension pneumothorax with higher pressures.

The rise and fall of the chest wall should indicate whether the tube is in the trachea. This can be confirmed by auscultation of the chest. Distension of the stomach indicates oesophageal intubation, necessitating resiting of the tube.

Box 27.3 Resuscitation equipment

- Resuscitaire with overhead radiant heater (switched on) and light, piped oxygen, manometer, suction and clock timer
- Two straight-bladed infant laryngoscopes, spare batteries and bulbs (size 0 and 1)
- Neonatal endotracheal tubes (2.0, 2.5, 3.0 and 3.5 mm) and connectors
- Neonatal airways (sizes 0, 00 and 000)
- Suction catheters (sizes 6, 8 and 10 FG)
- Neonatal bag and mask and facemasks of assorted sizes (clear, soft masks)
- Magill's forceps
- Endotracheal tube introducer
- Syringes (1 ml, 2 ml, 5 ml and 20 ml) and assorted needles
- Drugs

    Naloxone hydrochloride 1 ml ampoules 400 μg/ml (adult Narcan)

    Adrenaline (epinephrine) 1:10 000 and 1:1000

    Human albumin solution 4.5%

    THAM (tris-hydroxymethyl-amino-methane) 7%

    Sodium bicarbonate 4.2%

    Dextrose 10%

    Vitamin K_1 1 mg ampoules

    Normal saline 0.9%
- Stethoscope
- Cord clamps
- Warmed dry towels
- Adhesive tape for tube fixation

Mouth-to-face/nose resuscitation

In the absence of specialised equipment, assisted ventilation can be achieved by mouth-to-face resuscitation.

- With the baby's head in the 'sniffing' position, the operator places her mouth over the baby's mouth and nose.

■ Using only the air in her buccal cavity, she breathes gently into the baby's airway at a rate of 20 breaths per minute, allowing the infant to exhale between breaths.

It may be easier with larger babies to use mouth-to-nose resuscitation.

External cardiac massage

Chest compressions should be performed if the heart rate is less than 60 bpm, or between 60 and 100 bpm and falling despite adequate ventilation. The most effective way of performing chest compressions is to:

■ encircle the baby's chest with your fingers on the baby's spine and your thumbs on the lower mid-sternum (Fig. 27.1)
■ depress the chest at a rate of 100–120 times per minute, at a ratio of three compressions to one ventilation, and at a depth of one-third of the baby's chest.

(Excessive pressure over the lower end of the sternum may cause rib, lung or liver damage.)

Use of drugs

If the baby's response is slow or he/she remains hypotonic after ventilation is achieved, consideration will be given to the use of drugs. In specialist obstetric units, pulse oximetry may be employed to monitor hypoxia and blood obtained through the umbilical artery or vein to ascertain biochemical status. Results will enable appropriate administration of resuscitation drugs, as discussed below.

Naloxone hydrochloride

■ This should be used with caution and only in specific circumstances.
■ It is a powerful anti-opioid drug for the reversal of the effects of maternal narcotic drugs given in the preceding 3 hours.

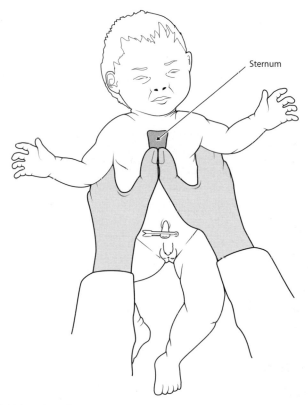

Sternum

Fig. 27.1 External cardiac massage.

- Ventilation should be established prior to its use.
- *It must not be given to apnoeic babies.*
- A dose of up to 100 µg/kg body weight may be administered intramuscularly for prolonged action.
- As opioid action may persist for some hours, the midwife must be alert for signs of relapse when a repeat dose may be required.
- *It should not be administered to babies of narcotic-addicted mothers, as this may precipitate acute withdrawal.*

Sodium bicarbonate

- This is not recommended for brief periods of cardiopulmonary resuscitation (CPR).

- Once tissues are oxygenated by lung inflation with 100% oxygen and cardiac compression, the acidosis will self-correct unless asphyxia is very severe.

- If the heart rate is less than 60 bpm despite effective ventilation, chest compression and two intravenous doses of adrenaline (epinephrine) then sodium bicarbonate 4.2% solution (0.5 mmol/ml) can be administered using 2–4 ml/kg (1–2 mmol/kg) by slow intravenous injection

- It should be given at a rate of 1 ml/minute in order to avoid rapid elevation of serum osmolality with the attendant risk of intracranial haemorrhage.

- *It should not be given prior to ventilation being established.*

- THAM 7% (tris-hydroxymethyl-amino-methane) 0.5 mmol/kg may be used in preference to sodium bicarbonate.

Adrenaline (epinephrine)

- This is indicated if the heart rate is less than 60 bpm despite 1 minute of effective ventilation and chest compression.

- An initial dose of 0.1–0.3 ml/kg of 1:10 000 solution (10–30 µg/kg) can be given intravenously; this may be repeated after 3 minutes for a further two doses.

- The Royal College of Paediatrics and Child Health (1997) recommends a higher dose of 100 µg/kg intravenously, if there is no response to the boluses. It is reasonable to try giving one dose of adrenaline 0.1 ml/kg of 1:1000 via the endotracheal tube, as this sometimes has an immediate effect.

Hypoglycaemia is not usually a problem unless resuscitation has been prolonged. A solution of dextrose 10% 3 ml/kg may be given intravenously to correct a blood sugar of less than 2.6 mmol/L.

Observations and after-care

Throughout the resuscitation procedure the baby's response is monitored and recorded. An accurate written record detailing the resuscitation events is essential. The endotracheal tube may be left in place for a few minutes after the baby starts to breathe spontaneously. Suction may be applied through the endotracheal tube as it is removed.

Box 27.4 Resuscitation action plan

A	Anticipation	Assessment (Apgar)	Airway — clear debris
B	Breathing	Bag + mask	Endotracheal tube
C	Circulation	Cardiac massage	Caring — warmth, comfort
D	Doctor	Drugs	Documentation
E	Explanation	Family	
F	Follow-up care	Environment	

Box 27.5 Key points for practice

- Anticipation of problems
- Checking of resuscitation equipment
- Starting clock
- Suctioning
- Keeping baby warm
- Apgar score
- Bag and mask ventilation
- Endotracheal ventilation
- Cardiac massage
- Drugs
- Other problems

Explanation must be given to the parents about the resuscitation and the need for transfer to hospital (if the baby was born at home) or to the neonatal unit. The principles of resuscitation of the newborn are applicable wherever and whenever apnoea occurs. The midwife must be able to implement emergency care whilst awaiting medical assistance (Boxes 27.4 and 27.5).

Chapter 28

The Normal Baby

General Characteristics

Appearance

Salient points relating to the newborn baby's general appearance are listed in Box 28.1.

Box 28.1 The appearance of the newborn baby

- Weight is highly variable but is normally around 3.5 kg
- Length is in the region of 50 cm from the crown of the head to the heels
- Occipitofrontal head circumference is 34–35 cm
- In an attitude of flexion, with arms extended, babies' fingers reach upper thigh level
- Vernix caseosa, a white sticky substance, is present on the baby's skin at birth
- Lanugo, downy hair, covers areas of the skin
- Colour is according to ethnic origin
- Cartilage of the ears is well formed
- Milia, distended glands in the skin, are often found over nose and cheeks

Physiology

Respiratory system

- The normal baby has a respiratory rate of 30–60 breaths per minute.

- Breathing is diaphragmatic, the chest and abdomen rising and falling synchronously.

- The breathing pattern is erratic. Respirations are shallow and irregular, being interspersed with brief 10- to 15-second periods of apnoea. This is known as periodic breathing.

- Babies are obligatory nose breathers and do not convert automatically to mouth breathing when nasal obstruction occurs.

- Babies have a lusty cry, which is normally loud and of medium pitch.

Cardiovascular system and blood

- The heart rate is rapid: 100–160 beats per minute.

- Blood pressure fluctuates from 50–55/25–30 mmHg to 80/50 mmHg in the first 10 days of life.

- The total circulating blood volume at birth is 80 ml/kg body weight.

- The haemoglobin level is high (13–20 g/dl), of which 50–85% is fetal Hb.

- Breakdown of excess red blood cells in the liver and spleen predisposes to jaundice in the first week.

- Vitamin K-dependent clotting factors II (prothrombin), VII, IX and X are low.

- Platelet levels equal those of the adult but there is a reduced capacity for adhesion and aggregation.

Temperature regulation

The baby's normal core temperature is 36.5–37.3°C. A healthy, clothed, term baby will maintain this body temperature satisfactorily, provided the environmental temperature is sustained between 18 and 21°C, nutrition is adequate and movements are not restricted by tight swaddling.

Renal system

The glomerular filtration rate is low and tubular reabsorption capabilities are limited. The baby is not able to concentrate or dilute urine very well in response to variations in fluid intake nor compensate for high or low levels of solutes in the blood. The first urine is passed at birth or within the first 24 hours, and thereafter with increasing frequency as fluid intake rises.

- The urine is dilute, straw-coloured and odourless.
- Cloudiness caused by mucus and urates may be present initially until fluid intake increases.
- Urates may cause pink staining, which is insignificant.

Gastrointestinal system

The mucous membrane of the mouth is pink and moist. The teeth are buried in the gums and ptyalin secretion is low. Small epithelial pearls are sometimes present at the junction of the hard and soft palates. Sucking pads in the cheeks give them a full appearance. Sucking and swallowing reflexes are coordinated.

The stomach has a small capacity (15–30 ml), which increases rapidly in the first weeks of life. The cardiac sphincter is weak, predisposing to regurgitation or posseting. Gastric acidity, equal to that of the adult within a few hours after delivery, diminishes rapidly within the first few days and by the 10th day the baby is virtually achlorhydric, which increases the risk of infection. Gastric emptying time is normally ½–3 hours.

The gut is sterile at birth but is colonised within a few hours. Bowel sounds are present within 1 hour of birth. Meconium, present in the large intestine from 16 weeks' gestation, is passed within the first 24 hours of life and is totally excreted within 48–72 hours.

- This first stool is blackish-green in colour, is tenacious and contains bile, fatty acids, mucus and epithelial cells.

- From the 3rd–5th days the stools undergo a transitional stage and are brownish-yellow in colour.

- Once feeding is established, yellow faeces are passed.

The consistency and frequency of stools reflect the type of feeding.

- Breast milk results in loose, bright yellow and inoffensive acid stools. The baby may pass 8–10 stools a day or alternatively pass stools as infrequently as every 2 or 3 days.

- The stools of the bottle-fed baby are paler in colour, semiformed and less acidic, and have a slightly sharp smell.

Physiological immaturity of the liver results in low production of glucuronyl transferase for the conjugation of bilirubin. This, together with a high level of red cell breakdown and stimulation of hepatic blood flow, may result in a transient jaundice which is manifest on the 3rd–5th days. Glycogen stores are rapidly depleted, so early feeding is required to maintain normal blood glucose levels (2.6–4.4 mmol/l). Feeding stimulates liver function and colonisation of the gut, which assists in the formation of vitamin K.

Immunological adaptations

Neonates demonstrate a marked susceptibility to infections. The baby has some immunoglobulins at birth. There are three main immunoglobulins — IgG, IgA and IgM.

- Of these only IgG is small enough to cross the placental barrier. It affords immunity to specific viral infections. At birth the baby levels of IgG are equal to or slightly higher than those of the mother. This provides passive immunity during the first few months of life.

■ IgM and IgA do not cross the placental barrier but can be manufactured by the fetus. Levels of IgM at term are 20% those of the adult, taking 2 years to attain adult levels. (Elevation of IgM levels at birth is suggestive of intrauterine infection.) Breast milk, especially colostrum, provides the baby with IgA passive immunity.

The thymus gland, where lymphocytes are produced, is relatively large at birth and continues to grow until 8 years of age.

Reproductive system: genitalia and breasts

■ In boys the testes are descended into the scrotum by 37 weeks. The urethral meatus opens at the tip of the penis and the prepuce is adherent to the glans.

■ In girls born at term the labia majora normally cover the labia minora. The hymen and clitoris may appear disproportionately large.

■ In both sexes withdrawal of maternal oestrogens results in breast engorgement sometimes accompanied by secretion of 'milk' by the 4th or 5th day. Baby girls may develop pseudomenstruation for the same reason. Both boys and girls have a nodule of breast tissue around the nipple.

Skeletomuscular system

The muscles are complete, subsequent growth occurring by hypertrophy rather than by hyperplasia. The long bones are incompletely ossified to facilitate growth at the epiphyses. The bones of the vault of the skull also reveal lack of ossification. This is essential for growth of the brain and facilitating moulding during labour. Moulding is resolved within a few days of birth.

- The posterior fontanelle closes at 6–8 weeks.

- The anterior fontanelle remains open until 18 months of age, making assessment of hydration and intracranial pressure possible by palpation of fontanelle tension.

Psychology and Perception

The newborn baby is alert and aware of his or her surroundings when awake.

Special senses

Vision

Babies are sensitive to bright lights, which cause them to frown or blink. They demonstrate a preference for bold black and white patterns and the shape of the human face, focusing at a distance of approximately 15–20 cm. No tears are present in the eyes of the newborn; therefore they become infected easily.

Hearing

Newborn babies eyes turn towards sound. On hearing a high-pitched sound they first blink or startle and then become agitated, and are comforted by low-pitched sounds. They prefer the sound of the human voice to other sounds.

Smell and taste

Babies prefer the smell of milk to that of other substances and show a preference for human milk. They turn away from unpleasant smell and show preference for sweet taste, as demonstrated by vigorou and sustained sucking and a speedy grimacing response to bitter, salty or sour substances.

Touch

Babies are acutely sensitive to touch, enjoying:

- skin-to-skin contact
- immersion in water
- stroking, cuddling and rocking movements.

Sleeping and waking

Sleeping and waking rhythms show marked variations. Initially, waking periods are related to hunger, but within a few weeks the waking periods last longer and meet the need for social interaction.

Crying

The crying repertoire of babies distinguishes different needs and is the way in which they communicate discomfort and summon assistance. With experience it is possible to differentiate the cry and identify the need, which may be hunger, thirst, pain, general discomfort (for example, wanting a change of position or feeling too cold or too hot), boredom, loneliness or a desire for physical and social contact.

Examination at Birth

Overall symmetry should be verified and skin blemishes or abrasions noted.

Colour and respirations

Babies are obligatory nose breathers; bilateral nasal obstruction is of major significance if due to bilateral choanal atresia, which is a major medical emergency. Observe the colour of the baby's skin and mucous membranes. In the normal baby, the lips and mucous membranes are pink and well perfused.

Face, head and neck

Each eye should be visualised to confirm that it is present and that the lens is clear. The eyes open spontaneously if the baby is held in an upright position. Any slight oedema or bruising is noted but may be insignificant. The normal space between the eyes is up to 3 cm.

The skull should be palpated to determine the degree of moulding by the amount of overriding of the bones at the sutures and fontanelles.

- The bones should feel hard in a term baby.
- A wide anterior fontanelle and splayed sutures may indicate hydrocephalus or immaturity.
- An oedematous swelling, caput succedaneum, may be noted overlying the part that was presenting.

The short thick neck of the baby must be examined to exclude the presence of swellings and to ensure that rotation and flexion of the head is possible.

The mouth

The mouth can be opened easily by pressing against the angle of the jaw. This allows visual inspection of the tongue, gums and palate.

- The palate should be high-arched and intact, and the uvula should be central.
- Epithelial pearls (Epstein's pearls) may be observed. They are of no significance, though occasionally mistaken for infection, and they disappear spontaneously.
- Feel the palate for any submucous cleft. A normal baby will respond by sucking the finger.
- A tight frenulum will give the appearance of tongue-tie; no treatment is necessary for this.

The ears

The ears are inspected, noting their position.

- The upper notch of the pinna should be level with the canthus of the eye.
- Patency of the external auditory meatus is verified.
- Accessory auricles, small tags of tissue, are sometimes noted lying in front of the ear.

Ear abnormalities can be associated with chromosomal anomalies and syndromes, and should be reported to a paediatrician.

Chest and abdomen

- Chest and abdominal movements are synchronous. The respirations may still be irregular at this stage.
- The space between the nipples should be noted, widely spaced nipples being associated with chromosomal abnormality.
- The shape of the abdomen should be rounded.
- Haemostasis of the umbilical cord is vital. A blood loss of 30 ml from a baby is equivalent to almost 0.5 L of blood from an adult.
- Normally, three cord vessels are present. Absence of one of the arteries is occasionally associated with renal anomalies and must be reported to the paediatrician.

Genitalia and anus

If the sex is uncertain, the paediatrician will initiate investigations.

Limbs and digits

- The hands should be opened fully, as any accessory digits may be concealed in the clenched fist.
- The feet are examined for any deformity such as talipes equinovarus, as well as looking for extra digits.

- The axillae, elbows, groins and popliteal spaces should also be examined for abnormalities.
- Normal flexion and rotation of the wrist and ankle joints should be confirmed.

Spine

With the baby lying prone, the midwife should inspect and palpate the baby's back. Any swellings, dimples or hairy patches may signify an occult spinal defect.

Temperature

The baby's temperature may be taken, normally in the axilla (underarm), tympanum (ear) or groin. The normal baby's skin temperature should range from 36.5 to 37.3°C.

Documentation

The midwife records her findings in the case notes. Any abnormalities are brought to the attention of the paediatrician, or GP if birth took place at the woman's home, along with the receiving midwife in the postnatal ward.

Observation and General Care

The name bands must remain on the baby until discharge from hospital. It is recommended that the presence of two legible, matching, correct name bands is verified daily, on transfer to other wards, and on discharge from hospital.

During the first few hours after birth, the midwife should observe the baby frequently for any colour changes, patency of airway and haemorrhage from the umbilical cord. Temperature should also be monitored to ensure that it is maintained within the normal range.

Neonatal care

In caring for the normal baby it is important to ensure protection from:

- airway obstruction
- hypothermia
- infection
- injury and accident.

Prevention of airway obstruction

It is important for a baby to sleep in the supine position (on the back) with the feet at the foot of the cot.

Prevention of hypothermia

- Where possible, the room temperature should be maintained at 18–21°C.
- Bath water should be warm (36°C), and wet clothing should be changed as soon as possible.
- It is essential also to avoid overheating.
- Parents should be advised to take account of environmental temperature when dressing their baby. Swaddling should be loose enough to permit movement of arms and legs.

Prevention of infection

- Members of staff who are liable to be a source of infection should not handle babies and friends and relatives who have colds or sore throats (especially children) should not visit.
- Hand washing before and after handling babies is essential.

Skin care

Promotion of skin integrity is enhanced by avoiding friction against hard fabrics or soiled or wet clothing, and by minimising the length of time the skin is in contact with irritants such as gastric contents, urine and stool.

The timing of the first bath is not critical, although it has been suggested that removal of blood and liquor reduces the risk of transmission of HIV and other organisms to staff.

Daily bathing is not essential.

- The baby's eyes do not need to be cleansed unless a discharge is present.
- Attention should be paid to the washing and drying of skin flexures to prevent excoriation.
- The buttocks must be washed and dried carefully at every napkin change. Sore buttocks may occur if the stools are loose, if there is protracted delay in changing a soiled napkin or if the skin is traumatised by over-enthusiastic rubbing. Regular use of a barrier cream is recommended by some but may interfere with the 'one-way' membrane in disposable nappies.

Cleanliness of the umbilical cord is essential.

- Hand washing is required before and after handling the cord.
- No specific cord treatment is required, although a wide variety of preparations have been used to promote early separation. Cleansing with tap water and keeping the cord dry have been shown to promote separation.
- The cord clamp may be removed on the third day, provided the cord is dry and necrosed.

Vaccination and immunisation

- BCG vaccination may be given during the early neonatal period in some areas where early protection is desirable.
- Vaccination against hepatitis B and poliomyelitis may also be given in some parts of the world.

Prevention of injury and accident

Advice should also be given to parents about baby care and safety in the home. This should address such issues as:

- bed sharing
- the use of cat nets
- fireguards
- cooker guards
- stair gates
- pram brakes
- car seats.

'Smoking', 'back to sleep' and 'feet-to-foot' advice should be included.

Assessing the baby's well-being

At every contact the mother is asked about the baby's health and feeding. Examination of the baby is at the discretion of the midwife and when the mother has any concerns, having been given information about recognising problems and the baby's capabilities.

- Weight loss is normal in the first few days but more than 10% body weight loss is abnormal and requires investigation.
- Most babies regain their birth weight in 7–10 days, thereafter gaining weight at a rate of 150–200 g per week.

Full examination within 72 hours of birth

This is usually performed by a competent professional (usually paediatrician or midwife) (Box 28.2).

Blood tests

Certain inborn errors of metabolism and endocrine disorders are detected by means of a blood test, obtained from a heel prick made with a stilette on the lateral aspect of the heel to avoid nerves and

Box 28.2 Examination of the baby within 72 hours of birth

Appearance
- Activity
- Behaviour
- Breathing
- Colour
- Cry
- Posture

Skin
- Colour
- Texture
- Rashes
- Birthmarks

Head
- Symmetry and facial features
- Face
- Fontanelles
- Mouth
- Eyes
- Ears
- Neck

Neck, limbs and joints
- Proportions
- Symmetry
- Digits
- Movements

Heart
- Position
- Rate
- Rhythm
- Sounds
- Murmurs
- Femoral pulses

Lungs
- Rate
- Effort
- Sounds

Abdomen
- Shape
- Palpation for organ enlargement
- Umbilical cord

Genitalia and anus
- Sex clear
- Complete and patent
- Testes descended or not
- Meconium within 24 hours
- Urinary output

Spine
- Length felt for integrity and skin cover

Central nervous system
- Behaviour
- Tone
- Movements
- Posture
- Reflexes as appropriate

Hips
- Barlow and Ortolani's manœuvres
- Symmetry of limbs

Feeding
- Ask mother, carers

Measurements
- Weight
- Length
- Head circumference

blood vessels. Blood is dripped on to circles on an absorbent card, on to which full details of the baby's identity are entered.

- For detection of phenylketonuria, hypothyroidism and cystic fibrosis the baby must have had at least 4–6 days of milk feeding, and if for any reason the baby or mother is receiving antibiotics, this information should be recorded on the card.
- Some centres also test routinely for galactosaemia.

Promoting Family Relationships

Parent–infant attachment

Parents develop their relationship with their babies in individual ways and at their own pace. Some mothers feel somewhat distant from their baby at first; others experience an overwhelming protective urge and intense absorption in their babies.

It is suggested that the parents' relationship with one another is enhanced when the father is encouraged to be involved in discussions, choices and decisions about baby care and to share the responsibility for care.

Promoting confidence and competence

Total care should be delegated to the parents as soon as possible. In hospital, especially, procedures can be rendered unnecessarily complicated for new mothers. Teaching the principles and discussing individual care can help to overcome these anxieties.

Promoting communication

The increasing interest in baby massage in recent years capitalises on the knowledge that the baby is sensitive and responsive to touch.

- Grapeseed or equivalent oil is used rather than baby oils, which stick to the skin.
- Aromatherapy oils should not be used, as the extent of their absorption is not known.

Chapter 29

Infant Feeding

Anatomy and Physiology of the Breast

The breasts are compound secreting glands, composed mainly of glandular tissue, which is arranged in lobes.

- Each lobe is divided into lobules that consist of alveoli and ducts.

- The alveoli contain acini cells, which secrete the components of milk and are surrounded by myoepithelial cells, which contract and propel the milk out.

- Small lactiferous ducts, carrying milk from the alveoli, unite to form larger ducts.

- Myoepithelial cells are oriented longitudinally along the ducts; under the influence of oxytocin, these smooth muscle cells contract and the tubule becomes shorter and wider.

- The nipple is composed of erectile tissue and plain muscle fibres, which have a sphincter-like action in controlling the flow of milk.

- Surrounding the nipple is an area of pigmented skin called the areola, which contains Montgomery's glands. These produce a sebum-like substance, which acts as a lubricant during pregnancy and throughout breastfeeding.

- The breast is supplied with blood from the internal and external mammary arteries with corresponding venous drainage.
- Lymph drains freely between the two breasts and into lymph nodes in the axillae and the mediastinum.

During pregnancy, oestrogens and progesterone induce alveolar and ductal growth, as well as stimulating the secretion of colostrum. When the levels of placental hormones fall, this allows the already high levels of prolactin to initiate milk secretion. Continued production of prolactin is caused by the baby feeding at the breast, with concentrations highest following night feeds.

Prolactin is particularly important in the initiation of lactation. As lactation progresses, the milk removal becomes the driving force behind milk production. This is now known to be due to a protein feedback inhibitor of lactation. This protein accumulates in the breast as the milk accumulates and it exerts negative feedback control on the continued production of milk. Removal of this autocrine inhibitory factor, by removing the milk, allows milk production to be stepped up again.

Milk release is under neuroendocrine control. Tactile stimulation of the breast also stimulates the oxytocin, causing contraction of the myoepithelial cells. This process is known as the 'let-down' or 'milk ejection' reflex and makes the milk available to the baby. This occurs in discrete pulses throughout the feed and may well trigger the bursts of active feeding.

In the early days of lactation this reflex is unconditioned. Later, it becomes a conditioned reflex, which can be enhanced or suppressed by environmental factors.

Properties and Components of Breast Milk

Human milk varies in its composition. The most dramatic change in the composition of milk occurs during the course of a feed.

- At the beginning of the feed the baby receives a high volume of relatively low-fat milk.

- As the feed progresses, the volume of milk decreases but the proportion of fat in the milk increases, sometimes to as much as five times the initial value.

The baby's ability to obtain this fat-rich milk is *not* determined by the length of time spent at the breast, but by the quality of attachment to the breast. The baby needs to be well attached so that he or she can use the tongue to maximum effect, stripping the milk from the breast, rather than relying solely on the mother's milk ejection reflex.

Fats and fatty acids

For the human infant, with a unique and rapidly growing brain, it is the fat and not the protein in human milk that has particular significance.

- Ninety-eight per cent of the lipid in human milk is in the form of triglycerides: three fatty acids linked to a single molecule of glycerol.

- Over 100 fatty acids have so far been identified, about 46% being saturated fat and 54% unsaturated fat.

- Fat provides the baby with more than 50% of calorific requirements.

- It is utilised very rapidly because *the milk itself* contains the enzyme (bile salt-stimulated *lipase*) needed for fat digestion, but in a form that only becomes active when it reaches the infant's intestine.

- Pancreatic lipase is not plentiful in the newborn, so a baby who i not fed human milk is less able to digest fat.

Carbohydrate

- The carbohydrate component of human milk is provided chiefly by lactose, which supplies the baby with about 40% of calorific requirements.

- Lactose is converted into galactose and glucose by the action of the enzyme lactase and these sugars provide energy to the rapidly growing brain.
- Lactose enhances the absorption of calcium and also promotes the growth of lactobacilli which increase intestinal acidity, thus reducing the growth of pathogenic organisms.

Protein

Human milk contains less protein than any other mammalian milk and this accounts in part for its more 'transparent' appearance. Human milk is whey-dominant (the whey being mainly alpha-lactalbumin) and forms soft, flocculent curds when acidified in the stomach.

Vitamins

All the vitamins required for good nutrition and health are supplied in breast milk, although the actual amounts vary from mother to mother.

Fat-soluble vitamins

Vitamin A

This is present in human milk as retinol, retinyl esters and beta-carotene. Colostrum contains twice the amount present in mature human milk, and it is this which gives colostrum its yellow colour.

Vitamin D

This is the name given to two fat-soluble compounds:

- calciferol (vitamin D2)
- cholecalciferol (vitamin D3).

Vitamin D3 plays an essential role in the metabolism of calcium and phosphorus in the body and prevents rickets in children. Adults can obtain these substances from dietary sources and the conversion of -dehydrocholesterol in the skin to vitamin D3 from exposure to sunlight.

- For light-skinned babies, exposure to sunlight for 30 minutes per week wearing only a nappy, or 2 hours per week fully clothed but without a hat, will keep vitamin D requirements within the lower limits of the normal range.
- The babies of dark-skinned mothers living in temperate zones and preterm babies may be at risk of vitamin D deficiency.

Vitamin E

Although vitamin E is present in human milk, its role is uncertain. It appears to prevent the oxidisation of polyunsaturated fatty acids and may prevent certain types of anaemia to which preterm infants are susceptible.

Vitamin K

This vitamin (83% of which is present as alpha-tocopherol) is essential for the synthesis of blood-clotting factors. It is present in human milk and absorbed efficiently. Because it is fat soluble, it is present in greater concentrations in colostrum and in the high-fat hind-milk, although the increased volume of milk as lactation progresses means that the infant obtains twice as much vitamin K from mature milk as from colostrum.

Water-soluble vitamins

Unless the mother's diet is seriously deficient, breast milk will contain adequate levels of all the vitamins. An improved diet is always more beneficial than artificial supplements. With some vitamins, particularly vitamin C, a plateau may be reached where increased maternal intake has no further impact on breast milk composition.

Minerals and trace elements

Iron

Normal term babies are usually born with a high haemoglobin level (13–20 g/dl), which decreases rapidly after birth. The iron recovered from Hb breakdown is utilised again. Babies also have ample iron stores, sufficient for at least 4–6 months. Although the amounts of iron are lower than those found in formula, the bio-availability of iron in breast milk is very much higher:

- 70% of the iron in breast milk is absorbed.
- Only 10% is absorbed from formula.

Zinc

A deficiency of this essential trace mineral may result in failure to thrive and typical skin lesions.

- Although there is more zinc present in formula than in human milk, the bio-availability is greater in human milk.
- Breastfed babies maintain high plasma zinc values when compared with formula-fed infants, even when the concentration of zinc is three times that of human milk.

Calcium

- Calcium is more efficiently absorbed from human milk than from formula milks because of human milk's higher calcium: phosphorus ratio.
- Infant formulas, which are based on cow's milk, inevitably have a higher phosphorous content than human milk.

Other minerals

Human milk has significantly lower levels of calcium, phosphorus, sodium and potassium than formula. Copper, cobalt and selenium are present at higher levels. The higher bio-availability of these minerals and trace elements ensures that the infant's needs are met whilst also imposing a lower solute load on the neonatal kidney than do breast milk substitutes.

Anti-infective factors

Leucocytes

During the first 10 days of life there are more white cells per ml in breast milk than there are in blood. Macrophages and neutrophils are amongst the most common leucocytes in human milk and they surround and destroy harmful bacteria by their phagocytic activity.

Immunoglobulins

Five types of immunoglobulin have been identified in human milk: IgA, IgG, IgE, IgM and IgD. Of these the most important is IgA, which appears to be both synthesised and stored in the breast. Although some IgA is absorbed by the infant, much of it is not. Instead it 'paints' the intestinal epithelium and protects the mucosal surfaces against entry of pathogenic bacteria and enteroviruses. It affords protection against:

- *E. coli*
- salmonellae
- shigellae
- streptococci
- staphylococci
- pneumococci
- poliovirus
- the rotaviruses.

Lysozyme

This kills bacteria by disrupting their cell walls. The concentration of lysozyme increases with prolonged lactation.

Lactoferrin

This binds to enteric iron, thus preventing potentially pathogenic *E. coli* from obtaining the iron needed for survival. It also has antiviral activity (HIV, CMV, HSV), acting by interfering with virus absorption and/or penetration.

Bifidus factor

The bifidus factor in human milk promotes the growth of Gram-positive bacilli in the gut flora, particularly *Lactobacillus bifidus*, which discourages the multiplication of pathogens.

Hormones and growth factors

Epidermal growth factor (and insulin-like growth factor) found in breast milk and colostrum stimulate the baby's digestive tract to mature more quickly and strengthen the barrier properties of the gastrointestinal epithelium. Once the initially leaky membrane lining the gut matures, it is less likely to allow the passage of large molecules and becomes less vulnerable to microorganisms. The timing of the first feed also has a significant effect on gut permeability, which drops markedly if the first feed takes place soon after birth.

Management of Breastfeeding

The first feed

Early feeding contributes to the success of breastfeeding. The first feed should be supervised by the midwife. If it proceeds without pain and if the baby is allowed to terminate the feed spontaneously, both mother and baby will have been helped to begin the learning process necessary for good breastfeeding.

Attachment and positioning

There are two main positions for the mother to adopt while she is breastfeeding:

- lying on her side
- sitting up — back upright and at a right angle to her lap.

The baby's body should be *turned towards* the mother's body so that he or she is coming up to her breast at the same angle as her breast is coming down to him (Fig. 29.1). If the baby's nose is opposite the

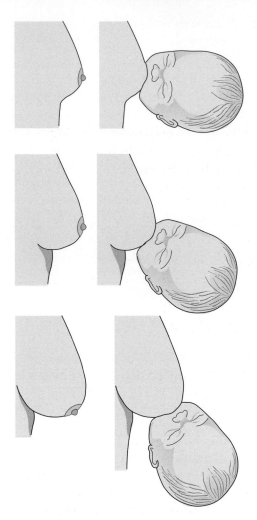

Fig. 29.1 The baby's body in relation to the mother's body, depending on the angle of the breast.
(From an original drawing by Hilary English.)

mother's nipple before the baby is brought to the breast and his/her neck is slightly extended, the baby's mouth will be in the correct relationship to the nipple.

In attaching the baby to the breast:

- the baby should be supported across the shoulders to allow slight extension of the neck
- encourage the baby to open the mouth wide by gently but persistently moving it against the mother's nipple
- aim the bottom lip as far away from the base of the nipple as is possible to draw breast tissue as well as the nipple into the mouth with the tongue
- the baby's lower jaw moves up and down, following the action of the tongue
- swallowing is visible and audible
- the mother may be startled by the physical sensation but should not experience pain.

Feeding behaviour

When babies first go to the breast, they feed vigorously, with few pauses. As the feed progresses, pausing occurs more frequently and lasts longer. Pausing is an integral part of the baby's feeding rhythm and should not be interrupted. The change in the pattern probably relates to milk flow. The fore-milk, which is obtained first, is more generous in quantity but lower in fat than the hind-milk delivered at the end, which is thus higher in calories. An excessive quantity of fore-milk is the most common cause of colic in breastfed babies; the problem is resolved by improving attachment and allowing babies to release the first breast when they have had sufficient milk.

The baby *should be offered* the second breast after being given the opportunity to bring up wind. Sometimes in the early days the baby will not need to feed from the second breast.

Provided that the baby starts each feed on alternate sides, both breasts will be used equally. If the baby does not release the breast or will not settle after a feed, the most likely reason is that he or she was not correctly attached to the breast and was therefore unable to strip the milk efficiently.

Other reasons for coming off the breast are:

- The baby may need to let go and pause if the milk flow is very fast.
- The baby may have swallowed air with the generous flow of milk that occurs at the beginning of a feed and needs an opportunity to burp.

There is no justification for imposing either one breast per feed or both breasts per feed as a feeding regime.

Timing and frequency of feeds

Term babies know better than anyone else how often and for how long they need to be fed.

- It is not unusual in the first day or two for the baby to feed infrequently, and to have 6–8-hour gaps between good feeds, each of which may be quite long. This is normal and provides the mother with the opportunity to sleep if she needs to.
- As the milk volume increases, the feeds tend to become more frequent and a little shorter. It is unusual for a baby to feed less often than six times in 24 hours from the 3rd day, and most babies ask for between six and eight feeds per 24 hours by the time they are a week old.
- Babies who feed infrequently may be consuming less milk than they need, and/or they may be unwell.
- Babies who feed very often (10–12 feeds in 24 hours after the first week) may be poorly attached.

The feeding technique and the weight should be monitored. However mother–baby pairs develop their own unique pattern of feeding and provided the baby is thriving and the mother is happy, there is n need to change it.

Expressing breast milk

Although all breastfeeding mothers should know how to hand-express milk, *routine* expression of the breasts should not be part of the normal management of lactation.

The situations where expressing is appropriate are listed in Box 29.1.

Care of the breasts

- Daily washing is all that is necessary for breast hygiene. The normal skin flora are beneficial to the baby.

- Brassieres may be worn in order to provide comfortable support and are useful if the breasts leak and breast pads (or breast shells) are used.

Breast problems

Sore and damaged nipples

- The cause is almost always trauma from the hard palate of the baby's mouth and tongue, which results from incorrect attachment of the baby to the breast. Correcting this will provide immediate relief from pain and will also allow rapid healing to

---

Box 29.1 Appropriate situations for expressing breast milk

- There is concern about the interval between feeds in the early newborn period (expressed colostrum should always be given in preference to formula to healthy term babies)
- There are problems in attaching the baby to the breast
- The baby is separated from the mother, owing to prematurity or illness
- There is concern about the baby's rate of growth or the mother's milk supply (expressing to top up with the mother's own milk may be necessary in the short term while the cause of the problem is resolved)
- Later in lactation, the mother may need to be separated from her baby for periods (occasionally or regularly)

take place. Epithelial growth factor, contained in fresh human milk and saliva, may aid this process.

■ 'Resting' the nipple is not advised as, although this enables healing to take place, it makes the continuation of lactation much more complicated.

■ Nipple shields should be used with extreme caution, and never before the mother has begun to lactate.

Other causes of soreness

Infection with *Candida albicans* (thrush) can occur, although it is not common during the first week. The sudden development of pain, when the mother has had a period of trouble-free feeding, is suggestive of thrush. The nipple and areola are often inflamed and shiny, and pain typically persists throughout the feed. The baby may show signs of oral or anal thrush. Both mother and baby should receive concurrent fungicidal treatment.

One breast only

It is perfectly possible to feed a baby well using just one breast, as each breast works independently.

Anatomical variations

These are described in Box 29.2.

Problems with breastfeeding

Engorgement

This condition occurs around the 3rd or 4th day postpartum. The breasts are hard (often oedematous), painful and sometimes flushed. The mother may be pyrexial. Engorgement is usually an indication that the baby is not in step with the stage of lactation. Engorgement may occur if feeds are delayed or restricted or if the baby is unable to feed efficiently because he or she is not correctly attached to the breast.

Box 29.2 Anatomical nipple variations

Long nipples

- These can lead to poor feeding because the baby is able to latch on to the nipple without drawing breast tissue into his or her mouth
- The mother may need to be shown how to help the baby to draw in a sufficient portion of the breast

Short nipples

- As the baby has to form a teat from both the breast and nipple, short nipples should not cause problems
- The mother should be reassured

Abnormally large nipples

- If the baby is small, his/her mouth may not be able to get beyond the nipple and on to the breast
- Lactation could be initiated by expressing, either by hand or by pump, provided that the nipple fits into the breast cup
- As the baby grows and the breast and nipple become more protractile, breastfeeding may become possible

Inverted and flat nipples

- If the nipple is deeply inverted it may be necessary to initiate lactation by expressing
- Attempts to attach the baby to the breast are delayed until lactation is established and the breasts have become soft and the breast tissue more protractile

---

Management should be aimed at enabling the baby to feed well. In severe cases the only solution will be hand expression. This will reduce the tension in the breast and *will not* cause excessive milk production. The mother's fluid intake should not be restricted, as this has no direct effect on milk production.

Deep breast pain

In most cases this responds to improvement in breastfeeding technique and is thus likely to be due to raised intraductal pressure caused by inefficient milk removal.

Although it may occur during the feed, it typically occurs afterwards and thus can be distinguished from the sensation of the letdown reflex, which some mothers experience as a fleeting pain. Very rarely, deep breast pain may be the result of ductal thrush infection.

Mastitis

Mastitis means inflammation of the breast. In the majority of cases it is the result of milk stasis, not infection, although infection may supervene. Typically, one or more adjacent segments are inflamed and appear as a wedge-shaped area of redness and swelling. In some cases flu-like symptoms, including shivering attacks or rigors, may occur.

Non-infective (acute intramammary) mastitis

This condition results from milk stasis. It may occur during the early days as the result of unresolved engorgement or at any time when poor feeding technique results in the milk from one or more segments of the breast not being efficiently removed by the baby. It occurs much more frequently in the breast that is opposite the mother's preferred side for holding her baby. It is extremely important that breastfeeding from the affected breast continues; otherwise milk stasis will increase further and provide ideal conditions for pathogenic bacteria to replicate.

Infective mastitis

The main cause of superficial breast infection is damage to the epithelium, which allows bacteria to enter the underlying tissues. The damage results from incorrect attachment of the baby to the breast which has caused trauma to the nipple. The mother therefore urgently needs help to improve her technique, as well as the appropriate antibiotic. Multiplication of bacteria may be enhanced by the use of breast pads or shells. In spite of antibiotic therapy, absces formation may occur. Infection may also enter the breast via the milk ducts if milk stasis remains unresolved.

Breast abscess

A fluctuant swelling develops in a previously inflamed area. Pus may be discharged from the nipple. Simple needle aspiration may be effective or incision and drainage may be necessary. It may not be possible to feed from the affected breast for a few days but milk removal should continue and breastfeeding should recommence as soon as practicable to reduce the chances of further abscess formation. A sinus that drains milk may form but it is likely to heal in time.

Blocked ducts

Lumpy areas in the breast are not uncommon — the mother is usually feeling distended glandular tissue. If they become very firm and tender (and sometimes flushed), they are often described as 'blocked ducts'. The solution is to improve milk removal (improved attachment, and possibly milk expression as well) and to treat the accompanying pain and inflammation. Massage, which is often advocated to clear the imagined 'blockage', may make matters worse by forcing more milk into the surrounding tissue.

White spots

Very occasionally, a ductal opening in the tip of the nipple may become obstructed by a white granule or by epithelial overgrowth.

- White granules appear to be caused by the aggregation and fusion of casein micelles, to which further materials become added. This hardened lump may obstruct a milk duct as it slowly makes its way down to the nipple, where it may be removed by the baby during a feed or expressed manually.
- Epithelial overgrowth seems to be the more common cause of a physical obstruction. A white blister is evident on the surface of the nipple, and it effectively closes off one of the exit points in

the nipple, which leads from one or more milk-producing sections of the breast.

This problem may also be resolved if the baby feeds. Alternatively, after the baby has fed (and the skin is softened), the spot may be removed with a clean fingernail, a rough flannel or a sterile needle.

True blockages of this sort tend to recur, but once the woman understands how to deal with them, progression to mastitis can be avoided.

Feeding difficulties due to the baby

Cleft lip

Provided that the palate is intact, the presence of a cleft in the lip should not interfere with breastfeeding because the vacuum that is necessary to enable the baby to attach to the breast is created between the tongue and the hard palate, not the breast and the lips.

Cleft palate

Babies are only able to obtain milk as the result of the mother's milk ejection reflex. Because of the cleft, the baby is unable to create a vacuum and thus form a teat out of the breast and nipple. The use of an orthodontic plate has limited success. The mother should be encouraged to put the baby to the breast — for comfort, pleasure or food — provided that she is aware that expressed breast milk will also be required.

Tongue-tie

If the baby cannot extend the tongue over the lower gum he or she is unlikely to be able to draw the breast deeply into the mouth, which is necessary for effective feeding. Sometimes this is because the tongue is short, and sometimes this is because the frenulum, the whitish strip of tissue which attaches the tongue to the floor of the mouth, is preventing it. As the baby lifts the tongue, the tip becomes heart-shaped as the frenulum pulls on it.

Blocked nose

Babies normally breathe through their noses. If there is an obstruction, they have great difficulty with feeding because they have to interrupt the process in order to breathe.

Down syndrome

Babies with this condition can be successfully breastfed, although extra help and encouragement may be necessary initially.

Prematurity

Preterm infants who are sufficiently mature to have developed sucking and swallowing reflexes may successfully breastfeed. Babies who are too immature to breastfeed may be able to cup-feed, as an alternative to being tube-fed. Less mature babies who are unable to suck or swallow at all will be dependent on artificial methods such as tube feeding and intravenous alimentation.

Contraindications to breastfeeding

Medication

Breastfeeding may have to be suspended temporarily following the administration of certain drugs or following diagnostic techniques. Breast milk expression must continue to maintain lactation. Most regions have drug centres where advice may be sought about the safety of drugs for lactating women.

Cancer

If the mother has cancer, the treatment she receives will make it impossible to breastfeed without harming the baby. However, if she wishes to, she could express and discard her milk for the duration of the treatment and resume breastfeeding later. If she has had a mastectomy, she may feed successfully from the other breast. Following a lumpectomy for cancer, she may also be able to breastfeed. She should seek advice from her surgeon.

HIV infection

HIV may be transmitted in breast milk.

- In developed countries, where artificial feeding is relatively safe, the mother may be advised not to breastfeed if she is HIV-positive.

- In countries where artificial feeding is a significant cause of infant mortality, exclusive breastfeeding may be the safer option.

Weaning from the breast

- When the mother or the baby decides to stop breastfeeding, feeds should be tailed off gradually.

- Breastfeeds may be omitted, one at a time, and spaced further apart.

- Adding supplementary foods should not begin until about 6 months of age.

- If the mother is using solid food to give the baby 'tastes' and the experience of different textures before weaning, these should be given after the breastfeed. Solid foods given before the breastfeed (weaning) will result in the baby taking less milk from the breast and thus less will be produced.

Complementary and supplementary feeds

Complementary feeds (or 'top-ups') are feeds given *after* a breastfeed Complementary feeds of breast milk substitutes are not recommended, except for medical indications.

- About 10% of newborns are at risk for hypoglycaemia, and may thus need a higher intake straight from birth than their mothers are able to provide. Where possible, this should be human milk, from a human milk bank. Donors will have been serologically tested for HIV and a negative result must be received before their milk can be accepted.

■ Babies who are well but sleepy, jaundiced, unsettled or difficult to attach should, if necessary, be given their mother's own expressed milk in addition to being offered the breast.

If complementary feeds are clinically indicated and the mother is unable to express sufficient milk, donor milk from a human milk bank could be used.

Supplementary feeds are feeds given *in place of* a breastfeed. There can be no justification for their use, except in extreme circumstances (such as severe illness or unconsciousness), because each breastfeed missed by the baby will interfere with the establishment of lactation and damage the mother's confidence.

Artificial feeding

Most breast milk substitutes (infant formula) are modified cow's milk. The two main components used are:

■ skimmed milk (a by-product of butter manufacture)

■ whey (a by-product of cheese manufacture).

Breast milk substitutes may contain fats from any source, animal or vegetable (except from sesame and cotton seeds), provided that they do not contain more than 8% trans-isomers of fatty acids. They may also contain, among other things, soya protein, maltodextrin, dried glucose syrup and gelatinised and precooked starch.

There are two main types of formula:

■ whey dominant

■ casein dominant.

Whey-dominant formulae

A small amount of skimmed milk is combined with demineralised whey. The ratio of proteins in the formulae approximates to the ratio of whey to casein found in human milk (60:40). Whey-dominant formula feeds only should be used up to 6 months. These feeds are more easily digested than the casein-dominant formulae.

Casein-dominant formulae

Although these are sold as being suitable for use from birth, more of the protein present is in the form of casein (20:80), which forms large relatively indigestible curds in the stomach. This will inevitably place greater metabolic demands on the infant.

Babies intolerant of standard formulae

- *Hydrolysate formulae.* If breastfeeding is not possible, there are (prescription-only) alternatives that carry less risk of allergy than standard formulae — hydrolysates — some of which are designed to treat an existing allergy. Others are designed for preventative use in bottle-fed babies who are at high risk of developing cow's milk protein allergy.

- *Whey hydrolysates.* These are made from the whey of cow's milk, (rather than whole milk) and these are potentially more useful for highly allergenic babies.

- *Amino acid-based formulae or elemental formulae.* This has a completely synthetic protein base providing the essential and non-essential amino acids, together with fat, maltodextrin, vitamins minerals and trace elements.

- *Soya-based formulae.* These are no longer recommended because of concerns about the possible effects of phyto-oestrogens compounds and the possibility of unavoidably high levels of manganese and aluminium.

Preparation of an artificial feed

All powdered formula available in the UK is now reconstituted usin 1 scoop (provided with the powder) to 30 ml water. Clear instruc tions about the volumes of powder and water are also printed on th container. Many of the major UK manufacturers of formula no produce ready-to-feed cartons. Reconstituted formula should b prepared as required due to the growth of pathogenic bacteria in stored reconstituted formula.

The water supply

It is essential that the water used is free from bacterial contamination and any harmful chemicals. It is generally assumed in the UK that boiled tap water will meet these criteria, but from time to time this is shown not to be the case. In some areas of the UK, mothers who are artificially feeding their babies have to be provided with a separate supply of water because the tap water is not suitable for babies' consumption.

If bottled water is used, a still, non-mineralised variety suitable for babies must be chosen and it should be boiled as usual. Softened water is usually unsuitable.

Sterilisation of feeding equipment

The effective cleaning of all utensils should be demonstrated and the method of sterilisation discussed.

- If boiling is to be used, full immersion is essential and the contents of the pan must be boiled for 10 minutes.

- If cold sterilisation using a hypochlorite solution is the method of choice, the utensils must be fully immersed in the solution for the recommended time.

- The manufacturer's advice should be followed with regard to rinsing items that have been removed from the solution. If the item is to be rinsed, previously boiled water should be used, not water direct from the tap.

- Both steam and microwave sterilisation is now possible, but the mother should check that her equipment can withstand it.

Bottle teats

The size of the hole in the teat causes much anxiety to mothers. It is probably a good idea to have several teats with holes of different sizes so that they can be changed throughout the feed as necessary. A useful test for the correct hole size is to turn the bottle upside down; the feed should drip at a rate of about one drop per second.

Feeding the baby with the bottle

Mothers should be warned about the dangers of 'bottle propping', and told that the baby must never be left unattended while feeding from a bottle. They should be advised of the need of the baby to relate to a small number of caregivers and that he or she should not be passed from person to person for feeding.

Modern formulae do not, when correctly prepared, cause hypernatraemia. There is therefore no need to give the babies extra water. The stools and vomit of a formula-fed baby have an unpleasant sour smell. The stools tend to be more formed than those of a breastfed baby and, unlike a breastfed baby, there is a real risk that an artificially fed baby may become constipated.

If, in an emergency, artificial feed has to be prepared from liquid pasteurised (doorstep) milk, it should be made as follows:

- two-thirds full cream milk,
- one-third water
- 1 level teaspoonful of sugar.

The milk should be boiled for 2 minutes so as not to over-concentrate it, before adding the previously boiled water and the sugar.

The Baby-Friendly Hospital Initiative

This is an initiative that was launched in 1991 by WHO and UNICEF to encourage hospitals to promote practices that are supportive of breastfeeding. It was focused around the 'Ten Steps' (Box 29.3), with which all hospitals that wish to achieve 'baby-friendly' status must comply. The evidence for the 10 Steps is contained in the WHO document of the same name, published in 1998.

Box 29.3 The Ten Steps

- Have a written breastfeeding policy that is routinely communicated to all health-care staff
- Train all health-care staff in the skills necessary to implement this policy
- Inform all pregnant women about the benefits and management of breastfeeding
- Help mothers initiate breastfeeding soon after birth
- Show mothers how to breastfeed and how to maintain lactation, even if they should be separated from their infants
- Give newborn infants no food or drink other than breast milk, unless medically indicated
- Practise rooming-in, allowing mothers and infants to remain together 24 hours a day
- Encourage breastfeeding on demand
- Give no artificial teats or dummies to breastfeeding infants
- Foster the establishment of breastfeeding support groups and refer mothers to them on discharge from hospital or clinic

Chapter 30

The Healthy Low-Birth-Weight Baby

Classification of Babies by Weight and Gestation

Definitions of low birth weight (LBW) are based upon weight alone and do not consider the gestational age of the baby. Likewise, definitions of gestational age disregard any considerations of birth weight. It is the *relationship* between these two separate considerations of weight (for assessment of growth) and gestational age (for assessment of maturity) that is of great importance and can be plotted on centile charts (Fig. 30.1). Growth charts should be derived from studies of local populations.

Weight

- Low-birth-weight (LBW) babies are those weighing below 2500 g at birth.

- Very low-birth-weight (VLBW) babies are those weighing below 1500 g at birth.

- Extremely low-birth-weight (ELBW) babies are those who weigh under 1000 g at birth.

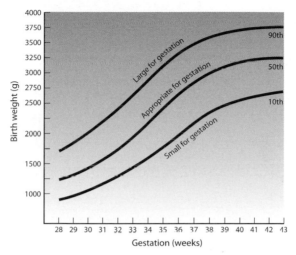

Fig. 30.1 A centile chart, showing weight and gestation.
(From Simpson 1997, with permission of Baillière Tindall.)

Gestational age

A preterm baby is born before completion of the 37th week of gestation, calculated from the first day of the last menstrual period.

Small for gestational age (SGA)

SGA babies are defined as having a birth weight below the 10th centile for gestational age or <2 standard deviations below mean (the 50th centile) for gestational age.

Intrauterine growth restriction (IUGR)

This is failure of normal fetal growth caused by multiple adverse effects on the fetus.

Causes of Intrauterine Growth Restriction

Fetal growth is regulated by maternal, placental and fetal factors and represents a mix of genetic mechanisms and environmental influences through which growth potential is expressed. The mechanisms that appear to limit fetal growth are multifactorial and can be maternal, fetal or placental, although several factors might be interrelated.

Asymmetric growth (sometimes called acute)

Fetal weight is reduced out of proportion to length and head circumference. This is thought to be caused by extrinsic factors, such as pregnancy-induced hypertension, that adversely affect fetal nutrition.

Appearance

See Box 30.1.

Symmetric growth (chronic)

This is due either to decreased growth potential of the fetus as a result of congenital infection or chromosomal/genetic defects (intrinsic), or to extrinsic factors that are active early in gestational life (e.g. the

---

Box 30.1 Appearance of the baby with asymmetric intrauterine growth restriction

- Head looks disproportionately large compared to the body
- Head circumference is usually within normal parameters
- Bones are within gestational norms for length and density
- Anterior fontanelle may be larger than expected, due to diminished membranous bone formation
- Abdomen looks 'scaphoid', or sunken due to shrinkage of the liver and spleen
- There is decreased subcutaneous fat deposition
- Skin is loose, which can give the baby a wizened, old appearance
- Vernix caseosa is frequently reduced or absent as a result of diminished skin perfusion
- Unless severely affected, these babies appear hyperactive and hungry with a lusty cry

---

effects of maternal smoking or poor dietary intake), or a combination of both intrinsic and extrinsic factors.

Appearance

See Box 30.2.

Symmetric growth (genetically small) babies are small normal babies and should be treated in accordance with their gestational age.

The Preterm Baby

Birth occurs before the end of the 37th gestational week, regardless of birth weight. Most of these babies are appropriately grown; some are SGA, while a small number are LGA. (These tend to be babies of mothers with diabetes.) See Box 30.3 for causes of preterm labour.

Characteristics of the preterm baby

The appearance at birth of the preterm baby will depend upon gestational age (Box 30.4).

Box 30.2 Appearance of the baby with symmetric intrauterine growth restriction

- Head circumference, length and weight are all proportionately reduced for gestational age
- Babies are diminutive in size
- They do not appear wasted, and have subcutaneous fat appropriate for their size
- Skin is taut
- Babies are generally vigorous and less likely to be hypoglycaemic or polycythaemic
- They may suffer major congenital abnormalities and can be a source of infection to carers, as a result of transplacental infection

---

Box 30.3 Causes of preterm labour

Spontaneous causes

- 40% unknown
- Multiple gestation
- Hyperpyrexia as a result of viral or bacterial infection
- Premature rupture of the membranes caused by maternal infection
- Maternal short stature
- Maternal age and parity.
- Poor obstetric history; history of preterm labour
- Cervical incompetence
- Poor social circumstances

Elective causes

- Pregnancy-induced hypertension, pre-eclampsia, chronic hypertension
- Maternal disease: renal, cardiac
- Placenta praevia, abruptio placenta
- Rhesus incompatibility
- Congenital abnormality
- IUGR

Box 30.4 Appearance of the preterm baby

- Posture appears flattened with hips abducted, knees and ankles flexed
- Babies are generally hypotonic with a weak and feeble cry
- Head is in proportion to the body
- The skull bones are soft with large fontanelles and wide sutures
- Chest is small and narrow and appears under-developed due to minimal lung expansion during fetal life
- Abdomen is prominent because the liver and spleen are large and abdominal muscle tone is poor
- Umbilicus appears low in the abdomen because linear growth is cephalocaudal (more apparent nearer to the head than the feet)

(Continued

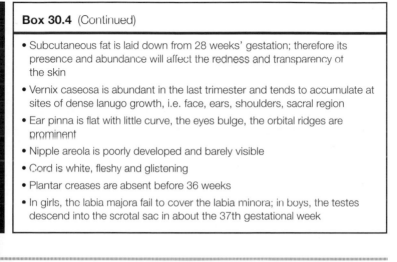

Box 30.4 (Continued)

- Subcutaneous fat is laid down from 28 weeks' gestation; therefore its presence and abundance will affect the redness and transparency of the skin
- Vernix caseosa is abundant in the last trimester and tends to accumulate at sites of dense lanugo growth, i.e. face, ears, shoulders, sacral region
- Ear pinna is flat with little curve, the eyes bulge, the orbital ridges are prominent
- Nipple areola is poorly developed and barely visible
- Cord is white, fleshy and glistening
- Plantar creases are absent before 36 weeks
- In girls, the labia majora fail to cover the labia minora; in boys, the testes descend into the scrotal sac in about the 37th gestational week

Management at Birth of the Healthy Low-Birth-Weight Baby

- Current cot availability in the NICU, transitional care unit (as applicable) and postnatal ward should be known.
- The ambient temperature of the delivery room should ideally be between 23°C and 25°C.
- The neonatal resuscitaire should be checked and ready for use.
- A second person skilled in resuscitation skills should be present.
- On cutting the cord, leave an extra length, in case access to the umbilical vessels be necessary later.
- The Apgar score is traditionally scored at 1 and 5 minutes.
- Labelling of the LBW baby is particularly important because separation of mother and baby could happen at any time if the baby's condition becomes unstable.
- A detailed but expedient examination of the baby should be carried out.

- Once it is established that the baby is healthy, the midwife may attempt to normalise care by emphasising to the parents the importance of preventing cold stress and promoting skin-to-skin contact for a period of up to 50 minutes.

- Ensure that the baby is thoroughly dried before skin-to-skin contact is attempted.

- The baby's axilla temperature should be maintained between 36.5°C and 37.3°C.

Care of the Healthy Low-Birth-Weight Baby

Many of the care issues relevant to the LBW baby apply to both the preterm and SGA infant.

Principles of thermoregulation

Thermoregulation is the balance between heat production and heat loss. The prevention of cold stress, which may lead to hypothermia (body temperature <36°C), is critical for the intact survival of the LBW baby. Newborn babies are unable to shiver, move very much or ask for an extra blanket, and therefore rely upon physical adaptations that generate heat by raising their basal metabolic rate and utilising brown fat deposits. As body temperature falls, tissue oxygen consumption rises as the baby attempts to raise its metabolic rate by burning glucose to generate energy and heat. Care measures should aim to provide an environment that supports thermoneutrality.

Thermoregulation and the healthy mature SGA baby

- Rapid heat loss due to the large head to body ratio and large surface area is exaggerated, particularly in the asymmetrically grown SGA baby.

- Wide sutures and large fontanelles add to the heat-losing tendency.

- These babies often have depleted stores of subcutaneous fat, which is used for insulation. Their raised basal metabolic rate helps them to produce heat, but their high energy demands in the presence of poor glycogen stores and minimal fat deposition can soon lead to hypoglycaemia and then hypothermia.

- Once the baby is thoroughly dried, a prewarmed hat will minimise heat loss from the head.

Thermoregulation and the healthy preterm baby

- All preterm babies are prone to heat loss because their ability to produce heat is compromised by their immaturity, so factors like their large surface area to weight ratio, their varying amounts of subcutaneous fat and their ability to mobilise brown fat stores will be affected by their gestational age.

- During cooling, the immature heat-regulating centres in the hypothalamus and medulla oblongata fail, to different degrees, to recognise and marshal adequately coordinated homeostatic controls.

- Preterm babies are often unable to increase their oxygen consumption effectively through normal respiratory function, and their calorific intake is often inadequate to meet increasing metabolic requirements.

- Furthermore, their open resting postures increase their surface area and insensible water losses.

- Babies under 2.0 kg may need incubator care when the baby is not in skin-to-skin contact with either parent. The warm conditions in an incubator can be achieved either by heating the air to 30–32°C (air mode) or by servo-controlling the baby's body temperature at a desired set point (36°C). In servo mode, a thermocouple is taped to the upper abdomen and the incubator heater maintains the skin at that site to a preset constant. Babies are clothed with bedding, in a room temperature of 26°C.

- Most preterm babies between 2.0 and 2.5 kg will be cared for in a cot, in a room temperature of 24°C.

Hypoglycaemia and the healthy LBW baby

- Hypoglycaemia refers to a low blood glucose concentration; it is more likely to occur in conditions where babies become cold or where the initiation of early feeding (within the first hour), is delayed.

- The aim is to maintain the true blood sugar above 2.6 mmol/dl. However, this does not mean that every LBW baby should be *routinely* screened. Well LBW babies who show no clinical signs of hypoglycaemia, are demanding and taking nutritive feeds on a regular basis, and are maintaining their body temperature do not need screening for hypoglycaemia.

- If a baby, despite being fed, presents with clinical signs of hypoglycaemia, a venous sample should be taken by the paediatrician to assess true blood sugar.

- A blood glucose that remains <2.6 mmol/dl, despite the baby's further attempts to feed by breast or to take colostrum by cup, may warrant transfer to the NICU, because glucose by intravenous bolus may be necessary to correct the metabolic disturbance.

- In addition, consideration should be given as to whether there may be some underlying medical condition.

Hypoglycemia and the healthy mature SGA baby

- Asymmetrically grown babies have reduced glycogen stores in liver and skeletal muscles.

- Their greater brain to body mass and a tendency towards polycythaemia increase their energy demands, which in turn increases glucose requirements.

- Mature SGA babies with an asymmetric growth pattern will usually feed within the first half an hour of birth and demand feeds 2–3-hourly thereafter.

- Their susceptibility to hypoglycaemia is relatively short-lived and is limited to the first 48 hours following birth.

■ If the baby is taking formula milk, feeds are usually calculated at 90 ml/kg on the first day, with 30 ml increments per day thereafter.

Hypoglycaemia and the preterm baby

■ The preterm baby may be sleepier, and attempts to take the first feed may reflect gestational age.

■ Total feed requirements (60 ml/kg on the first day, with 30 ml/kg increments per day thereafter) may not be taken directly from the breast and supplementary feeds can be given by cup.

Feeding the low-birth-weight baby

Both preterm and SGA babies benefit from human milk because it contains long-chain polyunsaturated omega 3 fatty acids, which are thought to be essential for the myelination of neural membranes and retinal development. Preterm breast milk has:

■ a higher concentration of lipids, protein, sodium, calcium and immunoglobulins

■ a low osmolarity

■ lipases and enzymes that improve digestion and absorption.

Sucking and swallowing reflexes are present by 28 weeks' gestation, but the baby is unable to coordinate these activities until 34–36 weeks. Preterm babies are limited in their ability to suck by their weak musculature and flexor control, which is important for firm lip and jaw closure. Before 32 weeks, most healthy preterm babies will need to be tube-fed on a regular basis, usually on a 3-hourly regime with breast milk, hind-milk or formula milk.

Tube feeding has the advantage that the tube can be left in situ during a cup feed or breastfeed and has been shown to eliminate the need to introduce bottles into a breastfeeding regime. However, several problems have been identified with tube feeding:

■ Nasal and oral gastric tubes encourage milk lipid adherence to their inside surfaces and reduce the amount of fat calories available to the baby.

- Babies are preferential nose breathers and the presence of a nasogastric tube will take up part of their available airway.

- Prolonged use has been associated with delay in the development of sucking and swallowing reflexes simply because the mouth is bypassed.

Cup feeding has been used therefore in favour of tube feeding:

- to provide the baby with a positive oral experience

- to stimulate saliva and lingual lipases to aid digestion

- to accelerate the transition from naso/oral gastric feeding to breastfeeding without the introduction of bottles and teats.

Certain behaviours, such as licking and lapping, are well established *before* sucking and swallowing.

- Babies between 30 and 32 weeks' gestation can be given expressed breast milk (EBM) by cup.

- Between 32 and 34 weeks' gestation, cup feeding can act as the main method of feeding, with the baby taking occasional complete breastfeeds.

- From 35 weeks onwards, cup feeding can be gradually replaced by complete breastfeeding.

An unrushed feed can take up to an hour to complete. Feeding frequency can vary between 6 and 10 feeds per day.

The Care Environment: Promoting Health and Development

The ideal environment should provide a cycle of day and night, regular nourishment, rest, stimulation and loving attention. The mother desire to be involved is seen as an *essential* element in the success caring for LBW babies on postnatal wards.

Handling and touch

Kangaroo care (KC) is used to promote closeness between a baby and mother and involves placing the nappy-clad baby upright between the maternal breasts for skin-to-skin contact. The LBW baby remains beneath the mother's clothing for varying periods of time that suit the mother.

Noise and light hazards

- Noise should be kept to a minimum.
- In dimmed lighting conditions, preterm babies are more able to improve their quality of sleep and alert status.
- Reduced light levels at night will help to promote the development of circadian rhythms and diurnal cycles.
- Screens to shield adjacent babies from phototherapy lights are essential.

Sleeping position

Preterm babies have reduced muscle power and bulk, with flaccid muscle tone; therefore their movements are erratic, weak or flailing. Without support they may, to differing degrees, develop head, shoulder and hip flattening, which in turn can lead to poor mobility.

- Nesting the more immature preterm babies into soft bedding, in addition to the use of close flexible boundaries, helps to keep their limbs in midline flexion.
- However, it is vital that they are nursed in a supine position to prevent asphyxia.

Sudden infant death syndrome (SIDS)

There is a need to remind parents constantly of the risk factors and safety procedures (feet-to-foot sleeping position, smoke-free room) associated with SIDS, alongside teaching them to keep their babies warm. However, the Health Education Council leaflet, 'Don't let your infant get too hot', may cause some confusion. The midwife needs to explain how the issues apply to individual families and take into consideration time of year, gestational age and postnatal age when care is transferred to the community midwife. Parental training on 'what to do if my baby stops breathing' should be offered to parents but the decision to receive training should be their choice.

The prevention of infection

LBW babies, particularly preterm ones, are especially vulnerable to infections caused by immaturity of their host defence systems.

The provision of neonatal care: the question of venue and facilities

The decision to transfer a healthy LBW baby to a postnatal ward, a transitional unit or a NICU will depend upon the baby's gestational age and weight. In addition, the availability of facilities and level of staffing are also taken into account.

Chapter 31

Recognising the Ill Baby

Assessment of the Infant

Immediately after birth, all infants should be examined for any gross congenital abnormalities or evidence of birth trauma. They should also have their weight and gestational age plotted on a standard growth chart.

History

Maternal health

Any disease in the mother can have an effect on the pregnancy. Influencing factors include:

- pregnancy-induced hypertension
- history of epilepsy
- maternal diabetes
- history of substance abuse
- history of sexually transmitted diseases.

Fetal well-being and health

The following are examples of significant questions that a midwife may ask herself, as they may have a critical influence on the well-being of the infant:

- What was the estimated date of birth?
- Was this a twin pregnancy?
- Was the baby presenting by the breech?
- Is the baby preterm?
- Is the infant SGA?
- Was there poor growth in utero?
- Was any evidence of congenital abnormality picked up on scanning, such as enlarged heart or bowel obstruction?

Perinatal and birth complications

Labour and birth may also have an effect on the general welfare of the newborn infant in the following ways:

- prolonged rupture of membranes
- abnormal fetal heart rate pattern
- meconium staining
- difficult or rapid birth
- caesarean section and the reason for this.

Physical Assessment

The skin

The presence of meconium on the skin, usually seen in the nail bed and around the umbilicus, is frequently associated with infants who have cardiorespiratory problems. The skin of all babies should be examined for:

- pallor
- plethora

- cyanosis
- jaundice
- rashes.

Pallor

A pale, mottled baby is an indication of poor peripheral perfusion. At birth this can be associated with low circulating blood volume or with circulatory adaptation and compensation for perinatal hypoxaemia. The anaemic infant's appearance is usually pale pink, white or in severe cases where there is vascular collapse, grey. Other presenting signs are:

- tachycardia
- tachypnoea
- poor capillary refill.

The most likely causes of anaemia in the newborn period are listed in Box 31.1.

Pallor can also be observed in infants who are hypothermic or hypoglycaemic. Problems associated with pallor include:

- anaemia and shock
- respiratory disorders
- cardiac anomalies
- sepsis (where poor peripheral perfusion might also be observed).

Box 31.1 Common causes of anaemia in the newborn period

- A history in the infant of haemolytic disease of the newborn
- Twin-to-twin transfusions in utero (which can cause one infant to be anaemic and the other polycythaemic)
- Maternal antepartum or intrapartum haemorrhage

Plethora

The baby's colour may indicate an excess of circulating red blood cells (polycythaemia). This is defined as a venous haematocrit greater than 70%. Newborn infants can become polycythaemic if they are recipients of:

- twin-to-twin transfusion in utero
- a large placental transfusion.

Other infants at risk are:

- SGA babies
- infants of diabetic mothers
- babies with Down syndrome
- neonatal hypothyroidism.

Hypoglycaemia is commonly seen in plethoric infants because red blood cells consume glucose. The infant can exhibit a neurological disorder; irritability, jitteriness and convulsions can occur. Other problems that may manifest are:

- apnoea
- respiratory distress
- cardiac failure
- necrotising enterocolitis.

Cyanosis

The mucous membranes are the most reliable indicators of central colour in all babies, and if the tongue and mucous membrane appear blue, this indicates low oxygen saturation levels in the blood usually of respiratory or cardiac origin. Episodic central cyanotic attacks may be an indication that the infant is having a convulsion. Peripheral cyanosis of the hands and feet is common during the first 24 hours of life; after this time it may be a non-specific sign of illness.

Jaundice (see ch. 35)

Early-onset jaundice (occurring in the skin and sclera within the first 12 hours of life) is abnormal and needs investigating. If a jaundiced baby is unduly lethargic, is a poor feeder, vomits or has an unstable body temperature, this may indicate infection and action should be taken to exclude this.

Surface lesions and rashes

Rashes (Box 31.2) are quite common in newborn babies but most are benign and self-limiting.

Box 31.2 Surface lesions and rashes in the newborn baby

Milia

- White or yellow papules seen over the cheeks, nose and forehead
- Invariably disappear spontaneously over the first few weeks of life

Miliaria

- Clear vesicles on the face, scalp and perineum, caused by retention of sweat in unopened sweat glands
- Appear on the chest and around areas where clothes can cause friction
- Treatment is to care for the infant in a cooler environment or remove excess clothing

Petechiae or purpura rash

- Can occur in neonatal thrombocytopenia, a condition of platelet deficiency that usually presents with a petechial rash over the whole of the body
- There may also be prolonged bleeding from puncture sites and/or the umbilicus and bleeding into the gut
- Thrombocytopenia may be found in infants with:
  Congenital infections, both viral and bacterial
  Maternal idiopathic thrombocytopenia

(Continued)

Box 31.2 (Continued)

Drugs (administered to mother or infant)

Severe Rhesus haemolytic disease

Bruising

- Can occur extensively following breech extractions, forceps and ventouse deliveries
- Bleeding can cause a decrease in circulating blood volume, predisposing the infant to anaemia or, if the bruising is severe, hypotension

Erythema toxicum

- A rash that consists of white papules on an erythematous base
- Occurs in about 30–70% of infants
- Is benign and should not be confused with a staphylococcal infection, which will require antibiotics
- Diagnosis can be confirmed by examination of a smear of aspirate from a pustule, which will show numerous eosinophils (white cells indicative of an allergic response, rather than infection)

Thrush

- A fungal infection of the mouth and throat
- Very common in neonates, especially if they have been treated with antibiotics
- Presents as white patches seen over the tongue and mucous membranes and as a red rash on the perineum

Herpes simplex virus

- If acquired in the neonatal period, this is a most serious viral infection
- Transmission in utero is rare; the infection usually occurs during birth
- 70% of affected infants will produce a rash, which appears as vesicles or pustules

Umbilical sepsis

- Can be caused by a bacterial infection
- Until its separation, the umbilical cord can be a focus for infection by bacteria that colonise the skin of the newborn
- If periumbilical redness occurs or a discharge is noted, it may be necessary to commence antibiotic therapy in order to prevent an ascending infection

Bullous impetigo

- A condition which makes the skin look as though it has been scalded
- Caused by streptococci or staphylococci

Box 31.2 (Continued)

- Presents as widespread tender erythema, followed by blisters that break, leaving raw areas of skin
- Particularly noticeable around the napkin area but may also cause umbilical sepsis, breast abscesses, conjunctivitis and, in deep infections, involvement of the bones and joints

Other factors that affect the appearance of the skin

If the infant is dehydrated, the skin looks dry and pale and is often cool to touch. If gently pinched, it will be slow in retracting. Other signs of dehydration are pallor or mottled skin, sunken fontanelle or eyeball sockets, and tachycardia.

Respiratory system

It is important to observe the baby's breathing when he or she is at rest and when active. The midwife should always start by observing skin colour and then carry out a respiratory inspection, taking into account whether the baby is making either an extra effort or insufficient effort to breathe.

Respiratory inspection

The respiration rate should be between 30 and 60 breaths per minute but will vary between levels of activity. Newborn infants are primarily nose breathers and obstructions of the nares may lead to respiratory distress and cyanosis. The chest should expand symmetrically. If there is unilateral expansion and breath sounds are diminished on one side, this may indicate that a pneumothorax has occurred. Infants at risk of pneumothorax or other air leaks are:

- preterm infants with respiratory distress
- term infants with meconium-stained amniotic fluid
- infants who require resuscitation at birth.

Increased work of breathing

- Tachypnoea is an abnormal respiratory rate at rest above 60 breaths per minute.

- Note any inspiratory pulling in of the chest wall above and below the sternum or between the ribs (retraction).

- If nasal flaring is also present, this may indicate that there has been a delay in the lung fluid clearance or that a more serious respiratory problem is developing.

- Grunting, heard either with a stethoscope or audibly, is an abnormal expiratory sound. The grunting baby forcibly exhales against a closed glottis in order to prevent the alveoli from collapsing.

These infants may require help with their breathing, either by intubation or continuous positive airway pressure ventilation (CPAP).

Apnoea

Apnoea is cessation of breathing for 20 seconds or more. It is associated with pallor, bradycardia, cyanosis, oxygen desaturation or a change in the level of consciousness.

Disorders that can cause apnoea, other than the type found in preterm babies, are listed in Box 31.3.

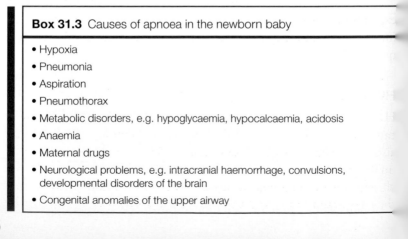

Box 31.3 Causes of apnoea in the newborn baby

- Hypoxia
- Pneumonia
- Aspiration
- Pneumothorax
- Metabolic disorders, e.g. hypoglycaemia, hypocalcaemia, acidosis
- Anaemia
- Maternal drugs
- Neurological problems, e.g. intracranial haemorrhage, convulsions, developmental disorders of the brain
- Congenital anomalies of the upper airway

Body temperature

The normal body temperature range for term infants is a skin temperature of 36.5–37.3°C.

Hypothermia

Hypothermia is defined as a core temperature below 36°C. This can cause complications such as:

- increased oxygen consumption
- lactic acid production
- apnoea
- decrease in blood coagulability
- hypoglycaemia (most common).

In preterm infants, cold stress may also cause a decrease in surfactant secretion and synthesis.

When neonates are exposed to cold, they will at first become very restless; then, as their body temperature falls, they adopt a tightly flexed position to try to conserve heat. The sick or preterm infant will tend to lie supine in a frog-like position with all surfaces exposed, which maximises heat loss.

Hypoglycaemia is a common feature of infants with increased energy expenditure associated with thermoregulation and this can cause the infant to have jittery movements of the limbs, even though he or she is quiet and often limp.

Hyperthermia

Hyperthermia is defined as a core temperature above 38°C. The usual cause of hyperthermia is overheating of the environment but it can also be a clinical sign of sepsis, brain injury or drug therapy. If infants are too warm, they become restless and may have bright red cheeks. They will attempt to regulate their temperature by increasing their respiratory rate, and this can lead to an increased fluid loss by

evaporation through the airways. Other problems caused by hyperthermia are:

- hypernatraemia
- jaundice
- recurrent apnoea.

Cardiovascular system

The normal heart rate of a newborn baby is 110–160 bpm with an
average of 130 bpm. Cardiovascular dysfunction should be suspected
in infants who commonly present with lethargy and breathlessness
during feeding.

It can be very difficult to identify infants with congenital heart disease because the clinical picture of tachycardia, tachypnoea, pallor or
cyanosis may be suggestive of a respiratory problem or sepsis.

Persistent pulmonary hypertension of the newborn is usually seen in
term or post-term infants who have a history of hypoxia or asphyxia at
birth. The infants are slow to take their first breath or are difficult to
ventilate. Respiratory distress and cyanosis are seen before 12 hours of
age. Hypoxaemia is usually profound and may suggest cyanotic heart
disease. Risk factors include:

- meconium-stained amniotic fluid
- nuchal cord
- placental abruption
- acute blood loss
- maternal sedation.

Cyanosis can be a prominent feature in some cardiac defects but no
all. Box 31.4 lists signs that may be indicative of congenital hear
disease.

Cardiac shock may resemble early septicaemia, pneumonia or men
ingitis. The first indication of an underlying cardiac lesion may be th
presence of a murmur heard on routine examination. However, a sof

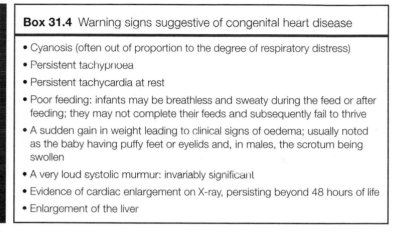

> **Box 31.4** Warning signs suggestive of congenital heart disease
>
> - Cyanosis (often out of proportion to the degree of respiratory distress)
> - Persistent tachypnoea
> - Persistent tachycardia at rest
> - Poor feeding: infants may be breathless and sweaty during the feed or after feeding; they may not complete their feeds and subsequently fail to thrive
> - A sudden gain in weight leading to clinical signs of oedema; usually noted as the baby having puffy feet or eyelids and, in males, the scrotum being swollen
> - A very loud systolic murmur: invariably significant
> - Evidence of cardiac enlargement on X-ray, persisting beyond 48 hours of life
> - Enlargement of the liver

localised systolic murmur with no evidence of any symptoms of cardiac disease is usually of no significance.

Central nervous system

Abnormal postures, which include neck retraction, frog-like postures, hyperextension or hyperflexion of the limbs or jittery or abnormal involuntary movements, along with a high-pitched or weak cry, could be indicative of neurological impairment and need investigation.

Neurological disorders

Neurological disorders found at or soon after birth may be either prenatal or perinatal in origin. They include:

- congenital abnormalities: hydrocephaly, microcephaly, encephalocele, chromosomal anomalies
- hypoxic–ischaemic cerebral injuries
- birth traumas: skull fractures, spinal cord and brachial plexus injuries, subdural and subarachnoid haemorrhage
- infections passed on to the fetus (toxoplasmosis, rubella, cytomegalovirus (CMV), syphilis).

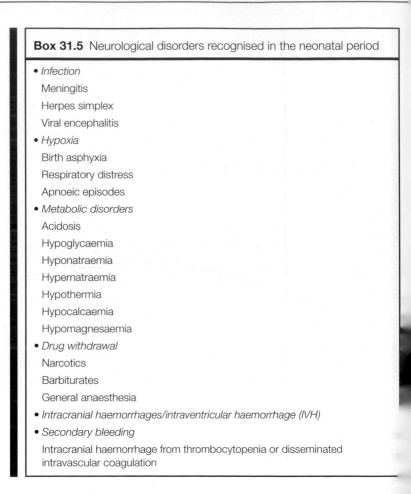

Box 31.5 Neurological disorders recognised in the neonatal period

- *Infection*
  Meningitis
  Herpes simplex
  Viral encephalitis
- *Hypoxia*
  Birth asphyxia
  Respiratory distress
  Apnoeic episodes
- *Metabolic disorders*
  Acidosis
  Hypoglycaemia
  Hyponatraemia
  Hypernatraemia
  Hypothermia
  Hypocalcaemia
  Hypomagnesaemia
- *Drug withdrawal*
  Narcotics
  Barbiturates
  General anaesthesia
- *Intracranial haemorrhages/intraventricular haemorrhage (IVH)*
- *Secondary bleeding*
  Intracranial haemorrhage from thrombocytopenia or disseminated intravascular coagulation

Neurological disorders that appear in the neonatal period need to be recognised promptly in order to minimise brain damage. The most common are listed in Box 31.5.

Seizures

Seizures in the newborn period can be extremely difficult to diagnose, as they are often very subtle and easily missed (Table 31.1).

Table 31.1 Neonatal seizure chart

Type	Affected infants
Subtle	
Apnoea usually seen with abnormal eye movements, tonic horizontal deviation, blinking, fluttering eyelids, jerking, drooling, sucking, tonic posturing or unusual movements of limbs (rowing, pedalling or swimming)	Most frequent type and most common in preterm infants
Clonic	
Jerking activity	
Multifocal: movements of one body part followed by encephalopathy or inborn errors of metabolism	Term infants: hypoxic–ischaemic
Focal: movement of one part	Disturbance of the entire cerebrum
Tonic	
Posturing similar to decerebrate posture in adults	Preterm infants with intraventricular haemorrhage
Myoclonic	
Single or multiple jerks of upper and lower extremities	Possible prediction of myoclonic spasms in early infancy

The most common causes of seizure activity are:

- asphyxia
- metabolic disturbance
- intracranial/intraventricular haemorrhage
- infection
- malformation/genetic defect.

Hypotonia (floppy infant)

The term hypotonia describes the loss of body tension and tone. As a result, the infant adopts an abnormal posture which is noticeable on handling.

The causes of hypotonia include:

- maternal sedation
- birth asphyxia
- prematurity
- infection
- Down syndrome
- metabolic problems, e.g. hypoglycaemia, hyponatraemia, inborn errors of metabolism
- neurological problems, e.g. spinal cord injuries (sustained by difficult breech or forceps delivery), myasthenia gravis related to maternal disease, myotonic dystrophy
- endocrine, e.g. hypothyroidism
- neuromuscular disorders.

Renal/genitourinary system

Urinary infections typically present with lethargy, poor feeding, increasing jaundice and vomiting. Urine that only dribbles out, rather than being passed forcefully, may be an indication of a problem with posterior urethral valves. Urine that is cloudy in appearance or smelly may be an indication of a urinary tract infection.

Renal problems may present as a failure to pass urine. The normal infant usually passes urine 4–10 hours after birth. Normal urine output for a term baby in the first day of life should be 2–4 ml/kg/hour. Urine output of less than 1 ml/kg/hour (oliguria) should be investigated.

Common causes of reduced urine output include:

- inadequate fluid intake
- increased fluid loss due to hyperthermia, use of radiant heaters and phototherapy units
- birth asphyxia
- congenital abnormalities
- infection.

Gastrointestinal tract

Oesophageal atresia can be diagnosed antenatally because the fetus is unable to swallow the amniotic fluid, giving rise to polyhydramnios in the mother. If, however, the condition is not identified antenatally, the infant usually presents with copious saliva, which causes gagging, choking, pallor or cyanosis. In infants who are inadvertently fed milk this may cause a severe respiratory arrest due to milk aspiration.

Intestinal obstructions may be caused by atresias, malformations or structural damage anywhere below the stomach. In the newborn period, gastrointestinal disorders often present with:

- vomiting
- abdominal distension
- failure to pass stools
- diarrhoea with or without blood in the stools.

However, vomiting in the postnatal period can be caused by factors other than gastrointestinal obstructions. Early vomiting may be caused by the infant swallowing meconium or maternal blood at delivery. This can cause a gastritis, which will eventually settle. Some infants may require a gastric lavage if the symptoms are severe.

All vomit should be checked for the presence of bile or blood. Observe the infant for other signs such as abdominal distension, watery or blood-stained stools and temperature instability.

The infant who has an infection can often display signs of gastrointestinal problems, usually poor feeding, vomiting and/or diarrhoea. Diarrhoea caused by gastroenteritis is usually very watery and may sometimes resemble urine. Loose stools can also be a feature of infants being treated for hyperbilirubinaemia with phototherapy.

Some of the more commonly seen gastrointestinal problems include:

- duodenal atresia
- malrotation of the gut
- volvulus

- meconium ileus
- necrotising enterocolitis
- imperforate anus
- rectal fistulas
- Hirschsprung's disease.

Duodenal atresia

Duodenal atresia usually presents with bile-stained vomiting within 24 hours of birth. Abdominal distension is not usually present, but often visible peristalsis is seen over the stomach. Insertion of a nasogastric tube may reveal a large amount of bile in the stomach and there is usually a history of polyhydramnios and a delay in passing meconium.

Malrotation of the gut

Malrotation may present as a mechanical bowel obstruction caused by the abnormal attachments (Ladd's bands). The infant usually has no problems in the first few days of life, then presents with bilious vomiting and abdominal distension.

Volvulus

Volvulus can occur in infants who have an incomplete rotation of the gut. Diagnosis can be delayed because the obstruction is intermittent, twisting enough to cause obstruction, then untwisting causing relief. As a result of venous impairment and mucosal injury, there may be blood passed per rectum. Bilious vomiting also occurs. These infants are commonly gravely ill.

Meconium ileus

The infant with meconium ileus often has cystic fibrosis. Clinical signs include marked abdominal distension. Meconium is not passed, but occasionally small pellet-type stools, pale in colour, are mistakenly identified as bowel action. Vomiting gradually increases, mainly gastric secretions and feed, but later becomes bilious.

Necrotising enterocolitis (NEC)

NEC is an acquired disease of the small and large intestine caused by ischaemia of the intestinal mucosa. It occurs more often in preterm infants, but may also occur in term infants who have been asphyxiated at birth or infants with polycythaemia and hypothermia (commonly found in SGA infants). NEC may present with vomiting or, if gastric emptying is being monitored, the aspirate is large and bile-stained. The abdomen becomes distended, while stools are loose and may have blood in them. In the early stages of NEC, the infant can display non-specific signs of temperature instability, unstable glucose levels, lethargy and poor peripheral circulation. As the illness progresses, the infant becomes apnoeic and bradycardic and may need ventilating.

Imperforate anus

All infants should be checked at birth for this.

Rectal fistulas

The midwife should look for the presence of meconium in the urine, or in female infants, meconium being passed per vaginam.

Hirschsprung's disease

Hirschsprung's disease should be suspected in term infants with delayed passage of meconium, certainly beyond the first 24 hours of life. It is caused by an absence of ganglion cells in the distal rectum. The area of aganglionosis varies and may include the lower rectum, colon and small intestine. An incomplete obstruction occurs above the affected segment. Abdominal distension and vomiting are clinical signs, with the vomit becoming bile-stained if meconium is not passed.

Metabolic disorders (see ch. 36)

Metabolic disorders, such as galactosaemia and phenylketonuria, present in the newborn period with vomiting, weight loss, jaundice and lethargy.

Chapter 32

Respiratory Problems

Pathophysiology

Anatomical influences

Neonates are susceptible to respiratory compromise resulting from:

- Their stage of lung development and contributing lack of maturation in the other body systems. The gestation of the baby at birth has implications for their susceptibility to some disease processes, like hyaline membrane disease (HMD), in which surfactant production is inhibited.

- An increased work of breathing owing to the high compliance of the neonatal lung, which results from the cartilaginous nature of the rib structure. This flexibility allows for some collapse of the airways with each breath, which would not occur with a rigid rib structure. Subsequently, with each breath, the baby needs to generate larger pressures within the lung to prevent respiratory compromise through airway collapse.

- An altered diaphragmatic muscle structure from the adult. The neonatal diaphragm is more susceptible to fatigue due to the composition and location of the muscle within the neonatal chest

- The size of neonatal airways. This is smaller, which generates higher resistance to airflow and a smaller area through which perfusion can occur.
- The tendency for pulmonary blood flow to bypass areas of hypoxia, across the alveolar bed, consequently reducing alveolar perfusion.

Signs of respiratory compromise

These are listed in Box 32.1.

Box 32.1 Signs of respiratory compromise

Grunting
- An audible noise heard on expiration
- Appears when there is the partial closure of the glottis as the breath is expired
- The baby is attempting to preserve some internal lung pressure and prevent the airways from collapsing at the end of the breath

Retractions
- Chest distortions occur due to an increase in the need to create higher inspiratory pressures in a compliant chest
- Appear as intercostal, subcostal or sternal recession across the thorax

Asynchrony
- The breathing appears as a 'see-saw' pattern as the abdominal movements and the diaphragm work out of unison
- A result of increased muscle fatigue and the compliant chest wall

Tachypnoea
- This is a compensatory rise in the respiratory rate (above 60 breaths per minute) initiated from the respiratory centre and aims to remove the hypoxia and hypercarbia

Nasal flaring
- An attempt to minimise the effect of the airway's resistance by maximising the diameter of the upper airways
- The nares are seen to flare open with each breath

(Continued)

> **Box 32.1** (Continued)
>
> **Apnoea**
> - Occurs as the conclusion of increasing respiratory fatigue in the term baby
> - The preterm baby may experience apnoea of prematurity due to the immature respiratory centre, as well as apnoea from respiratory fatigue

Common Respiratory Problems

Pneumothorax

Pneumothoraces are known to occur spontaneously in 1% of the newborn population either during or after birth; however, only one-tenth of this 1% will be symptomatic. The cause at birth is the result of the large pressures generated by the baby's first breaths. These may range up to 40–80 cm of water. This leads to alveolar distension and rupture, allowing air to leak to a number of sites of which the potential space between the lung pleura is one.

Babies receiving assisted ventilation also have an increased susceptibility to a pneumothorax due to:

- maldistribution of the ventilated gas in the lungs
- high ventilation settings
- infant–ventilator breathing interactions.

Presumptive diagnosis:

- reduced breath sounds on the affected side
- displaced heart sounds
- distorted chest/diaphragm movement with respiration
- distension of the chest on the affected side.

Emergency treatment involves either a needle aspiration or the placement of a chest drain.

Transient tachypnoea of the newborn (TTN)

TTN is frequently seen as a diagnosis of exclusion of other possible respiratory causes. The chest X-ray may show a streaky appearance with fluid apparent in the horizontal fissure, confirming the diagnosis and also accounting for the colloquialism of 'wet lung'.

The most common predisposing factor for TTN is a caesarean section, as the thorax has not been squeezed whilst the baby descends along the birth canal. This results in lower thoracic pressures after birth. Although these babies require initial care on a neonatal unit, their stay is usually of a short duration with the provision of oxygen and observation.

Infection/pneumonia

Pneumonia in the neonate is difficult to diagnose, as secretions are difficult to obtain and the radiological appearances can be hard to distinguish.

- Pneumonia presenting before 48 hours of age has normally been acquired either at or before birth
- Presentation after 48 hours indicates infection resulting from hospitalisation.

All infants with infection require antibiotics.

Meconium aspiration syndrome

A baby can develop meconium aspiration syndrome if stimulated to breathe or gasp, either before or after birth, if there is meconium in the airway that could be inhaled.

- The initial respiratory distress may be mild, moderate or severe, with a gradual deterioration over the first 12–24 hours in moderate or severe cases.
- The meconium becomes trapped in the airways and causes a ball-valve effect; the air can get in and the meconium blocks the airway during expiration, causing an accumulation of air behind the blockage.

- This accumulation can then lead to rupture of the alveoli and cause the baby to develop a pneumothorax.
- Where the meconium has contact with the lung tissue, a pneumonitis occurs.
- The surfactant is also broken down in the presence of meconium.

These factors combine with a previously hypoxic infant to produce a severe disease process. These babies will need full intensive care and ventilation to prevent further deterioration.

Respiratory distress syndrome (RDS)

RDS occurs as a result of insufficient production of surfactant, seen most frequently after a premature birth; however, other disorders such as maternal diabetes or meconium aspiration syndrome can also inhibit surfactant production. Surfactant is produced to reduce the surface tension within the alveoli, preventing their collapse at the end of exhalation. It is much harder to inflate collapsed alveoli, in terms of the pressure and exertion required, than to reinflate partially collapsed alveoli.

Diagnosis involves the following:

- Increasing respiratory distress and work of breathing are noted.
- The X-ray shows a ground glass appearance across the lung fields, whilst severe disease is represented by a 'white-out' (Fig. 32.1).

Treatment includes:

- oxygen therapy
- surfactant administration directly into the lungs
- ventilatory support for the most severely affected.

Cardiac Disease

Cardiac defects (Box 32.2), whilst not a respiratory disease, presen with respiratory symptoms.

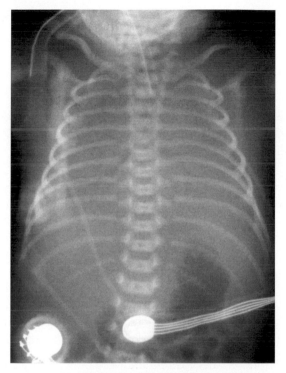

Fig. 32.1 X-ray showing the lungs of a baby with respiratory distress syndrome.

Box 32.2 Cardiac lesions

Right-sided lesions

- The most frequently seen lesions are transposition of the great arteries, tetralogy of Fallot and pulmonary atresia or stenosis

- These infants typically present as 'blue' babies. On examination there is little to note other than the presence of cyanosis

- Their respiratory distress, if present, is mild and consists of tachypnoea alone

- These babies will remain cyanotic in the presence of 100% oxygen

(Continued)

Box 32.2 (Continued)

Left-sided lesions

- The most frequently seen left-sided lesions are hypoplastic left heart syndrome and coarctation of the aorta
- These frequently present with neonatal heart failure
- Initially, the baby may appear irritable, lethargic, sweaty and uninterested in feeding
- The presence of 'effortless' tachypnoea may be seen, characterised by the lack of any other sign of respiratory compromise; for example, no grunting is heard, there is no head bobbing and recession is minimal
- As the heart failure progresses, the infant shows signs of cardiogenic shock and will go on to require full resuscitative measures if left unsupported

---

When a cardiac condition is suspected, common practice involves the administration of an infusion of prostaglandin to maintain the patency of the arterial duct. This may then necessitate the elective intubation and ventilation of a baby who has previously appeared to be breathing adequately without assistance. This assisted mechanical ventilation is provided without oxygen, even if the saturation monitor records saturation percentages in the eighties or seventies, as additional oxygen can stimulate the arterial duct to close. The patency of the arterial duct is needed to keep the blood flowing through the heart and around the peripheral circulation.

Care of the Respiratorily Compromised Baby

Respiratory care

The following assist in observations of the baby:

- saturation monitors
- transcutaneous monitors
- arterial catheter readings.

When satisfactory oxygenation is not being achieved, additional oxygen can be delivered:

- via a nasal cannula
- into a headbox
- from high-frequency oscillation (HFOV)
- by conventional mechanical ventilation (CMV)
- with continuous positive airway pressure (CPAP).

Some ventilation techniques are available at specialised centres only. These include continuous negative end-expiratory pressure (CNEEP) and extra corporeal membrane oxygenation (ECMO).

Cardiovascular support

Cardiac failure in a neonate is rare, as the majority of arrests are respiratory in origin. However, neonates may require support to maintain a normal heart rate or stroke volume. Maintenance of an adequate blood pressure — for example, the mean equivalent to the gestational age — may need pharmaceutical support whilst a bradycardia (a heart rate below 80) may be a sign of various influences such as a blocked endotracheal tube or sepsis.

Occasionally, the transition from a fetal to an adult circulation is compromised and the baby develops persistent pulmonary hypertension of the newborn. The use of nitric oxide as the vasodilator, delivered with the ventilation gases, works directly upon the pulmonary vessels with minimal effect on the systemic circulation.

Nutrition and hydration

A preterm baby has few nutritional reserves and will need supplementation soon after birth to meet the continual demand for glucose from the brain. Whilst the ideal would be to establish oral breast milk feeding, this is not possible for a sick neonate, as the presence of the endotracheal tube or the absence of a suck reflex prevents oral feeding.

The majority of infants will receive a glucose-based intravenous infusion. This allows milk feeds to be given via a nasogastric, orogastric or nasojejunal tube, increasing the volumes as the baby's condition allows. Sick or immature babies need a cautious introduction to milk, whether expressed breast milk or formula feeds, as they are susceptible to necrotising enterocolitis (NEC). When it is expected to take more than 4–5 days before full feeding is established, total parenteral nutrition (TPN) is needed to ensure all nutritional requirements can be met. Whilst some babies may need TPN for many weeks, it can have some undesirable side-effects upon the liver, giving rise to a conjugated hyperbilirubinaemia or cholestasis. Prolonged TPN is sometimes needed in very immature babies with gastroschisis and those with NEC.

The causes of NEC are multifactorial:

- Delayed feeding causes a lowered immune response to potential pathogens.
- Administration of antibiotics can alter the dominant gut flora, as can formula milk.
- Bacterial infection can occur following episodes of hypoxia.
- Polycythaemia reduces the arterial blood flow through the mesenteric circulation and causes mucosal ischaemia; reperfusion leads to oedema, haemorrhage, ulceration and necrosis.

Signs and symptoms include:

- a painful distended abdomen
- blood in the stool
- poor feed tolerance
- air within the gut wall, leading to a perforation, hypovolaemic shock or disseminated intravascular coagulation.

Treatment involves:

- antibiotics and medical management initially
- surgery if there is a perforation or a failure to respond to the medical therapy.

The disease can be fatal; long-term problems for those who do recover can include short gut syndrome and gut stenosis.

A safe environment

The respiratorily compromised baby needs all its energy to maintain satisfactory oxygenation and hence particular care is needed to:

■ protect from infection

■ maintain a thermoneutral environment

■ minimise stressors

■ detect and treat pain and distress.

The family

The midwife and neonatal staff have important roles in assisting parental attachment by maintaining regular, reliable and effective communication about the baby and giving advice on how parents can participate in the baby's care.

Chapter 33

Trauma during Birth, Haemorrhage and Convulsions

Trauma to Skin and Superficial Tissues

Skin

Damage to the skin may result from forceps blades, vacuum extractor cups, scalp electrodes and scalpels.

- Abrasions and lacerations should be kept clean and dry.
- If there are signs of infection, antibiotics may be required.
- Deeper lacerations may require closure with butterfly strips or sutures.

Superficial tissues

Trauma to soft tissue involves oedematous swellings and/or bruising. The oedema consists of serum and blood (serosanguineous fluid).

Caput succedaneum

This is an oedematous swelling under the scalp and above the periosteum (Fig. 33.1 and Box 33.1). A 'false' caput succedaneum ca

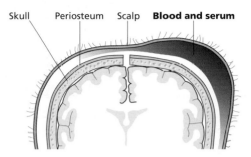

Skull   Periosteum   Scalp   **Blood and serum**

Fig. 33.1 Caput succedaneum.

Box 33.1 Features of a caput succedaneum

- Is present at birth
- Does not usually enlarge
- Can 'pit' on pressure
- Can cross a suture line
- Involves oedema that may move to the dependent area of the scalp
- Usually resolves by 36 hours of life
- Has no longer-term consequences

also occur if a vacuum extractor cup is used; the resulting oedematous deformity is known as a 'chignon'.

The baby will usually experience some discomfort.

Other injury

When the face presents, it becomes congested and bruised, and the eyes and lips become oedematous. In a breech presentation the fetus will develop bruised and oedematous genitalia and buttocks.

Uncomplicated oedema and bruising usually resolve within a few days of life. However, if there is significant trauma during a vaginal breech birth, there can be serious complications such as:

- hyperbilirubinaemia
- excessive blood loss, resulting in hypovolaemia, shock, anaemia and disseminated intravascular coagulation

■ damage to muscles, resulting in difficulties with micturition and defecation.

Muscle trauma

Injuries to muscle result from tearing or from disruption of the blood supply.

Torticollis

Excessive traction or twisting can cause tearing to one of the sternomastoid muscles during the birth of the anterior shoulder of a fetus with a cephalic presentation, or during rotation of the shoulders when the fetus is being born by vaginal breech. A small lump can be felt on the affected sternomastoid muscle. It appears painless for the baby. The muscle length is shortened; therefore the neck is twisted on the affected side.

The management of torticollis involves stretching of the affected muscle, achieved under the guidance of a physiotherapist. The swelling will usually resolve over several weeks.

Nerve trauma

Commonly, there is trauma to the facial nerve or to the brachial plexus nerves.

Facial nerve

Damage to the facial nerve usually results from its compression against the ramus of the mandible by a forceps blade, resulting in a unilateral facial palsy. The eyelid on the affected side remains open and the mouth is drawn over to the normal side. If the baby cannot form an effective seal on the breast or teat, there may be some initial feeding difficulties. Spontaneous resolution usually occurs within 7–10 days.

Brachial plexus

Trauma to this group of nerves usually results from excessive lateral flexion, rotation or traction of the head and neck during vaginal breech birth or when shoulder dystocia occurs. These injuries can be unilateral or bilateral. There are three main types of injury:

- *Erb's palsy.* There is damage to the upper brachial plexus involving the fifth and sixth cervical nerve roots. The baby's affected arm is inwardly rotated, the elbow is extended, the wrist is pronated and flexed, and the hand is partially closed. This is commonly known as the 'waiter's tip position'. The arm is limp, although some movement of the fingers and arm is possible.

- *Klumpke's palsy.* There is damage to the lower brachial plexus involving the seventh and eighth cervical and the first thoracic nerve roots. The upper arm has normal movement but the lower arm, wrist and hand are affected. There is wrist drop and flaccid paralysis of the hand with no grasp reflex.

- *Total brachial plexus palsy.* There is damage to all brachial plexus nerve roots with complete paralysis of the arm and hand, lack of sensation and circulatory problems. If there is bilateral paralysis, spinal injury should be suspected.

All types of brachial plexus trauma will require further investigations such as X-ray and ultrasound scanning (USS), and assessment of the joints. Passive movements of the joints and limb can then be initiated under the direction of a physiotherapist. At approximately 1 month of age, magnetic resonance imaging (MRI) can offer specific data on nerve damage.

Spontaneous recovery within days to weeks is expected for most babies. Follow-up is recommended. Babies with no functional recovery by 4 months of age may require surgical repair.

Fractures

Fractures are rare but the most commonly affected bones are:

- clavicle
- humerus

- femur
- skull bones.

Haemorrhage

Haemorrhage can be due to:

- trauma
- disruptions in blood flow

or can be related to:

- coagulopathies
- other causes.

Blood volume in the term baby is approximately 80–100 ml/kg and in the preterm baby 90–105 ml/kg; therefore even a small haemorrhage can be potentially fatal.

Haemorrhage due to trauma

Cephalhaematoma

A cephalhaematoma is an effusion of blood under the periosteum that covers the skull bones (Fig. 33.2 and Box 33.2). During a vaginal

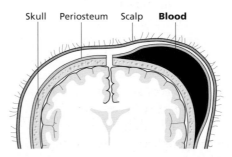

Fig. 33.2 Cephalhaematoma.

> **Box 33.2** Features of a cephalhaematoma
>
> - Is not present at birth
> - Appears after 12 hours
> - Involves swelling that grows larger over subsequent days and can persist for weeks
> - Is circumscribed and firm
> - Does not pit on pressure
> - Does not cross a suture and is fixed

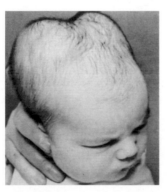

Fig. 33.3 Bilateral cephalhaematoma.

birth, if there is friction between the fetal skull and the maternal pelvic bones, such as in cephalopelvic disproportion or precipitate labour, the periosteum is torn from the bone, causing bleeding underneath. Cephalhaematomas can also be caused during vacuum-assisted births. More than one bone may be affected, causing multiple cephalhaematomas to develop (Fig. 33.3).

No treatment is necessary and the swelling subsides when the blood is reabsorbed. Erythrocyte breakdown in the extravasated blood may result in hyperbilirubinaemia. A ridge of bone may later be felt round the periphery of the swelling, owing to the accumulation of osteoblasts.

Subaponeurotic and subdural haemorrhage

Less common types of haemorrhage due to trauma are:

- subaponeurotic haemorrhage
- subdural haemorrhage.

These are usually associated with precipitate or difficult births or instrumental deliveries. The most common cause of subdural haemorrhage in a term baby is a tentorial tear.

Haemorrhage due to disruptions in blood flow

Subarachnoid haemorrhage

- A primary subarachnoid haemorrhage involves bleeding directly into the subarachnoid space. Preterm babies, those who suffer hypoxia at birth and term babies who suffer traumatic births are vulnerable.
- A secondary haemorrhage involves the leakage of blood into the subarachnoid space from an intraventricular haemorrhage.

The baby may have generalised convulsions from the second day of life and preterm babies may have apnoeic episodes; otherwise they appear normal and some exhibit no signs. If a lumbar puncture is performed, the cerebrospinal fluid will be uniformly blood-stained. Management involves control of the consequences of asphyxia and of convulsions. The condition is usually self-limiting.

Periventricular/intraventricular haemorrhage

Periventricular/intraventricular haemorrhage (PVH/IVH) primarily affects babies of less than 32 weeks' gestation and those weighing less than 1500 g, although term babies can be affected.

- A small PVH can have a 'silent' onset and is only detectable on USS.
- If the haemorrhage is larger or extends, the clinical features may gradually appear and worsen. These may include apnoeic episodes.

which become more frequent and severe, episodes of bradycardia, pallor, falling haematocrit, tense anterior fontanelle, metabolic acidosis and convulsions. The baby may be limp or unresponsive.

■ If the PVH/IVH is large and sudden in onset, the baby may present with apnoea and circulatory collapse.

The care of at-risk babies is focused on prevention of PVH/IVH: for example, antenatal administration of steroids to the mother, artificial surfactant after birth or antibiotic therapy in the management of preterm premature rupture of the membranes.

The neurological prognosis for babies with small haemorrhages is usually good. Babies who suffer a massive haemorrhage may die within 48 hours of the onset and those who survive are likely to develop significant neurological and intellectual impairment.

Haemorrhage related to coagulopathies

These haemorrhages occur because of a disruption in the baby's blood-clotting abilities.

Vitamin K deficiency bleeding

Vitamin K deficiency bleeding (VKDB) can occur up to 12 months of age, although it more commonly occurs between birth and 8 weeks of life. Several proteins require vitamin K to be converted into active clotting factors. A deficiency of vitamin K leads to a deficiency of these clotting factors and resultant bleeding. Neonates are deficient in vitamin K and therefore vulnerable to VKDB.

■ Early VKDB (first 24 hours) is rare and principally affects babies born to women who, during pregnancy, have taken warfarin, phenobarbital or phenytoin for treatment of their medical conditions. Babies who are more susceptible to developing classical VKDB (1–7 days) are listed in Box 33.3.

■ Late VKDB (1–12 months) almost exclusively occurs in breastfed babies. However, babies who have liver disease or a condition

> **Box 33.3** Babies susceptible to vitamin K deficiency bleeding
>
> - Those who have experienced birth trauma
> - Those who have experienced asphyxia
> - Those who have experienced postnatal hypoxia
> - Those who are preterm
> - Those who are of low birth weight
> - Those who have been given antibiotic therapy
> - Those who cannot maintain enteral feeding or feed poorly

that disrupts the absorption of vitamin K_1 from the bowel — for example, cystic fibrosis — may develop late VKDB.

Bleeding may be evident superficially as bruising or haemorrhage from the umbilicus, puncture sites, the nose and the scalp. Severe jaundice for more than 1 week and persistent jaundice for more than 2 weeks are warning signs. Gastrointestinal bleeding is manifested as melaena and haematemesis. In early and late VKDB, there may be serious extracranial and intracranial bleeding. With severe haemorrhage, circulatory collapse occurs. Diagnosis is confirmed by blood tests.

Babies who have VKDB require careful investigation and monitoring to assess their need for treatment. With all forms of VKDB, the baby will require administration of vitamin K_1, 1–2 mg intramuscularly. VKDB is a potentially fatal condition; therefore prophylactic administration of vitamin K has become the norm in many countries. However, there is debate about the need for vitamin K_1 prophylaxis for 'normal risk' babies and about the most appropriate route of administration.

Current evidence recommends:

- a single 1 mg dose of vitamin K_1 intramuscularly at birth

or

- oral administration on the first day and between 4 and 7 days of life; if the baby is breastfed, a further dose is required at 30 days.

Box 33.4 Babies susceptible to thrombocytopenia

- Those who have a severe congenital or acquired infection, e.g. syphilis, CMV, rubella, toxoplasmosis or bacterial infection
- Those whose mother has idiopathic thrombocytopenia, purpura, systemic lupus erythematosus or thyrotoxicosis
- Those whose mother takes thiazide diuretics
- Those who have isoimmune thrombocytopenia
- Those who have inherited thrombocytopenia

Thrombocytopenia

Thrombocytopenia is a low count of circulating platelets ($<100\,000/\mu L$). Babies who are at risk are listed in Box 33.4.

A petechial rash appears soon after birth, presenting in a mild case with a few localised petechiae. In a severe case there is widespread and serious haemorrhage from multiple sites. Diagnosis is based on history, clinical examination and the presence of a reduced platelet count.

- In mild cases no treatment is required.

- In immune-mediated thrombocytopenia, intravenous immunoglobulin administration is helpful.

- In severe cases, where there is haemorrhage and a very low platelet count, transfusion of platelet concentrate may be required.

Disseminated intravascular coagulation (consumptive coagulopathy)

Disseminated intravascular coagulation (DIC) is an acquired coagulation disorder associated with the release of thromboplastin from damaged tissue, stimulating abnormal coagulation and fibrinolysis.

Inherited coagulation factor deficiencies

The X-linked recessive conditions such as haemophilia (factor VIII deficiency) and Christmas disease (factor IX deficiency) rarely cause problems in the neonatal period but may present with excessive bleeding after birth trauma or surgical intervention, such as circumcision.

Haemorrhage related to other causes

Umbilical haemorrhage

This usually occurs as a result of a poorly applied cord ligature. A purse-string suture should always be inserted if umbilical bleeding does not stop after 15 or 20 minutes.

Vaginal bleeding

A small temporary discharge of blood-stained mucus occurring in the first days of life, often referred to as pseudomenstruation, is due to the withdrawal of maternal oestrogen.

Haematemesis and melaena

These signs usually present when the baby has swallowed maternal blood during birth or from cracked nipples during breastfeeding. The diagnosis must be differentiated from other serious causes.

- If the cause is swallowed blood, the condition is self-limiting, requiring no specific treatment.
- However, if the cause is cracked nipples, appropriate treatment for the mother must be implemented.

Haematuria

Haematuria can be associated with coagulopathies, urinary tract infections and structural abnormality of the urinary tract. Birth trauma may cause renal contusion and haematuria. Occasionally, after suprapubic aspiration of urine, transient mild haematuria may be observed. Treatment of the primary cause should resolve the haematuria.

Convulsions

A convulsion is a sign of neurological disturbance, not a disease. It can present quite differently in the neonate and can be difficult to recognise.

Convulsive movement can be differentiated from jitteriness or tremors in that, with the latter two, the movements:

- are rapid, rhythmic and equal
- are often stimulated or made worse by disturbance
- can be stopped by touching or flexing the affected limb
- are normal in an active, hungry baby and are usually of no consequence, although their occurrence should be documented.

Convulsive movements:

- tend to be slower and less equal
- are not necessarily stimulated by disturbance
- cannot be stopped by restraint
- are always pathological.

Subtle convulsions include movements such as:

- blinking or fluttering of the eyelids
- staring
- clonic movements of the chin
- horizontal or downward movements of the eyes
- sucking
- drooling
- sticking the tongue out
- cycling movements of the legs
- apnoea.

Both term and preterm babies can experience subtle convulsions. These movements should be differentiated from the normal ones associated with rapid eye movement sleep.

If the baby has tonic convulsions, there will be:

- extension or flexion of the limbs
- altered patterns of breathing
- maintenance of eye deviations.

Tonic convulsions are more common in preterm babies.

Term babies demonstrate multifocal clonic convulsions and the movements include random jerking movements of the extremities.

Term babies also experience focal clonic convulsions in which localised repetitive clonic jerking movements are seen. An extremity, a limb or a localised muscle group can be affected.

Myoclonic convulsions are the least common but affect term and preterm babies. The movements are single or multiple flexion jerks of the feet, legs, hands or arms, which should not be confused with similar movements in a sleeping baby.

During a convulsion the baby may have:

- tachycardia
- hypertension
- raised cerebral blood flow
- raised intracranial pressure.

All of these predispose to serious complications.

There are many conditions that cause newborn convulsions, as shown in Table 33.1.

Immediate treatment of a convulsion involves:

- seeking the assistance of a doctor
- ensuring a clear airway and adequate ventilation
- turning the baby to the semiprone position, with the head neither hyperflexed nor hyperextended.

The prognosis depends on the cause of convulsion, the type of convulsion and the EEG tracing.

Table 33.1 Selected causes of neonatal convulsions

Category	Selected causes
Central nervous system	Intracranial haemorrhage
	Intracerebral haemorrhage
	Hypoxic–ischaemic encephalopathy
	Kernicterus
	Congenital abnormalities
Metabolic	Hypo- and hyperglycaemia
	Hypo- and hypercalcaemia
	Hypo- and hypernatraemia
	Inborn errors of metabolism
Other	Hypoxia
	Congenital infections
	Severe postnatally acquired infections
	Neonatal abstinence syndrome
	Hyperthermia
Idiopathic	Unknown

Chapter 34

Congenital Abnormalities

Definition and Causes

By definition, a congenital abnormality is any defect in form, structure or function that is present at birth. Identifiable defects can be categorised in four ways:

- chromosome and gene abnormalities
- teratogenic causes
- multifactorial causes
- unknown causes.

Chromosome and gene abnormalities

Each human cell carries 44 chromosomes (autosomes) and two sex chromosomes. Each chromosome comprises a number of genes. The fertilised zygote should have 22 autosomes and one sex chromosome from each parent.

Genetic disorders (Mendelian inheritance)

Genes are composed of DNA and each is concerned with the transmission of one specific hereditary factor. Genetically inherited factors may be dominant or recessive.

- *A dominant gene* will produce its effect even if present in only one chromosome of a pair. An autosomal dominant condition can usually be traced through several generations: for example, achondroplasia, osteogenesis imperfecta, adult polycystic kidney disease or Huntington's chorea.

- *A recessive gene* needs to be present in both chromosomes before producing its effect: for example, cystic fibrosis or phenylketonuria.

- *In an X-linked recessive inheritance* the condition affects males almost exclusively, although females can be carriers. X-linked recessive inheritance is responsible for conditions such as haemophilia A and B and Duchenne muscular dystrophy.

Teratogenic causes

A teratogen is any agent that raises the incidence of congenital abnormality. The list of known and suspected teratogens is continually growing (Box 34.1).

Multifactorial causes

These stem from a genetic defect in addition to one or more teratogenic influences.

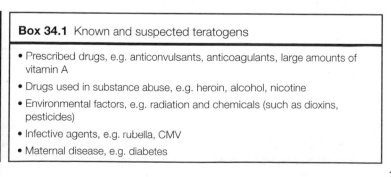

Box 34.1 Known and suspected teratogens

- Prescribed drugs, e.g. anticonvulsants, anticoagulants, large amounts of vitamin A
- Drugs used in substance abuse, e.g. heroin, alcohol, nicotine
- Environmental factors, e.g. radiation and chemicals (such as dioxins, pesticides)
- Infective agents, e.g. rubella, CMV
- Maternal disease, e.g. diabetes

Unknown causes

In spite of a growing body of knowledge, the specific cause of around 80% of abnormalities remains unspecified.

Fetal alcohol syndrome

The following characteristics are recognisable:

- a growth-restricted infant with microcephaly
- flat facies
- close-set eyes
- epicanthic folds
- small upturned nose
- thin upper lip
- low-set ears.

Being able to establishing a direct link between a teratogen and a complex clinical pattern such as this is the exception rather than the rule.

Gastrointestinal Malformations

Most of the abnormalities affecting this system call for prompt surgical intervention.

Gastroschisis and exomphalos

Gastroschisis (Fig. 34.1) is a paramedian defect of the abdominal wall with extrusion of bowel that is not covered by peritoneum.

Exomphalos (Fig. 34.2) or omphalocele is when the bowel or other viscera protrude through the umbilicus. Very often, these babies have other abnormalities: for example, heart defects.

Immediate management of both is as follows:

- Cover the herniated abdominal contents with clean cellophane wrap (Clingfilm) or warm sterile saline swabs.
- Aspirate stomach contents.

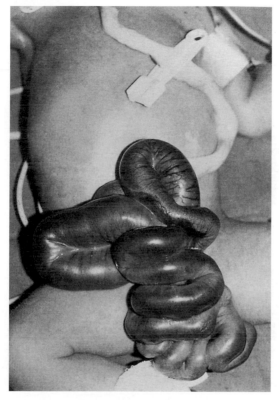

Fig. 34.1 Gastroschisis showing prolapsed intestine to the right of the umbilical cord. (From Rennie & Roberton 1999, with permission of Churchill Livingstone.)

- Reduce heat loss.
- Expedite transfer to a surgical unit.

Atresias

Oesophageal atresia

Oesophageal atresia occurs when there is incomplete canalisation of the oesophagus in early intrauterine development. It is commonly

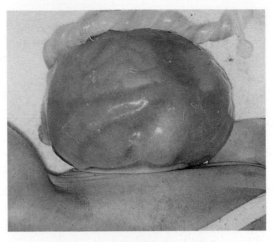

Fig. 34.2 Omphalocele defect with bowel visible through sac in the lower part and abnormally lobulated liver in the sac in the upper part.
(From Rennie & Roberton 1999, with permission of Churchill Livingstone.)

associated with tracheo-oesophageal fistula. The most common type of abnormality is where the upper oesophagus terminates in a blind upper pouch and the lower oesophagus connects to the trachea. This abnormality should be suspected in the presence of maternal polyhydramnios. At birth the baby has copious amounts of mucus coming from the mouth.

- The midwife should attempt to pass a wide orogastric tube but it may travel less than 10–12 cm.

- Radiography will confirm the diagnosis.

- The baby must be given no oral fluid but a wide-bore oesophageal tube should be passed into the upper pouch and connected to gentle continuous suction. Usually a double-lumen 10fg (replogle) tube is used and the baby nursed head-up.

- He or she should be transferred immediately to a paediatric surgical unit and continuous suction must be available throughout the transfer.

Duodenal atresia

This is persistent vomiting within 24–36 hours of birth.

A characteristic double bubble of gas may be seen on radiological examination. Prognosis is good if the baby is otherwise healthy, but this abnormality is often associated with other problems, such as Down syndrome.

Rectal atresia and imperforate anus

An imperforate anus should be obvious at birth on examination of the baby but a rectal atresia might not become apparent until it is noted that the baby has not passed meconium.

Should a baby fail to pass meconium in the first 24 hours, three other possibilities should be considered:

- malrotation/volvulus
- meconium ileus (cystic fibrosis)
- Hirschsprung's disease.

Pyloric stenosis

Pyloric stenosis arises from a genetic defect which causes hypertrophy of the muscles of the pyloric sphincter. The characteristic clinical presentation is projectile vomiting, usually around 6 weeks of age but possibly earlier.

Cleft lip and cleft palate

Cleft lip may be unilateral or bilateral and is very often accompanied by cleft palate.

Clefts may affect the hard palate, soft palate, or both. Some defects will include alveolar margins and sometimes the uvula. The palate is examined by means of a good light source rather than by digital palpation.

- If the defect is limited to unilateral cleft lip, mothers who had intended to breastfeed should be encouraged to do so.

- Where there is the additional problem of cleft palate, arranging for the baby to be fitted with an orthodontic plate may facilitate breastfeeding but this obviously does not afford the same stimulus as nipple to palate contact.

- Cup or spoon feeding is an alternative method, and for those who wish to bottle-feed there is a wide variety of specially shaped teats available to accommodate the different sizes and positions of palate defects.

Pierre Robin syndrome

Pierre Robin syndrome is characterised by micrognathia (hypoplasia of the lower jaw), abnormal attachment of muscles controlling the tongue, which allows it to fall backward and occlude the airway, and a central cleft palate. Maintenance of a clear airway is paramount. In order to achieve this, the baby is nursed prone and some may require the insertion of an oral airway. Nasal and nasopharyngeal constant positive airways pressure may be necessary for some time after birth. This is one of the few exceptions to the rules given in the 'Back to sleep' campaign, which is aimed at reducing cot deaths. Feeding can be problematic. There is a high risk of aspiration occurring. Suction catheter and oxygen equipment should be ready to hand. An orthodontic plate may be fitted to facilitate feeding.

Abnormalities Relating to Respiration

Diaphragmatic hernia

This abnormality consists of a defect in the diaphragm, which allow herniation of abdominal contents into the thoracic cavity. The exten to which lung development is compromised as a result depends o the size of the defect and the gestational age at which herniation first occurred.

At birth:

- the baby is cyanosed
- difficulty is experienced in resuscitation
- heart sounds may be displaced to the right
- the abdomen may have a flat or scaphoid appearance.

Chest X-ray will confirm the diagnosis. Continuous gastric suction should be commenced. Prognosis relates to the degree of pulmonary hypoplasia. There is also the possibility of coexistent abnormalities, such as cardiac defects or skeletal anomalies.

Choanal atresia (Fig. 34.3)

Choanal atresia describes a unilateral or bilateral narrowing of the nasal passage(s) with a web of tissue or bone occluding the nasopharynx. Tachypnoea and dyspnoea are cardinal features, particularly when a bilateral lesion is present.

Diagnosis rests on the following criteria:

- The baby mouth-breathes and finds feeding impossible without cyanosis.
- Nasal catheters cannot be passed into the pharynx.
- If a mirror or cold spoon is held under the nose, no steam will collect.
- The baby's colour will improve with crying.
- Maintaining a clear airway is essential; an oral airway may have to be used to effect this.

Laryngeal stridor

This is a noise made by the baby, usually on inspiration; it is exacerbated by crying. Most commonly, the cause is laryngomalacia, which is due to laxity of the laryngeal cartilage. The stridor may take up to

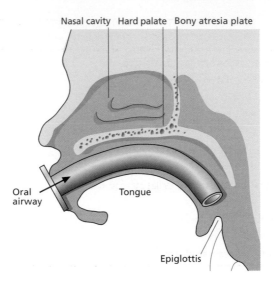

Fig. 34.3 Choanal atresia.
A bony plate blocks the nose. (From Rennie & Roberton 1999, with permission of Churchill Livingstone.)

2 years to resolve. If it is accompanied by signs of dyspnoea or feeding problems, further investigations such as bronchoscopy or laryngoscopy become necessary to rule out a more sinister cause.

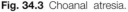

Congenital Cardiac Defects

Postnatal recognition

Clinically, babies with cardiac anomalies can be divided into two groups: those with central cyanosis and those without, i.e. cyanotic and acyanotic congenital heart disease.

Cardiac defects presenting with cyanosis

Defects included in this group are listed in Box 34.2 in order of frequency.

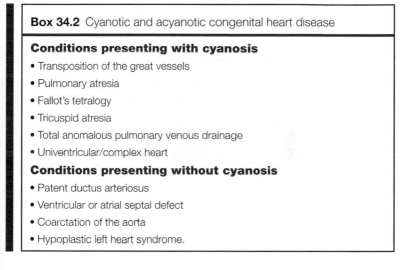

Box 34.2 Cyanotic and acyanotic congenital heart disease

Conditions presenting with cyanosis

- Transposition of the great vessels
- Pulmonary atresia
- Fallot's tetralogy
- Tricuspid atresia
- Total anomalous pulmonary venous drainage
- Univentricular/complex heart

Conditions presenting without cyanosis

- Patent ductus arteriosus
- Ventricular or atrial septal defect
- Coarctation of the aorta
- Hypoplastic left heart syndrome.

The persistence of central cyanosis (that is, cyanosis of the lips and mucous membranes), tachypnoea and tachycardia may be the first signs that a cardiac defect is present. If there is cyanosis, administration of oxygen to these babies will be ineffective in improving their colour and oxygen saturation monitoring will show no improvement. Indeed, giving 100% oxygen may encourage closure of the ductus arteriosus, the patency of which is literally a lifeline for some of these babies.

Acyanotic cardiac defects

Anomalies subsumed under this heading are listed in Box 34.2 in order of frequency.

Signs of cardiac failure

Signs of cardiac failure include:

- tachypnoea
- tachycardia
- incipient cyanosis, especially following the exertion of crying or feeding.

These signs will become more evident, sometimes dramatically so, with the closure of the ductus arteriosus if either coarctation of the aorta or hypoplastic left heart syndrome is present. Detailed examination may disclose heart murmurs and diminution or absence of femoral pulses in both conditions. In this event resuscitation with prostaglandin usually stabilises the baby and allows time for further assessment.

- While coarctation of the aorta is usually amenable to surgical correction, hypoplastic left heart syndrome is still a major surgical challenge with a poor long-term outcome.

- Patent ductus arteriosus, ventricular septal defects and atrial septal defects seldom entail medical or surgical intervention in early neonatal life, but do require careful follow-up for signs of developing heart failure; surgery or interventional cardiology may be necessary at a later stage.

Not all heart murmurs heard at the first examination are significant.

Central Nervous System Abnormalities

Anencephaly

This major abnormality describes the absence of the forebrain and vault of the skull. It is a condition that is incompatible with sustained life, but occasionally such a baby is born alive.

Spina bifida aperta

Spina bifida aperta results from failure of fusion of the vertebral column.

- There is no skin covering the defect, which allows protrusion of the meninges (*meningocele*). The meningeal membrane may be flat or appear as a membranous sac with or without cerebrospinal fluid but it does not contain neural tissue (Fig. 34.4).

- *Meningomyelocele* does involve the spinal cord (Figs 34.4 and 34.5). This lesion may be enclosed or the meningocele may rupture and expose the neural tissue. Meningomyelocele usually gives rise to neural damage, producing paralysis distal to the

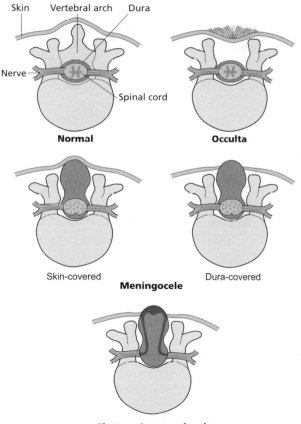

Fig. 34.4 Various forms of spina bifida.
(After Wallis S, Harvey D 1979. Copyright Emap Public Sector 1979. Reproduced by permission of *Nursing Times*.)

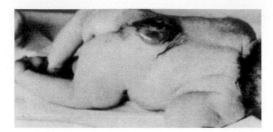

Fig. 34.5 Baby with meningomyelocele.

defect and impaired function of urinary bladder and bowel. The lumbosacral area is the most common site for these to present, but they may appear at any point along the vertebral column.

■ When the defect is at the level of the base of the skull, it is known as an *encephalocele*. An encephalocele may contain brain tissue.

Immediate management involves covering open lesions with a non-adherent dressing.

Spina bifida occulta

Spina bifida occulta (Fig. 34.4) is the most minor type of defect where the vertebra is bifid. There is usually no spinal cord involvement. A tuft of hair or sinus at the base of the spine may be noted on first examination of the baby.

Hydrocephalus

This condition arises from a blockage in the circulation and absorption of cerebrospinal fluid, which is produced from the choroid plexuses within the lateral ventricles of the brain. The large lateral ventricles increase in size and eventually compress the surrounding brain tissue. It is a not infrequent accompaniment to the more severe spina bifida lesions because of a structural defect around the area of the foramen magnum known as the Arnold–Chiari malformation. Hydrocephaly may either be present at birth or develop following surgical closure of a myelomeningocele. In the absence of myelomeningocele, aqueduc stenosis is the most common cause of hydrocephalus. The risk of cerebral impairment may be minimised by the insertion of a ventriculoperitoneal shunt. As the baby grows, this will need to be replaced. The midwife must be alert for the signs of increased intracranial pressure:

- large tense anterior fontanelle
- splayed skull sutures
- inappropriate increase in occipitofrontal circumference
- sun-setting appearance to the eyes
- irritability or abnormal movements.

Microcephaly

This is where the occipitofrontal circumference is more than 2 standard deviations below normal for gestational age. The disproportionately small head may be associated with intrauterine infection, e.g. rubella, fetal alcohol syndrome or some trisomic disorders. Most babies will be mentally impaired with evidence of cerebral palsy and often seizures.

Musculoskeletal Deformities

Polydactyly and syndactyly

- In polydactyly the extra digit(s) may be fully formed or may simply be extra tissue attached by a pedicle.
- Syndactyly (webbing) more commonly affects the hands. It can appear as an independent anomaly or as a feature of a syndrome such as Apert syndrome.

Limb reduction anomalies

Postulated causes include:

- amniotic band syndrome
- environmental teratogens

- iatrogenic trauma, perhaps at the time of chorionic villus sampling
- failure of formation (arrest of development), e.g. thalidomide, an antiemetic.

Talipes

- Talipes equinovarus (TEV, club foot) is when the ankle is bent downwards (plantarflexed) and the front part of the foot is turned inwards (inverted).
- Talipes calcaneovalgus describes the opposite position where the foot is dorsiflexed and everted.

Possible causes are:

- multiple pregnancy
- macrosomic fetus
- oligohydramnios
- association with spina bifida
- family history
- gender: statistically, more boys than girls are born with talipes.

In the mildest form the foot may easily be turned to the correct position and exercised in this way several times a day. More severe forms will require manipulation, splinting and/or surgical correction.

Developmental hip dysplasia

Congenital hip dysplasia is an abnormality more commonly found where there has been a history of oligohydramnios or breech presentation. It more often occurs in primigravida pregnancies and there is a higher percentage of girls born with this defect. The left hip is more often affected than the right. The dysplastic hip may present in one of three ways:

- dislocated
- dislocatable
- subluxation of the joint.

Examination of the hip should be carried out using either Ortolani's test or Barlow's test. It is usual for the baby to have a splint or harness, such as the Pavlik harness, that will keep the hips in a flexed and abducted position of about 60°.

Achondroplasia

Achondroplasia is an autosomal dominant condition where the baby is generally small with a disproportionately large head and short limbs.

Osteogenesis imperfecta

This autosomal dominant disorder of collagen production has at least four forms and leads to unduly brittle bones in the affected fetus and infant.

Abnormalities of the Skin

Vascular naevi

These defects in the development of the skin can be divided into two main types, which commonly overlap.

Capillary malformations

These are due to defects in the dermal capillaries. The most commonly observed are stork marks. These are usually found on the nape of the neck. They are generally small and will fade. No treatment is necessary.

Port wine stain

This is a purple–blue capillary malformation affecting the face and is twice as common in girls. It does not regress with time; laser treatment and the skilful use of cosmetics will help to disguise it.

Should the malformation appear to mimic the distribution of a branch of the trigeminal nerve, further malformations in the meninges may be suspected. This is known as Sturge–Weber syndrome.

Capillary haemangiomata ('strawberry marks')

Capillary haemangiomata are not usually noticeable at birth but appear as red raised lesions in the first few weeks of life. These lesions are particularly common in preterm infants and especially in girls. They can appear anywhere on the body. Although the lesion will grow bigger for the first few months, it will then regress and usually disappear completely by the age of 5–6 years. No treatment is normally required.

Pigmented naevi (melanocytic)

These are brown, sometimes hairy, marks on the skin which vary in size and may be flat or raised. A percentage of this type of birthmark may become malignant. Surgical excision may be recommended to preempt this.

Genitourinary System

At birth the first indication that there is an abnormality of the renal tract may be:

- a single umbilical artery in the umbilical cord
- the abnormal facies associated with Potter syndrome
- no passage of urine within 24 hours
- constant dribbling urine
- poor urine stream.

Dribbling of urine is a sign of nerve damage such as occurs with neural tube defects, whilst a poor urine stream may indicate lower urinary tract obstruction (posterior urethral valve).

Posterior urethral valve(s)

This is an abnormality affecting boys. The presence of valves in the posterior urethra prevents the normal outflow of urine. Back pressure from the distended bladder will ultimately cause hydronephrosis. Treatment involves surgical intervention.

Polycystic kidneys

These are likely to cause problems during the birth due to an increase in abdominal girth. On abdominal examination the kidneys will be palpable. Radiological or ultrasound investigations confirm the diagnosis. The prognosis is poor, with renal failure the likely outcome.

Hypospadias

The urethral meatus opens on to the under-surface of the penis. The meatus can be placed at any point along the length of the penis and in some cases will open on to the perineum. This abnormality often coexists with chordee, in which the penis is short and bent and the foreskin is only present on the dorsal side. Some babies will require surgery in the neonatal period to 'release' the chordee and enlarge the urethral meatus.

Cryptorchidism

Undescended testes may be unilateral or bilateral. If on examination of the baby after birth the scrotum is empty, the undescended testes may be found in the inguinal pouch.

Ambiguous genitalia

If there is any doubt, a gender must not be assigned to the baby. Examination of the baby may reveal any of the signs listed in Box 34.3.

There are a number of causes of ambiguous genitalia, all of which need expert clarification.

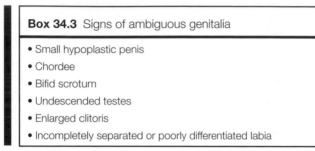

Box 34.3 Signs of ambiguous genitalia

- Small hypoplastic penis
- Chordee
- Bifid scrotum
- Undescended testes
- Enlarged clitoris
- Incompletely separated or poorly differentiated labia

Congenital adrenal hyperplasia

One of the reasons for ambiguous genitalia is an autosomal recessive condition called congenital adrenal hyperplasia. The adrenal gland is stimulated to overproduce androgens because of a deficiency of an enzyme called 21-hydroxylase, which is necessary for normal steroid production from cholesterol. The condition is not always recognised in boys in the neonatal period.

Intersex

This is where the internal reproductive organs are at variance with the external appearance of the genitalia. Ultrasound examination will help identify the nature of internal reproductive organs. True hermaphroditism is extremely rare. Following chromosomal studies to determine genetic make-up, hormone assays and consideration of the potential for cosmetic surgery, the decision of gender attribution is made.

Commonly Occurring Syndromes

Trisomy 21 or Down syndrome

This arises as a non-disjunction process in the majority. Unbalanced translocation occurs in about 2.5% of cases, usually between

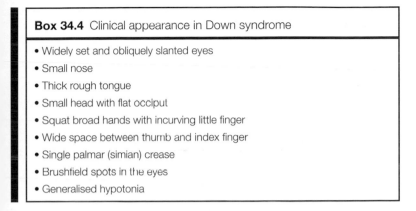

Box 34.4 Clinical appearance in Down syndrome

- Widely set and obliquely slanted eyes
- Small nose
- Thick rough tongue
- Small head with flat occiput
- Squat broad hands with incurving little finger
- Wide space between thumb and index finger
- Single palmar (simian) crease
- Brushfield spots in the eyes
- Generalised hypotonia

chromosomes 14 and 21. Mosaic forms also occur. There is no difference in clinical appearance, which are listed in Box 34.4.

Not all of the manifestations listed need be present and any of them can occur alone without implying chromosomal aberration. Babies born with Down syndrome also have a higher incidence of cardiac anomalies, leukaemia and hypothyroidism. The intelligence quotient is below average, at 40–80.

Investigations indicated include karyotyping and echocardiography, because of the increased risk of congenital heart disease. Some centres offer diagnosis using fluorescent in-situ hybridisation (FISH) techniques which provide an answer within 2 rather than the standard 5–7 days.

Trisomy 18 (Edwards syndrome)

This condition is found in about 1 in 5000 births. An extra 18th chromosome is responsible for the characteristic features. The lifespan of these children is short and the majority die during their first year.

- The head is small with a flattened forehead, a receding chin and frequently a cleft palate.

- The ears are low set and maldeveloped.
- The sternum tends to be short.
- The fingers often overlap each other and the feet have a characteristic rocker-bottom appearance.
- Malformations of the cardiovascular and gastrointestinal systems are common.

Trisomy 13 (Patau syndrome)

An extra copy of the 13th chromosome leads to multiple abnormalities. These children have a short life, only 5% living beyond 3 years.

- Affected infants are small and are microcephalic.
- Midline facial abnormalities, such as cleft lip and palate, are common and limb abnormalities are frequently seen.
- Brain, cardiac and renal abnormalities may coexist with this trisomy.

Potter syndrome

This collection of features is due to the compressive effects of oligohydramnios in renal agenesis or severe hypoplasia.

- The baby's face will have a flattened appearance, with low-set ears, an anti-mongoloid slant to the eyes with deep epicanthic folds, and a beaked nose.
- These babies are usually severely asphyxiated at birth because they have lung hypoplasia.

It is a syndrome incompatible with sustained life.

Turner syndrome (XO)

In this monosomal condition, only one sex chromosome exists: an X.

- The child is a girl with a short, webbed neck, widely spaced nipples and oedematous feet.

- The genitalia tend to be underdeveloped and the internal reproductive organs do not mature.
- The condition may not be diagnosed until puberty fails to occur.
- Congenital cardiac defects may also be found.
- Mental development is usually normal.

Klinefelter syndrome (XXY)

This is an abnormality that affects boys. It is not normally diagnosed until pubertal changes fail to occur.

Chapter 35

Jaundice and Infection

Jaundice is the yellow discoloration of the skin and sclera that results from raised levels of bilirubin in the blood (hyperbilirubinaemia).

Conjugation of Bilirubin

Bilirubin is a waste product from the breakdown of haem, most of which is found in red blood cells (RBCs). Ageing, immature or malformed RBCs are removed from the circulation and broken down in the reticuloendothelial system (liver, spleen and macrophages), and haemoglobin becomes the by-products of haem: globin and iron.

- Haem is converted to biliverdin and then to unconjugated bilirubin.
- Globin is broken down into amino acids that are reused by the body to make proteins.
- Iron is stored in the body or used for new red blood cells.

  Two main forms of bilirubin are found in the body:

- Unconjugated bilirubin is fat soluble and cannot be excreted easily either in bile or urine.
- Conjugated bilirubin has been made water soluble in the liver and can be excreted in either faeces or urine.

Three stages are involved in the processing of bilirubin:

- transport
- conjugation
- excretion.

Transport

Unconjugated bilirubin is transported in the plasma to the liver, bound to the plasma protein albumin. If not attached to albumin, it can be deposited into extravascular fatty and nerve tissues in the body. The skin and the brain are the two most common sites.

- Staining of the skin is known as *jaundice*.
- Damage to the brain as a result of bilirubin staining and toxicity is known as *kernicterus*.

Conjugation

Once in the liver, bilirubin is combined with glucose and *glucuronic acid*, and conjugation occurs in the presence of oxygen. *Uridine diphosphoglucuronyl transferase* (UDP-GT or *glucuronyl transferase*) is the major enzyme involved in bilirubin conjugation. The conjugated bilirubin is now water soluble and available for excretion.

Excretion

The conjugated bilirubin is excreted via the biliary system into the small intestine, where it is catabolised by normal intestinal bacteria to form urobilinogen, then oxidised into orange-coloured urobilin. Most of the conjugated bilirubin is excreted in the faeces but a small amount is excreted in urine.

Jaundice

In term neonates, jaundice appears when serum bilirubin concentrations reach 85–120 μmol/l (5–7 mg/dl).

Physiological jaundice

Physiological jaundice:

- *never* appears before 24 hours of life
- *usually* fades by 1 week of age.

  Bilirubin levels *never* exceed 200–215 μmol/l (12–13 mg/dl).

Causes

Neonatal physiological jaundice is the result of a discrepancy between RBC breakdown and the baby's ability to transport, conjugate and excrete unconjugated bilirubin. Neonates also have increased beta-glucuronidase enzyme activity in the gut, which hydrolyses conjugated bilirubin back into the unconjugated state. If feeding is delayed, bowel motility is decreased, further compromising excretion of unconjugated bilirubin.

Exaggerated physiological jaundice in breastfed infants

Although the exact mechanisms are unknown, current evidence suggests that two different processes cause jaundice in the breastfeeding baby:

- Breastfeeding or early-onset jaundice. It is thought that low fluid and calorie intake during colostrum production causes a slower intestinal transit time, which increases exposure to *beta-glucuronidase*; this in turn adds more unconjugated bilirubin to the system.

- Breast milk or later-onset jaundice.

Exaggerated physiological jaundice in preterm babies

This is characterised by bilirubin levels of 165 μmol/l (10 mg/dl) or greater by day 3 or 4, with peak concentrations on days 5–7 that return to normal over several weeks. Preterm babies are more at risk of kernicterus. Contributing factors include:

■ a delay in the expression of the enzyme UDP-GT

■ shorter red cell life

■ complications such as hypoxia, acidosis and hypothermia that can interfere with albumin-binding capacity.

Midwifery practice and physiological jaundice

It is important to distinguish between healthy babies with a normal physiological response who need no active treatment and those who require serum bilirubin testing. Parents should be advised to report:

■ excessive sleepiness

■ reluctance to feed

■ decrease in the number of wet nappies

■ pale stools and yellow or orange urine.

Early, frequent feeding assists newborns to cope with an increased bilirubin load.

Pathological jaundice

Pathological jaundice in newborns usually appears within 24 hours of birth, and is characterised by a *rapid rise* in serum bilirubin. Criteria are listed in Box 35.1.

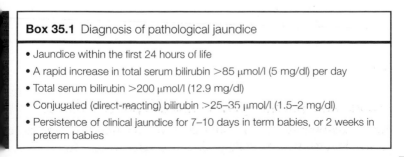

Box 35.1 Diagnosis of pathological jaundice

- Jaundice within the first 24 hours of life
- A rapid increase in total serum bilirubin >85 μmol/l (5 mg/dl) per day
- Total serum bilirubin >200 μmol/l (12.9 mg/dl)
- Conjugated (direct-reacting) bilirubin >25–35 μmol/l (1.5–2 mg/dl)
- Persistence of clinical jaundice for 7–10 days in term babies, or 2 weeks in preterm babies

Causes

The underlying aetiology of pathological jaundice is some type of interference with bilirubin production, transport, conjugation or excretion. Any disease or disorder that increases bilirubin production or that alters the transport or metabolism of bilirubin is superimposed upon normal physiological jaundice.

Production

Factors that increase haemoglobin destruction also increase bilirubin levels. Causes of increased haemolysis include:

- Rhesus anti-D, anti-A, anti-B and anti-Kell and ABO blood group incompatibility
- haemoglobinopathies — sickle-cell disease and thalassaemia
- spherocytosis — fragile RBC membrane
- extravasated blood — cephalhaematoma and bruising
- sepsis — can lead to increased haemoglobin breakdown
- polycythaemia — blood contains too many red cells, as in maternofetal or twin-to-twin transfusion.

Transport

Factors that lower blood albumin levels or decrease albumin-binding capacity include:

- hypothermia, acidosis or hypoxia (can interfere with albumin-binding capacity)
- drugs that compete with bilirubin for albumin-binding sites, e.g. aspirin, sulphonamides and ampicillin.

Conjugation

As well as immaturity of the neonate's enzyme system, other factors can interfere with bilirubin conjugation in the liver:

- dehydration, starvation, hypoxia and sepsis (oxygen and glucose are required for conjugation)

- TORCH infections (toxoplasmosis, others, rubella, cytomegalo-virus, herpes)
- other viral infections, e.g. neonatal viral hepatitis
- other bacterial infections, particularly those caused by *E. coli*
- metabolic and endocrine disorders that alter UDP-GT enzyme activity, e.g. Crigler–Najjar disease and Gilbert syndrome
- other metabolic disorders, such as hypothyroidism and galactosaemia.

Excretion

Factors that can interfere with bilirubin excretion include:

- hepatic obstruction caused by congenital anomalies
- obstruction from increased bile viscosity
- saturation of protein carriers needed to excrete conjugated bilirubin into the biliary system
- infection, other congenital disorders, and idiopathic neonatal hepatitis (can also cause an excess of conjugated bilirubin).

Haemolytic Jaundice

Rhesus (RhD) isoimmunisation causes haemolytic disease of the newborn (HDN), which usually requires some form of obstetric intervention. Few antibodies to blood group antigens other than those in the Rh system cause severe HDN; fetal transfusion is unusual for multiple maternal antibody isoimmunisation without anti-D. ABO incompatibility is possibly the most frequent cause of mild to moderate haemolysis in neonates.

RhD incompatibility

RhD incompatibility can occur when a woman with Rh-negative blood type is pregnant with a fetus with Rh-positive blood type.

- The placenta usually acts as a barrier to prevent fetal blood entering the maternal circulation. However, during pregnancy or birth small amounts of fetal Rh-positive blood cross the placenta and enter the circulation of the mother, who has Rh-negative blood.

- The woman's immune system reacts by producing anti-D antibodies that cause sensitisation.

- In subsequent pregnancies these maternal antibodies can cross the placenta and destroy fetal erythrocytes.

- Usually, sensitisation occurs during the first pregnancy or birth, leading to extensive destruction of fetal red blood cells during subsequent pregnancies.

Rh isoimmunisation can result from any procedure or incident where maternal blood leaks across the placenta or from the inadvertent transfusion of Rh-positive blood to the woman.

Prevention of RhD isoimmunisation

This is by routine antenatal anti-D immunoglobulin (Ig) prophylaxis, within 72 hours of birth or after any other sensitising event. Anti-D Ig is a human plasma-based product that prevents the production of anti-D antibodies by the mother.

Administration of anti-D Ig

Anti-D Ig is administered to Rh-negative women who are pregnant with, or have given birth to, an Rh-positive baby. It destroys any fetal cells in the mother's blood before her immune system produces antibodies. The process for non-sensitised women is set out in Box 35.2.

Dose of anti-D Ig

Research evidence for the optimal dose is still limited but the doses listed in Box 35.3 are recommended.

Box 35.2 Administration of anti-D Ig to non-sensitised women

1. Women who are Rh-negative are screened for Rh antibodies (indirect Coombs' test). A negative test shows an *absence* of antibodies or sensitisation

2. Blood is retested at 28 weeks of pregnancy. In countries where antenatal prophylaxis is routine (at 28 and 34 weeks' gestation), the first injection of anti-D Ig is given just after this blood sample is taken

3. Where a policy of routine antenatal anti-D Ig prophylaxis is *not* in place, blood is retested for antibodies at 34 weeks of pregnancy

4. When anti-D Ig prophylaxis is given at 28 weeks, blood is not retested, as it difficult to distinguish passive anti-D Ig from immune anti-D

5. Following the birth, cord blood is tested for confirmation of Rh type, ABO blood group, haemoglobin and serum bilirubin levels and the presence of maternal antibodies on fetal red cells (direct Coombs' test). Again, a negative test indicates an absence of antibodies or sensitisation. The postnatal dose of anti-D Ig is *still given* if passive anti-D Ig is present

6. A Kleihauer acid elution test is also carried out on an anticoagulated maternal blood sample immediately after birth to estimate the number of fetal cells in a sample of maternal blood

7. Anti-D Ig must always be given as soon as possible, and in any case within 72 hours of any sensitising event and the birth. Anti-D Ig is injected into the deltoid muscle, from which absorption is optimal

Box 35.3 Recommended dosages of anti-D Ig

- 100 µg (500 IU) anti-D Ig at 28 and 34 weeks' gestation for women in their first pregnancy
- At least 500 IU for all non-sensitised Rh-negative woman following the birth of a Rh-positive infant
- 250 IU following sensitising events *up to* 20 weeks' gestation
- At least 500 IU following sensitising events *after* 20 weeks' gestation
- Larger doses for traumatic events and procedures such as caesarean birth, stillbirths and intrauterine deaths, abdominal trauma during the third trimester, or manual removal of the placenta (dose calculated on 500 IU of anti-D Ig suppressing immunisation from 4 ml of RhD-positive red blood cells)
- Larger doses for any other instance of inadvertent transfusion of Rh-positive red blood cells, e.g. from an incorrect blood transfusion of Rh-positive blood platelets

Ethical and legal issues

Anti-D Ig is a human plasma-based product. To give informed consent to its use, women need to know the possible consequences of treatment, as opposed to non-treatment, with anti-D Ig.

Management of RhD isoimmunisation

Effects of RhD isoimmunisation

- Destruction of fetal RBCs results in anaemia, possibly oedema and congestive cardiac failure.
- Fetal bilirubin levels also increase as more red cells are destroyed, with possible neurological damage as bilirubin is deposited in the brain.
- Lesser degrees of destruction result in haemolytic anaemia, while extensive haemolysis can cause hydrops fetalis and death in utero.

Antenatal monitoring and treatment of RhD isoimmunisation

Depending on the severity of Rh isoimmunisation, monitoring and treatment can include the following:

- Women who are Rh-negative are screened for Rh antibodies (indirect Coombs' test). A positive test indicates the *presence* of antibodies or sensitisation.
- RBCs obtained by chorionic villus sampling (using an immune rosette technique) can be Rh-phenotyped as early as 9–11 weeks' gestation.
- Maternal blood is retested frequently to monitor any increase in antibody titres. Sudden and unexpected rises in serum anti-D levels can result in hydrops fetalis.
- If antibody titres remain stable, ongoing monitoring is continued.
- If antibody titres increase, amniocentesis is used to evaluate changes in the optical density of amniotic fluid. Elevated optical

density measurements indicate a worsening of the isoimmunisation.

- High concentrations of anti-D antibodies in the mother, in the fetus and in the amniotic fluid indicate an active transport across the placenta and passive excretion into the amniotic fluid.
- Changes in fetal serum bilirubin levels are observed.
- The fetus is closely monitored by ultrasonography for oedema and hepatosplenomegaly.
- Intravenous immunoglobulin (IVIG) has the potential to maintain the fetus until intrauterine fetal transfusion (IUT) can be performed. IVIG works by blocking Fc-mediated antibody transport across the placenta, blocking fetal red cell destruction and reducing maternal antibody levels.
- IUT can be used from about 20 weeks of gestation to reduce the effects of haemolysis until the fetus is capable of survival outside the uterus.
- Early delivery depends on the ongoing severity of the haemolysis and the condition of the fetus.

Postnatal treatment of RhD isoimmunisation

- Babies with mild to moderate haemolytic anaemia and hyperbilirubinaemia may require careful monitoring but less aggressive management.
- Babies with hydrops fetalis are pale and have oedema and ascites; alternatively, they may be stillborn.
- Management of surviving infants aims to prevent further haemolysis, reduce bilirubin levels, remove maternal Rh antibodies from the baby's circulation, and combat anaemia.
- In some cases phototherapy can be effective but exchange transfusion is often required, and packed cell transfusion may be needed to increase Hb levels.
- Infants are at risk of ongoing haemolytic anaemia.

ABO incompatibility

ABO isoimmunisation usually occurs when the mother is blood group O and the baby is group A, or less often group B.

- Type A and B blood has a protein or antigen not present in type O blood.

- Individuals with type O blood develop antibodies throughout life from exposure to antigens in food, Gram-negative bacteria or blood transfusion, and by the first pregnancy may already have high serum anti-A and anti-B antibody titres.

- Some women produce IgG antibodies that can cross the placenta and attach to fetal red cells and destroy them.

First and subsequent babies are at risk; however, the destruction is usually much less severe than with Rh incompatibility. ABO incompatibility is also thought to protect the fetus from Rh incompatibility as the mother's anti-A and anti-B antibodies destroy any fetal cells that leak into the maternal circulation.

Treatment aims to:

- prevent further haemolysis
- reduce bilirubin levels
- combat any anaemia.

As with other causes of haemolysis, if babies require phototherapy it is usually commenced at a lower range of serum bilirubin levels ($140–165\,\mu$mol/l or $8–10\,$mg/dl). Babies with a high serum bilirubin level may require exchange transfusion.

Management of Jaundice

Phototherapy

Phototherapy is used to prevent the concentration of unconjugated bilirubin in the blood from reaching levels where neurotoxicity may occur. The neonate's skin surface is exposed to high-intensity light, which photochemically converts fat-soluble unconjugated bilirubin into water-soluble bilirubin that can be excreted in bile and urine. Treatment may be intermittent or continuous, with phototherapy interrupted only for essential care.

Indications for phototherapy

The commencement of phototherapy is based on serum bilirubin levels and the individual condition of each baby, particularly when jaundice occurs within the first 12–24 hours.

Side-effects of phototherapy

- Hyperthermia, increased fluid loss and dehydration.
- Damage to the retina from the high-intensity light.
- Lethargy or irritability, decreased eagerness to feed, loose stools.
- Rashes and skin burns.
- Alterations in infant state and neurobehavioural organisation.
- Isolation and lack of usual sensory experiences, including visual deprivation.
- A decrease in calcium levels, leading to hypocalcaemia.
- Low platelet counts and increased red cell osmotic fragility.
- Bronze baby syndrome, riboflavin deficiency and DNA damage.

Care of the baby needing phototherapy

See Box 35.4.

Exchange transfusion

Excess bilirubin is removed from the baby during a blood exchange transfusion. With HDN, sensitised erythrocytes are replaced with blood compatible with both the mother's and the infant's serum. With the exception of very premature babies and Rh incompatibility,

---

Box 35.4 Care of the baby needing phototherapy

Temperature
- Maintain a warm thermoneutral environment
- Observe for hypothermia or hyperthermia

Eyes
- Protect with eye shields, ensuring they do not occlude the nose and are not tight

Skin
- Clean with warm water and observe frequently for rashes, dryness and excoriation
- Creams and lotions are not used

Hydration
- Fluid intake and stool and urine output are monitored

Neurobehavioural status
- Observe sleeping and waking states, feeding behaviours, responsiveness, response to stress, and interaction with parents and other carers

Calcium levels
- Hypocalcaemia may be indicated by jitteriness, irritability, rash, loose stools, fever, dehydration and convulsions

Bilirubin levels
- Levels are usually estimated daily

---

exchange transfusion may now only be used when there is a risk of kernicterus.

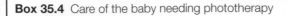

Neonatal Infection

Modes of acquiring infection

■ Through the placenta (transplacental infection).

■ From amniotic fluid.

- From their passage through the birth canal.
- From carers' hands, contaminated objects or droplet infection after birth.

Vulnerability to infection

Newborns are immunodeficient and prone to a higher incidence of infection. Preterm babies are even more vulnerable, as they have less well-developed defence mechanisms at birth (transfer of IgG mainly occurs after 32 weeks' gestation), and are more likely to experience invasive procedures. Full immunocompetence requires both innate (natural) and acquired immune responses.

At birth the baby has some immune protection from the mother but immunoglobulins are deficient. Maternal exposure and transfer of IgG across the placenta limit antibody levels. Breastfeeding increases the baby's immune protection through the transmission of secretory IgA in breast milk. During the early weeks of life the baby also has deficiencies in both the quantity and the quality of neutrophils.

Management of infection

Individual risk factors for infection

These include:

- a maternal history of prolonged rupture of membranes
- chorioamnionitis
- pyrexia during birth
- offensive amniotic fluid.

Physical assessment

This can include observation of:

- temperature instability
- lethargy or poor feeding, dehydration, starvation, hypothermia, acidosis or hypoxia

---

> **Box 35.5** Investigation of neonatal infection
>
> - A complete blood cell count
> - Testing of specimens of urine and meconium for specific organisms
> - Swabs from the nose, throat and umbilicus, and from any rashes, pustules or vesicles to test for specific organisms
> - MRI, CT scans and chest X-rays
> - A lumbar puncture to enable examination of cerebrospinal fluid (CSF)
> - Testing of amniotic fluid, placental tissue and cord blood for specific organisms

- bradycardia or tachycardia, and any apnoea
- urine and stool output and any vomiting
- central nervous system signs that require a complete neuro-developmental examination.

Investigations

See Box 35.5.

Management

The overall aim of management is to provide prompt and effective treatment that reduces the risk of septicaemia and life-threatening septic shock. Good management includes:

- caring for the baby in a warm thermoneutral environment and observing for temperature instability
- good hydration and the correction of electrolyte imbalance, with demand feeding if possible and intravenous fluids as required
- prompt systemic antibiotic or other drug therapy and local treatment of infection
- ongoing monitoring of the baby's neurobehavioural status
- reducing separation of mother and baby

- providing evidence-based information, support and reassurance to parents
- encouraging breastfeeding or expressing of milk, and informing women of the important role of breast milk in fighting infection.

Infections acquired before or during birth

The effects of sexually transmissible and reproductive tract infections are presented in chapter 15. Others of importance to midwives are discussed below.

Toxoplasmosis

- Toxoplasmosis is caused by *Toxoplasma gondii*, a protozoan parasite found in uncooked meat and cat and dog faeces.
- Infected neonates may be asymptomatic at birth, but can later develop retinal and neurological disease. Maternal-fetal transmission results from poor hygiene.
- Those with subclinical disease at birth can develop seizures, significant cognitive and motor deficits, and reduced cognitive function over time.

Varicella zoster

- Varicella zoster virus (VZV) is a highly contagious DNA virus of the herpes family, transmitted by respiratory droplets and contact with vesicle fluid; it causes varicella (chickenpox).
- It has an incubation period of 10–20 days and is infectious for 48 hours before the rash appears until vesicles crust over.

Incidence and effects during pregnancy

Maternal deaths have been associated with varicella infection during pregnancy. Fetal sequelae from primary maternal infection vary with the length of gestation at the time of the infection (Box 35.6).

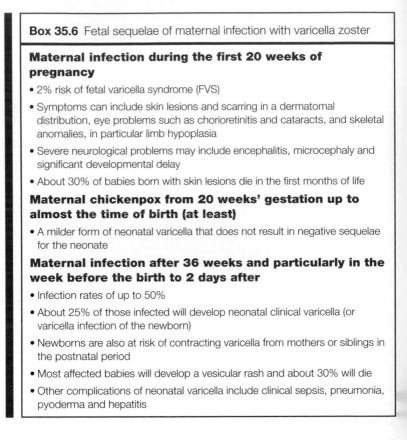

Box 35.6 Fetal sequelae of maternal infection with varicella zoster

Maternal infection during the first 20 weeks of pregnancy

- 2% risk of fetal varicella syndrome (FVS)
- Symptoms can include skin lesions and scarring in a dermatomal distribution, eye problems such as chorioretinitis and cataracts, and skeletal anomalies, in particular limb hypoplasia
- Severe neurological problems may include encephalitis, microcephaly and significant developmental delay
- About 30% of babies born with skin lesions die in the first months of life

Maternal chickenpox from 20 weeks' gestation up to almost the time of birth (at least)

- A milder form of neonatal varicella that does not result in negative sequelae for the neonate

Maternal infection after 36 weeks and particularly in the week before the birth to 2 days after

- Infection rates of up to 50%
- About 25% of those infected will develop neonatal clinical varicella (or varicella infection of the newborn)
- Newborns are also at risk of contracting varicella from mothers or siblings in the postnatal period
- Most affected babies will develop a vesicular rash and about 30% will die
- Other complications of neonatal varicella include clinical sepsis, pneumonia, pyoderma and hepatitis

Rubella

For most immunocompetent children and adults (including pregnant women), the rubella virus causes a mild and insignificant illness that is spread by droplet infection.

Incidence and effects during pregnancy

If primary rubella infection occurs during the first 12 weeks of pregnancy, maternal–fetal transmission rates are high. First-trimester infection can have the results listed in Box 35.7.

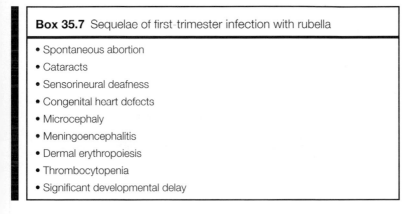

Box 35.7 Sequelae of first-trimester infection with rubella

- Spontaneous abortion
- Cataracts
- Sensorineural deafness
- Congenital heart defects
- Microcephaly
- Meningoencephalitis
- Dermal erythropoiesis
- Thrombocytopenia
- Significant developmental delay

Babies with congenital rubella are highly infectious and should be isolated from other infants and pregnant women (but not from their own mothers). Babies should always be followed up for several years, as some problems may not become apparent until they are older.

Ophthalmia neonatorum

Ophthalmia neonatorum is a notifiable condition. It involves a purulent discharge from the eyes of an infant within 21 days of birth. The condition is usually acquired during vaginal birth and causative organisms include:

- *Staphylococcus aureus*
- *Streptococcus pneumoniae*
- *Haemophilus influenzae*
- *Escherichia coli*
- *Klebsiella*
- *Pseudomonas*
- *Chlamydia trachomatis*
- *Neisseria gonorrhoeae.*

A swab must be taken for culture and sensitivity testing, and a doctor notified immediately. Chlamydial and gonococcal infections can cause:

- conjunctival scarring
- corneal infiltration
- blindness
- systemic spread.

Treatment includes:

- local cleaning and care of the eyes with normal saline
- appropriate drug therapy for the baby and also the mother if required.

Candida

- Candida is a Gram-positive yeast fungus that has a number of strains, including *C. albicans*, *C. parapsilosis*, *C. tropicalis* and *C. lusitaniae*.
- *C. albicans* is responsible for most fungal infections, including thrush in infants.
- Infection can affect the mouth (oral candidiasis), skin (cutaneous candidiasis) and other organs (systemic candidiasis).

Some infections acquired after birth

Eye infections

Mild eye infections are common in babies and can be treated with routine eye care and antibiotics if required. Other more serious conditions must be excluded.

Skin infections

Most neonatal skin infections are caused by *Staph. aureus*. In newborn infants the most likely skin lesions are septic spots or pustules, found either as a solitary lesion or clustered in the umbilical and buttock areas.

- For the well neonate with limited pustules, management includes regular cleansing with an antiseptic solution.
- Antibiotic therapy is given for more extensive pustules.

Meningitis

Neonatal meningitis is an inflammation of the membranes lining the brain and spinal column caused by organisms such as:

- *E. coli*
- group B streptococci
- *Listeria monocytogenes*
- (more unusually) *Candida* and herpes.

Very early signs may be non-specific, followed by those of meningeal irritation and raised intracranial pressure, such as:

- irritability
- bulging fontanelle
- increasing lethargy
- crying
- tremors
- twitching
- severe vomiting
- alterations in consciousness
- diminished muscle tone.

Diagnosis is usually confirmed by examination of CSF. Very ill babies will require intensive care, intravenous fluids and antibiotic therapy. Long-term neurological complications can occur in surviving infants.

Respiratory infections

These may be minor (nasopharyngitis and rhinitis) or more severe (pneumonia).

Gastrointestinal tract infections

In the newborn these can include gastroenteritis or the more severe necrotising enterocolitis. Causative organisms for gastroenteritis include:

- rotavirus
- *Salmonella*
- *Shigella*
- a pathogenic strain of *E. coli*.

The secretory IgA in breast milk offers important protection against these organisms, particularly rotavirus. The correction of fluid and electrolyte imbalance is an urgent priority.

Umbilical infection

Signs can include localised inflammation and an offensive discharge. Untreated infection can spread to the liver via the umbilical vein and cause hepatitis and septicaemia. Treatment may include:

- regular cleansing
- the administration of an antibiotic powder
- appropriate antibiotic therapy.

Urinary tract infections

Urinary tract infections can result from bacteria such as *E. coli*, or less often from a congenital anomaly that obstructs urine flow. The signs are usually those of an early non-specific infection. Diagnosis is usually confirmed through laboratory evaluation of a urine sample.

Chapter 36

Metabolic Disturbances, Inborn Errors of Metabolism, Endocrine Disorders and Drug Withdrawal

Metabolic Disturbances

Glucose homeostasis

Following birth there is a fall in glucose concentration. At the same time endocrine changes (decrease in insulin and a surge of catecholamines and release of glucagon) result in an increase in:

- glycogenolysis (breakdown of glycogen stores to provide glucose)
- gluconeogenesis (glucose production from the liver)
- ketogenesis (producing ketones, an alternative fuel)
- lipolysis (release of fatty acids from adipose), bringing about an increase in glucose and other metabolic fuel.

Problems arise in the newborn:

- when there is a lack of glycogen stores to mobilise (preterm and growth-restricted infants), *or*

- when there is excessive insulin production (infants of diabetic mothers), *or*
- when infants are sick and have a poor supply of energy and increased requirements.

Hypoglycaemia

The definition of hypoglycaemia is controversial. Pragmatically, however, a specific level is helpful for management purposes. The consensus would appear to favour a cut-off value in the newborn of 2.6 mmol/l.

Signs of hypoglycaemia are listed in Box 36.1.

Normal term babies

Healthy term babies are able to tolerate low blood glucose concentrations by using alternative fuels such as ketone bodies, lactate or fatty acids. Breastfed babies are a group who are particularly likely to have low blood glucose concentrations, probably because of the low energy content of breast milk in the first few postnatal days. Because of their ability to compensate, clinically well, appropriately grown term babies who are feeding do not require monitoring of their glucose concentration. Doing so would result in many infants being inappropriately treated.

Infants at risk of neurological sequelae of hypoglycaemia

- Preterm babies (of less than 37 weeks).
- Growth-restricted babies (less than third centile for gestation).

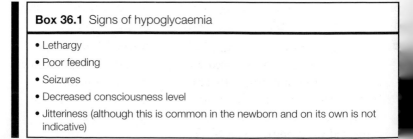

Box 36.1 Signs of hypoglycaemia

- Lethargy
- Poor feeding
- Seizures
- Decreased consciousness level
- Jitteriness (although this is common in the newborn and on its own is not indicative)

- Babies of diabetic mothers.
- Sick term babies, e.g. septic or following perinatal hypoxia–ischaemia.
- Babies with inborn errors of metabolism.

Diagnosis, prevention and treatment of hypoglycaemia

Term infants who are admitted to the postnatal ward and are feeding should not have measurements of blood glucose taken unless they are symptomatic. In particular, breastfeeding advice and intervention should not be based on blood glucose concentrations. Babies at risk of neurological complications of hypoglycaemia should be monitored.

Prevention is important and there should therefore be:

- adequate temperature control — keep the babies warm
- early feeding (within 1 hour of birth) with 100 ml/kg/day if formula feeding
- frequent feeding (3-hourly or less)
- blood glucose check immediately before the second feed and then 4–6-hourly.

As long as there are no symptoms, there is no advantage to checking the blood glucose concentration earlier than this, as it is likely to be low and the appropriate treatment at that stage is to feed the baby. If there are symptoms, the glucose should be checked and treatment given immediately. Breastfed babies are particularly difficult in this situation because it is important to avoid supplemental feeding with formula to promote successful breastfeeding; the risks associated with significant hypoglycaemia in at-risk infants outweigh this consideration.

- If the blood glucose concentration is <2.6 mmol/l, then feed should be given at an increased volume and decreased frequency (2-hourly or even hourly). This may require supplementary feeding with formula milk in infants who are breastfed, and/or nasogastric tube (NGT) feeding. Breast milk can also be expressed to be given via an NGT.

- If the blood glucose concentration remains low despite these measures and there is an adequate feed volume intake then intravenous treatment with dextrose is required. It is important in this situation that enteral feeding is continued, as feed contains much more energy than 10% glucose and promotes ketone body production and metabolic adaptation.

- If the blood glucose concentration is >2.6 mmol/l before the second and the third feed, then glucose monitoring can be discontinued but feeding should continue at 3-hourly intervals.

- In infants where enteral feeding is contraindicated for some reason, then intravenous 10% dextrose at least 60 ml/kg/day should commence.

Hyperglycaemia

Hyperglycaemia is much less of a clinical problem than hypoglycaemia and occurs predominantly in preterm and severely growth-restricted babies. It is also seen in term infants in response to stress, especially following perinatal hypoxia–ischaemia, surgery or drugs (especially corticosteroids). In general, no treatment is required.

Electrolyte imbalances in the newborn

Postnatal weight loss, fluid and electrolyte changes

In the first few days after birth, all babies lose weight due to a loss of extracellular fluid.

In general, they are not weighed during this period; however, weighing can be very useful when babies are unwell or if there are concerns about intake and fluid and electrolyte balance.

Sodium

Sodium is normally excreted via the kidney, controlled by the renin–angiotensin system. This control mechanism is functional in the pre-term infant but loss of sodium may occur because of renal tubule unresponsiveness. Term breast milk has relatively little sodium (<1 mmol/kg/day), showing that the normal newborn can preserve sodium via the kidney in order to maintain growth. Normal sodium requirements are 1–2 mmol/kg/day in term infants and 3–4 mmol/kg/day in preterm infants.

Changes in serum sodium reflect changes in sodium and water balance. In order to assess changes in sodium concentration it is important to know an infant's weight:

- Hypernatraemia in the presence of a loss of weight suggests dehydration.
- When there is weight gain, hypernatraemia is due to fluid and sodium overload.

Hyponatraemia

The normal serum sodium concentration is 133–146 mmol/l. Hyponatraemia is due to either fluid overload or sodium depletion.

- Hyponatraemia in the presence of weight gain represents fluid overload.
- A low sodium with inappropriate weight loss represents sodium depletion.

The latter may be due to inadequate intake or excessive losses.

Hypernatraemia

Increased sodium concentration is almost always due to water depletion and loss of extracellular fluid, but can also rarely be due to an excessive sodium intake.

Potassium

Potassium is the major intracellular cation. Abnormalities in serum potassium concentration can cause significant arrhythmias. Potassium concentrations can be severely affected by measurement technique and any haemolysis of the blood sample, especially from capillary sampling, is likely to lead to a falsely high value.

Calcium

Calcium metabolism is closely linked to phosphate metabolism. Preterm infants need much higher concentrations of phosphate and calcium. These are given as intravenous supplements, by supplementing breast milk with fortifier, or by giving specific preterm milk formulae rather than term formula.

High serum calcium concentrations are unusual but there are rare, important causes of low serum calcium. The normal serum concentration is 2.2–2.7 mmol/l but this must be interpreted with the serum albumin concentration, as serum calcium is bound to albumin; therefore a low albumin concentration will lead to a falsely low serum value.

Calcium concentrations fall within 18–24 hours of birth as the infant's supply of placental calcium ceases, but accretion into bone continues.

Inborn Errors of Metabolism

Inborn errors of metabolism (IEM) are rare inherited disorders occurring in approximately 1 in 5000 births. They result mainly from enzyme deficiencies in metabolic pathways leading to an accumulation of substrate, which in turn causes toxicity. Early diagnosis and institution of therapy can reduce morbidity. It has been estimated that 20% of infants presenting with sepsis in the absence of risk factors have an IEM.

Inheritance is usually autosomal recessive and the following features should be sought:

- affected sibling
- previous stillbirth/neonatal death
- parental consanguinity
- symptoms associated with feeding, fasting or a surgical procedure
- improvement when feeds stopped and relapse on restarting.

Clinical examination, however, is usually normal. The features below may be seen in isolation with many diagnoses. However, multiple features indicate that an underlying IEM should be seriously considered (Box 36.2).

■ Principles of emergency management are to reduce load on affected pathways by removing toxic metabolites and stimulating residual enzyme activity.

■ Hypoglycaemia is corrected, adequate ventilatory support and hydration are maintained, convulsions are treated, and significant metabolic acidosis is treated with intravenous sodium bicarbonate, and electrolyte abnormalities are corrected.

■ In general, antibiotics are frequently given, as infection may have precipitated metabolic decompensation; occasionally, dialysis may also be required.

Box 36.2 Clinical features of inborn errors of metabolism

- Septicaemia
- Hypoglycaemia
- Metabolic acidosis
- Convulsions
- Coma
- Cataracts
- Cardiomegaly
- Jaundice/liver disease
- Severe hypotonia
- Unusual body odour
- Dysmorphic features
- Abnormal hair
- Hydrops fetalis
- Diarrhoea

Phenylketonuria (PKU)

- This is an autosomal recessive disorder (1 in 10 000 incidence in the UK).

- It is caused by absence or reduction of an enzyme in the liver that converts phenylalanine to tyrosine (phenylalanine hydroxylase).

- Babies are well at birth but begin to be affected during the first few weeks.

- It is diagnosed by blood test, 5–8 days after birth, commonly collected on the Neonatal Screening Test Card.

- If untreated, PKU leads to severe mental retardation (IQ <30) due to build-up of phenylpyruvic acid, which is toxic to the brain.

- It is treated by a diet specifically restricted in phenylalanine. Affected women need to return to a strict diet in pregnancy.

Galactosaemia

- This is an autosomal recessive disorder (incidence of 1 in 60 000).

- It is caused by an absence or severe deficiency of the enzyme galactose-1-phosphate uridyltransferase (Gal-1-P UT) that converts galactose to glucose.

- As milk's main sugar, lactose, contains glucose and galactose, babies with this condition rapidly become affected.

- The build-up of galactose-1-phosphate is harmful and can quickly cause cataracts and brain injury.

- It is treated with lactose-free formula.

The clinical signs and symptoms of the disorder are those of liver failure and renal impairment.

Affected babies may also present with septicaemia (particularly with *E. coli*) due to damage to intestinal mucosa. Galactosaemia should also be considered in babies with unresponsive hypoglycaemia and prolonged or severe jaundice.

Regarding diagnosis:

- Urine-reducing substances (i.e. galactose) are present but the urine test for glucose is negative.

- Assay is made of the enzyme level (Gal-1-P UT) within red blood cells.

Endocrine Disease in the Newborn

Thyroid disorders

The thyroid gland produces hormones that have an effect on the metabolic rate in most tissues. They are also essential for normal neurological development. Thyroid-stimulating hormone (TSH) is produced by the anterior pituitary gland and this stimulates production of T3 and T4 by the thyroid gland with a feedback mechanism to the anterior pituitary.

Hypothyroidism

- Causes include abnormalities in gland formation, defects in hormone synthesis and rarely secondary pituitary causes.

- Babies tend to be large and to have a large posterior fontanelle, coarse features and often an umbilical hernia.

- Untreated babies develop impaired motor development, growth failure, a low IQ, impaired hearing and language problems.

- Screening is by measuring TSH (high) on a blood spot taken along with the screening test for PKU at 5–8 days of age.

- Screening does not detect pituitary causes, as they have a low TSH.

Hyperthyroidism

- This is rare; it is due to maternal Graves' disease.

- It can lead to preterm labour, low birth weight, stillbirth and fetal death.

- Symptoms are uncommon and may be present at birth or delayed till 4–6 weeks.
- Symptoms include irritability, jitteriness, tachycardia, prominent eyes, sweating, excessive appetite and weight loss.
- Babies with symptoms are treated with antithyroid medication.

Adrenal disorders

The adrenal cortex produces three groups of hormones — glucocorticoids, mineralocorticoids and sex hormones; these have distinct functions. Glucocorticoids regulate the general metabolism of carbohydrates, proteins and fats on a long-term basis. They have a particular role in modifying the metabolism in times of stress. Mineralocorticoids regulate sodium, potassium and water balance. The sex hormones are responsible for normal development of the genitalia and reproductive organs.

Adrenocortical insufficiency

- Causes are congenital hypoplasia, adrenal haemorrhage and enzyme defects.
- Its secondary cause is pituitary problems.
- Diagnosis rests on symptomatic hypoglycaemia, poor feeding, vomiting, poor weight gain and prolonged jaundice.
- Babies may have hyponatraemia, hypoglycaemia, hyperkalaemia and acidosis.
- Treatment is by intravenous therapy with glucose and electrolytes; replacement of corticosteroid and mineralocorticoid hormones is then required.

Adrenocortical hyperfunction

This may occur in the form of congenital adrenal hyperplasia. This is the name given to a group of inherited disorders that are due to deficiency of the enzymes responsible for hormone production within the adrenal gland. The most common enzyme deficiency results in an excess of androgenic hormones, but a deficiency of glucocorticoid and mineralocorticoids often also occurs. These disorders can cause abnormalities in the formation of the genitalia, leading to ambiguous genitalia (virilisation of females or inadequate virilisation of males), and symptoms of adrenal insufficiency (vomiting, diarrhoea, vascular collapse, hypoglycaemia and hyponatraemia, hyperkalaemia).

Treatment is by replacement of glucocorticoid and mineralocorticoid hormones. Virilised girls may also require surgical intervention to correct the genital abnormalities.

Pituitary disorders

Pituitary insufficiency is rare. It may occur in association with other abnormalities, particularly midline developmental defects. Presentation is with signs of glucocorticoid deficiency (hypoglycaemia), prolonged jaundice or signs of hypothyroidism. Growth hormone deficiency generally causes hypoglycaemia but no other signs in the newborn. Treatment is with replacement of the missing hormones.

Parathyroid disorders

The parathyroid glands are responsible for control of calcium metabolism, but abnormalities of the parathyroids are rare causes of hypocalcaemia or hypercalcaemia in the newborn. When hypoparathyroidism does occur it may be familial or may occur in association with deletions of chromosome 22 (22q11 deletion or DiGeorge syndrome).

Effects of Maternal Drug use During Pregnancy on the Newborn

Opiates and other drugs cross the placenta. The fetus during pregnancy is likely to be exposed to the same peaks and troughs of drug exposure as the mother. Withdrawal may be manifested before birth.

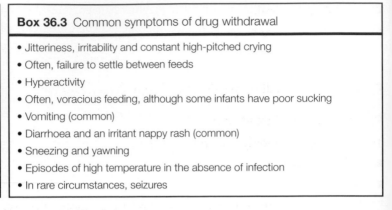

Box 36.3 Common symptoms of drug withdrawal

- Jitteriness, irritability and constant high-pitched crying
- Often, failure to settle between feeds
- Hyperactivity
- Often, voracious feeding, although some infants have poor sucking
- Vomiting (common)
- Diarrhoea and an irritant nappy rash (common)
- Sneezing and yawning
- Episodes of high temperature in the absence of infection
- In rare circumstances, seizures

Withdrawal symptoms

Each drug has a different half-life and this leads to different patterns of withdrawal symptoms. In general methadone produces symptoms for longer periods than heroin, but benzodiazepines may also contribute to this.

The symptoms most frequently seen are listed in Box 36.3. Infants assessed for signs of drug withdrawal using a scoring system are less likely to be inappropriately treated and may have a shorter hospital stay. It is important not to overtreat infants with drugs but babies who are withdrawing may appear to be in discomfort that needs to be relieved. The long-term effects of withdrawal symptoms are also unclear. The most useful sign is whether infants settle and sleep between feeding. If they do, then pharmacological treatment may be unnecessary.

Treatment

- Breastfeeding can be encouraged, as long as there is no evidence of HIV or on-going drug use that precludes this (cocaine, heroin). This includes methadone, as long as the dose is less than 20 mg/day.

- A quiet environment with reduced light and noise is helpful in keeping stimuli to a minimum.

- Swaddling is useful.
- Feeds may need to be given frequently. These infants will often take large volumes of milk; this is acceptable as long as vomiting is not a problem.
- Rocking and cradling are also useful adjuncts to treatment.

Pharmacological treatment

The two most commonly used treatments are:

- oral methadone
- oral morphine.

These appear to control withdrawal seizures much more effectively. They can be given in increasing doses if necessary until symptoms are controlled and then the dose may gradually be reduced.

If feeding and settling do not improve or profuse watery stools and profuse vomiting continue, other treatment needs to be considered. Alternative medication may sometimes be useful: for example, clonazepam for benzodiazepine use or chloral hydrate as a general sedative.

Cocaine

The effects of cocaine on the newborn are different. It can produce significant withdrawal symptoms but these are often less severe and less troublesome than with other drugs. However, it is associated with many other harmful effects on the fetus (Box 36.4).

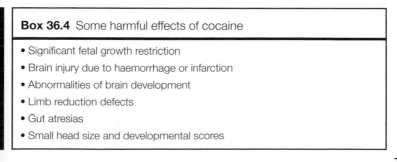

Box 36.4 Some harmful effects of cocaine

- Significant fetal growth restriction
- Brain injury due to haemorrhage or infarction
- Abnormalities of brain development
- Limb reduction defects
- Gut atresias
- Small head size and developmental scores

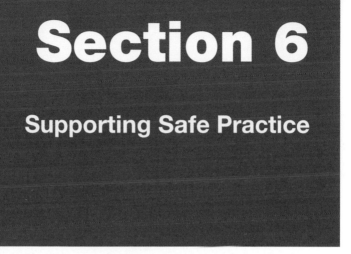

Section 6

Supporting Safe Practice

Chapter 37

Supervision of Midwives

The principal function of Supervisors of Midwives is the protection of the public, but the main ethos is support for midwives. Midwives have to notify their intention to practise midwifery each year to the Local Supervising Authority (LSA), and each LSA office maintains a database of all midwives practising within the LSA area. Information from the notifications of intention to practise is added to the details of registration on the Nursing and Midwifery Council (NMC) register.

A Supervisor of Midwives is an experienced practising midwife who has completed an approved programme of preparation and is appointed by the LSA. See Box 37.1 for the activities of a Supervisor of Midwives.

There is always a Supervisor of Midwives on call at any time who can be contacted if there are any practice concerns or if there has been a critical incident. For midwives to benefit from supervision, mutual respect between them and the supervisors is essential. Midwives should work in partnership with their supervisors and make the most of supervision, so that it can be effective not only for themselves but also for the mothers and babies for whom they care.

Local Supervising Authorities

The LSA has no management responsibility to NHS Trusts, but it acts as a focus for issues relating to midwifery practice. Its strength lies in its influence on quality in local midwifery services. All LSA officers have to be aware of the wider NHS picture and contemporary issues.

A practising midwife with experience as a Supervisor of Midwives performs the LSA 'Midwifery Officer' role in every LSA.

The duties of the LSA Midwifery Officer are detailed in Box 37.2.

Box 37.1 Activities of a Supervisor of Midwives

- Supporting best practice and ensuring evidence-based midwifery care
- Being a confident advocate for midwives and mothers
- Acting as an effective agent for change
- Providing leadership and guidance
- Acting as a role model
- Undertaking the role of mentor
- Empowering women and midwives
- Facilitating a supportive partnership with midwives
- Supporting midwives through dilemmas
- Helping midwives' personal and professional development
- Facilitating midwives' reflection on critical incidents
- Supporting midwives through supervised practice
- Maintaining an awareness of local, regional and national NHS issues
- Giving advice on ethical issues
- Liaising with clinicians, management and education
- Maintaining records of all supervisory activities
- Reporting to the LSA Midwifery Officer investigations of suboptimal care or misconduct

---

Box 37.2 Duties of the LSA Midwifery Officer

- Provides advice and guidance to Supervisors of Midwives
- Provides a framework of support for supervisory and midwifery practice
- Ensures each midwife meets the statutory requirements for practice

(Continued)

Box 37.2 (Continued)

- Selects and appoints Supervisors of Midwives and deselects if ever necessary
- Provides education and training for prospective Supervisors of Midwives
- Provides continuing education and training for Supervisors of Midwives
- Ensures appropriate ratios of midwives to Supervisors of Midwives in each Trust
- Provides advice on midwifery matters to health authorities
- Manages communications within supervisory systems
- Investigates cases of alleged misconduct
- Receives reports of maternal deaths
- Assesses the retraining requirements of non-practising midwives wishing to return to midwifery practice
- Leads the development of standards and audit of supervision
- Determines whether to suspend a midwife from practice, in accordance with the Nursing and Midwifery Council's Midwives Rules and Standards
- Prepares an annual report of supervisory activities within the report year, including audit outcomes and emerging trends affecting maternity services for Health Authorities and Trusts
- Maintains a list of current supervisors
- Provides a framework for supporting supervision and midwifery practice
- Publishes details of how to contact supervisors
- Publishes details of how the practice of midwives will be supervised
- Receives notifications of intention to practise
- Operates a system that ensures midwives meet statutory requirements for practice
- Ensures supervisors have access to education and training
- Leads the development of standards and audit of supervision
- Manages communications with supervisors
- Conducts regular meetings for supervisors to develop key areas of practice
- Facilitates inter-Trust activities, such as provision of cover by Supervisors of Midwives from other NHS Trusts
- May suspend a midwife, if appropriate
- Conducts investigations and initiates legal action in cases of practice by persons not qualified to do so under the Nursing and Midwifery Order 2001

Chapter 38

Complementary Medicine and Maternity Care

Women may have used complementary therapies prior to pregnancy, either by self-administering natural remedies or by consulting an independent practitioner, or they may wish to do so during pregnancy and for the birth. Expectant mothers are keen to use complementary therapies because they provide a range of additional strategies for pregnancy and labour at a time when pharmaceutical preparations are largely contraindicated and physiological discomforts are dismissed by the medical profession as 'minor disorders'. Also, many women wish to achieve as natural a birth as possible without recourse to drugs for pain relief in labour and may request the presence of a Complementary and Alternative Medicine (CAM) practitioner at the birth. Complementary medicine is based on the philosophy of holism and an appreciation of the innate interaction between the body, mind and spirit of the individual. Where women choose to consult independent complementary practitioners, they should ensure that the therapist has a thorough understanding of pregnancy physiopathology *and* the conventional maternity services. Mothers should also enquire whether or not the practitioner has current personal professional indemnity insurance cover, from which it is reasonable to assume that he or she has adequate qualifications to practise.

Any therapist who is unwilling to disclose this information should be rejected.

If the CAM practitioner is to be present during labour, he or she must acknowledge that the midwife or doctor, or both, legally remains the person responsible for the woman's care. When a midwife wishes to incorporate some aspect of complementary medicine within her own practice, she must nevertheless continue to work within the parameters laid down by the Nursing and Midwifery Council (UK) Midwives Rules and Standards.

Acupuncture

Acupuncture is based on the principle that the body has Qi or 'energy' lines, called meridians, flowing through it from top to hand or toe. Most of these pass through a major organ, after which the meridian is named. There are 12 major meridians, and 365 points on these in total. When the body, mind and spirit are in equilibrium, the energy flows along the meridians unimpeded and, to use the Chinese terminology, the 'Yin' and 'Yang' energies of the individual are balanced. However, when stressors of any sort affect the person, blockages occur at certain points (called acupuncture 'tsubos') on specific meridians. These points can be stimulated to release and rebalance the energies, either by the insertion of acupuncture needles or by other means. Sometimes thumb pressure is applied to the points (called acupressure, or the similar practice of *shiatsu*, the Japanese equivalent); on other occasions, heat is applied via moxa sticks (see moxibustion). Alternatively, suction can be used if the points are covered with special cups (cupping). Acupuncture needles may also be stimulated by mild electric pulsations; this is similar to transcutaneous nerve stimulation, which is used for pain relief in labour.

Certain acupuncture points are contraindicated during pregnancy as they may initiate labour; however, these points are good to stimulate for helping inefficient contractions in labour. Many antenatal conditions respond well to acupuncture or acupressure, including many of the physiological symptoms of pregnancy.

Uses

- *Moxibustion.* The use of moxibustion to attempt to turn a breech presentation is gaining popularity in the UK. In this technique, a stick of dried mugwort herb is used as a heat source over the bladder 67 acupuncture point on the outer edges of the little toes.

- *Labour.* Acupuncture is also useful in labour, especially for pain relief, induction and acceleration, and retained placenta.

Homeopathy

Homeopathy is considered by many of its practitioners to be a form of 'energy' medicine; it uses minute, highly diluted doses of substances that, if given in the full dose, would actually cause the symptoms being treated. Most homeopathic medicines are in tablet form but they do not work pharmacologically and will not interact with prescribed drugs, although certain drugs may inactivate the homeopathic tablet. Homeopathy treats the whole person and takes into account the personality of the individual, including the factors that make the symptoms better or worse. It sees as significant factors that may appear to be the most inconsequential of symptoms.

Although homeopathic remedies are available in pharmacies and health food stores, women should ensure they obtain accurate advice to help them make a decision regarding the most appropriate remedy for their condition. Only one tablet should normally be taken at one time. An increase in dosage means an increase in the frequency of administration, for the remedy acts as a stimulus to self-healing rather than as a chemical suppression or reversal of a symptom, as in the case of pharmaceutical drugs.

Uses

- *Arnica*. *Arnica montana*, found in tablet and cream form, is effective for the treatment of bruising, shock and trauma, both external and internal. Newly birthed mothers with perineal trauma would benefit from administration of arnica tablets to reduce trauma, although the cream should not be applied to the open wound, only to bruising surrounding the perineum. Similarly, in combination with homeopathic hypericum for wound healing, arnica can be useful for women who have had surgery such as caesarean section.

- *Pulsatilla*. Pulsatilla is also beneficial in pregnancy and seems to be suited to women with a mild and tearful disposition who are apprehensive. Haemorrhoids, varicosities and heartburn often respond well to a short course of pulsatilla, and slow progress in labour can be corrected in women with poor uterine contractions causing emotional distress, fainting and palpitations.

- *Other uses*. Homeopathy can be used for physiological discomforts of pregnancy, labour and the puerperium as well as some of the pathological conditions, although in an emergency some conflict could arise about the most appropriate system of medicine to use.

Herbal Medicine

The uses of herbal medicine in pregnancy and childbirth are summarised in Table 38.1.

Safety

There is a common misconception that just because herbal remedies are natural they are automatically safe. This is untrue. If herbal medicine (or any other form of complementary therapy) has the power to act therapeutically, it also theoretically has the power to harm if used

Table 38.1 Uses of herbal medicine for pregnancy and childbirth

Condition	Useful herbs
Nausea and vomiting	Peppermint, spearmint or camomile tea, ginger capsules or tea
Threatened miscarriage	Crampbark or chasteberry, raspberry leaf or lady's mantle
Varicose veins/haemorrhoids	Marigold or witch hazel compress
Constipation	Dandelion root or lime blossom
Heartburn and indigestion	Anise, caraway, lemon balm, camomile
Labour progress/exhaustion	Raspberry leaf, ginseng, rosemary
Contraction pain	Motherwort, skullcap
Perineal care	Comfrey, marigold, lavender
Engorgement/mastitis	Cabbage leaves, fennel

N.B. These are examples of herbal remedies that may be appropriate for certain conditions during the childbearing period; midwives should advise on using these remedies only if they are adequately and appropriately trained to do so.

incorrectly. All substances must be used appropriately — and expectant mothers may need expert help to select the necessary remedy for their particular condition. There are many herbal remedies that should be avoided during pregnancy or breastfeeding because they may induce uterine bleeding or miscarriage, or have other systemic effects on the mother or fetus.

St John's wort (*Hypericum perforatum*)

Uses

- St John's work is an antidepressant, especially useful for seasonal affective disorder.
- It is not recommended for pregnant and breastfeeding women, new mothers who have restarted the contraceptive pill and those taking certain medications such as anticoagulants and transplant antirejection drugs.

Raspberry leaf

Raspberry leaf is a popular herbal remedy that has long been advocated by pregnant women as a help in preparing for the birth. It is thought that certain constituents within the leaves of the raspberry have an effect on the uterine muscle, making it more efficient, possibly preventing postmaturity, easing discomfort in labour and enhancing uterine action. Qualified medical herbalists may use raspberry leaf to treat threatened miscarriage but midwives should advise women not to take it as a routine until the third trimester.

The tea, made from dried raspberry leaves, is more effective than tablets, although some brands of capsules can be opened to release the dried leaf from within, so that a tea can be made. Expectant mothers should start with just one cup of the tea or one tablet daily, giving themselves a few days to become accustomed to the effects before increasing the dose, to a maximum of four cups or tablets daily. The tea can be drunk during labour, as long as uterine activity is normal and no hypertonic contractions occur; it is best avoided if medical augmentation (e.g. oxytocin) is administered. Any tea or tablets that the mother may have left over after the birth can be taken postnatally to aid involution.

Osteopathy and Chiropractic

Both forms of treatment involve rebalancing of the neuromusculoskeletal system so that the whole body can be in alignment. Disorders, trauma or alterations in the body structure can cause imbalances in the whole system, which in turn can lead to a predisposition to other conditions. The main difference between osteopathy and chiropractic is that osteopaths are concerned with mobility of joints, whereas chiropractors deal with relative positions of joints. Different manipulative techniques are used and most chiropractors use more X-rays to aid diagnosis (although not for pregnant women). Osteopaths also use more soft tissue massage prior to manipulation.

Uses

- Both osteopathy and chiropractic are useful for treating a range of problems in pregnancy, including sickness, heartburn and constipation; they are notably valuable in the effective treatment of backache, sciatica and symphysis pubis diastasis.

- Other problems related to laxity of the joints caused by relaxin and progesterone, such as groin pain, legs 'giving way' and general pelvic instability, will also respond well to treatment.

- Chiropractic and osteopathy can also be useful in labour.

Craniosacral therapy

Craniosacral therapy, or cranial osteopathy, is gaining credibility and acceptance as a means of treating babies who are suffering the effects of excessive moulding following instrumental delivery; these effects include fractiousness, irritability, sleeplessness, poor feeding and, in older children, hyperactivity.

Aromatherapy

Aromatherapy is the use of highly concentrated essential oils extracted from plants. Essential oils enter the body by a variety of means, depending on the method of administration. The most frequently used modes of entry are via the skin, usually as massage, and also in the bath or in compresses or creams, via the mucous membranes in pessaries or suppositories, and via the respiratory tract in inhalations and vaporisers. All essential oils act in the same way as pharmaceutical drugs, being absorbed, metabolised and excreted via the same pathways; they are therefore likely to interact with prescribed medications.

Safety (see Box 38.1)

Essential oils can be very therapeutic when used appropriately, but also have the potential to be toxic if incorrectly administered or

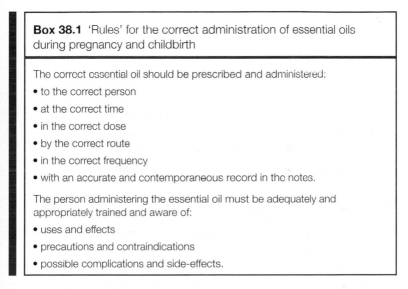

Box 38.1 'Rules' for the correct administration of essential oils during pregnancy and childbirth

The correct essential oil should be prescribed and administered:

• to the correct person
• at the correct time
• in the correct dose
• by the correct route
• in the correct frequency
• with an accurate and contemporaneous record in the notes.

The person administering the essential oil must be adequately and appropriately trained and aware of:

• uses and effects
• precautions and contraindications
• possible complications and side-effects.

abused. There are many oils that should be avoided during pregnancy, although some may be used in labour.

Uses

■ Lavender oil may relieve perineal discomfort after episiotomy.

■ Cypress oils are used in abdominal massage for constipation.

■ Camomile in the bath aids sleep.

■ All essential oils are antibacterial and some are also antifungal, antiviral or antimicrobial. Tea tree has gained credibility as an extremely effective combatant to candidal and other infections and is now also being used for people with HIV and for fighting meticillin-resistant *Staphylococcus aureus* (MRSA).

Reflexology

Reflexology, or reflex zone therapy, involves a precise manipulation of the feet, which are thought to represent a map of the whole body.

Every part of the body is reflected on one or both feet and therefore if specific parts of the feet are worked on, other areas of the body can be treated. Reflexology is a powerful therapy that can be very effective when used appropriately, although there are some contraindications, precautions and possible complications of treatment. Reflexology can also be performed on the hands, as well as the tongue, face and back. It is widely thought to work along the meridians used in acupuncture.

Uses

- Reflexology is used during pregnancy for relief of physiological discomforts as well as specific complaints, and in labour is invaluable for easing pain. Antenatal conditions that respond particularly well include constipation, headaches and migraine, sinus congestion, carpal tunnel syndrome, heartburn, insomnia, stress and anxiety, backache and sciatica.

- The destressing effects of the treatment can reduce hypertension and regulate cardiac function.

- Both postnatal and antenatal retention of urine may respond to reflexology.

- Stimulation of the foot zones corresponding to the pituitary gland can also assist the separation of a physiologically retained placenta. Similarly, lactation can be encouraged by treatment of these zones.

Coventry University Library

Appendix I

Drugs (Medicines)

Class of drug	Drug	Use and risk/contraindications
Anaesthetic	**Lidocaine hydrochloride**	Local anaesthetic used for perineal infiltration and nerve blocks
	Bupivicaine hydrochloride	Epidural and spinal anesthesia Contraindicated in hypovolaemia and local sepsis
Analgesia	**Non-steroidal anti-inflammatory drugs (NSAIDs)** (e.g. ibuprofen, indometacin, voltarol)	Relatively safe in the first trimester but have the potential to cause fetal renal dysfunction, premature closure of the ductus arteriosus, necrotising enterocolitis and intracerebral haemorrhage Safe in breastfeeding
	Opiate analgesics (e.g. pethidine, morphine, diamorphine, codeine, dihydrocodeine)	With long-term use there is a risk of neonatal withdrawal after birth. Risk of respiratory depression with large doses in labour
	Paracetamol	Recommended first-line analgesic agent in pregnancy Overdose can be potentially lethal to the mother and/or fetus

(Continued)

(Continued)

Class of drug	Drug	Use and risk/contraindications
Analgesia	Aspirin	Risk of maternal, fetal and neonatal bleeding with analgesic dose (e.g. 600 mg every 6 hours); therefore contraindicated in pregnancy Low-dose (75 mg daily) aspirin is used for treatment of recurrent miscarriage, thrombophilias (inherited risk of thromboembolism), and prevention of pre-eclampsia and intrauterine growth restriction Causes antiplatelet effect for around 10 days after administration and may prolong the bleeding time; therefore may be discontinued 3–4 weeks prior to expected birth
Antacid drugs	Ranitidine	To reduce the acidity of stomach acid in high-risk labours and prior to caesarean section or general anaesthetic
Antibiotics		To treat infection Caution should be exercised with some drugs during pregnancy
	Aminoglycosides (e.g. gentamicin, netilmicin)	Risk of ototoxicity but often used in serious maternal infection where benefit outweighs risk
	Chloramphenicol	Risk of 'grey baby syndrome' when used in second and third trimesters
	Erythromycin	Used if woman is penicillin-sensitive. Enhances effect of anticoagulants
	Metronidazole	Used to treat or prevent anaerobic infection Avoid large single doses when breastfeeding
	Nitrofurantoin	Risk of haemolysis in fetus at term — avoid during labour and delivery but safe at other times

Class of drug	Drug	Use and risk/ contraindications
	Penicillins	Not known to be harmful, trace amounts in breast milk
	Quinolones (e.g. ciprofloxacin, ofloxacin)	Risk of arthropathy in fetus — most of the evidence for this obtained from animal studies
	Tetracyclines (e.g. tetracycline, oxytetracycline, doxycycline)	Risk of discoloration and dysplasia of fetal bones and teeth, cataracts when used in second and third trimesters
Anticoagulants		History of a previous thromboembolic problem, an acute event, a known thrombophilia or heart valve replacement
	Heparin	Heparin does not cross the placenta and is not excreted into breast milk. Given intravenously or subcutaneously. Effectiveness is monitored by measuring the activated partial thromboplastin time (APTT). Side-effects include bleeding and bruising at the injection site, heparin-induced thrombocytopenia
	Low molecular weight (LMW) preparations (e.g. enoxaparin, dalteparin, tinzaparin)	Have a more predictable anticoagulant response and are usually given by once daily subcutaneous injection
	Warfarin	Women on warfarin should be converted to heparin as soon as they become pregnant and will continue on heparin throughout pregnancy. Considered safe in breastfeeding. The dose required is very variable

(Continued)

(Continued)

Class of drug	Drug	Use and risk/contraindications
		and is judged by monitoring the INR (international normalised ratio) in the blood
Anticonvulsants	**Carbamazepine** **Oxcarbazepine** **Phenytoin** **Valproate**	Increased risk of teratogenicity, particularly neural tube defects (NTDs). Benefits of treatment should outweigh risks Folic acid 5 mg should be taken daily. Risk of neonatal bleeding; prophylactic vitamin K is recommended for mother before birth in addition to the neonatal dose Small amounts in breast milk
	Magnesium sulphate	Treatment of eclampsia. Can be given intramuscularly or intravenously Care should be taken to avoid magnesium toxicity; clinical signs are loss of the patellar reflexes, a feeling of flushing, somnolence, slurred speech, respiratory difficulty and, in extreme cases, cardiac arrest. The 'antidote' to magnesium sulphate is calcium gluconate
Antiemetics		Non-pharmacological therapies should be tried first
	Metoclopramide	Not known to be harmful but use with caution in pregnancy and breastfeeding
Antihypertensive drugs		Pre-existing hypertension, pregnancy-induced hypertension or pre-eclampsia.
	ACE inhibitors (e.g. captopril, enalapril, lisinopril)	Contraindicated in pregnancy

Class of drug	Drug	Use and risk/ contraindications
	Beta-blockers (e.g. propranolol, atenolol, labetalol)	May cause intrauterine growth restriction, neonatal hypoglycaemia and bradycardia Considered safe in breastfeeding Contraindicated in women with asthma
	Calcium channel blockers (e.g. nifedipine, nicardipine)	Risk of serious hypotensive reactions, especially in association with magnesium sulphate Slow-release formulations should be used Risk of headache Small amounts in breast milk; avoidance recommended
	Hydralazine	Given by slow bolus injection or by infusion Avoid before third trimester Considered safe in breastfeeding
	Methyldopa	Given in 2–4 divided doses from a starting dose of 250 mg three times daily, up to a total of 3 g daily Considered safe in pregnancy and breastfeeding
Bronchodilators		To treat or prevent an asthma attack
	Inhaled bronchodilators (e.g. salbutamol, salmeterol, ipratropium), **inhaled cromoglicate, inhaled and oral corticosteroids and theophyllines**	Are all considered safe
Corticosteroids	**Prednisolone**	Pre-existing maternal disease such as asthma, rheumatoid arthritis

(Continued)

(Continued)

Class of drug	Drug	Use and risk/contraindications
Corticosteroids		and other inflammatory diseases Crosses the placenta in relatively small quantities; is considered safe for use in pregnancy Women who are on long-term steroid treatment should receive extra corticosteroids in labour, usually given as intravenous hydrocortisone
	Betamethasone and dexamethasone	Fetal lung maturation in actual or threatened preterm delivery Are generally given as intramuscular injections in divided doses over 24–48 hours; the most significant effect is noticed if 48 hours have elapsed between administration of the drug and birth
Diuretics	e.g. furosemide, bendroflumethiazide	Contraindicated in pregnancy
Drugs for diabetes mellitus	**Bovine insulin Metformin Sulphonylureas (oral hypoglycaemic agents)** (e.g. glibenclamide, gliclazide)	Glycaemic control Avoid in pregnancy
	Synthetic human insulins or pork-derived insulins	May be used in pregnancy
Folic acid		To reduce the risk of NTDs Recommended dose 400 µg daily Women at risk of NTDs and those taking antiepileptic drugs, 5 mg daily

Class of drug	Drug	Use and risk/contraindications
Hypnotics	**Benzodiazepines** (e.g. temazepam)	Avoid regular use during pregnancy and breastfeeding
Iron preparations		To treat iron deficiency anaemia
	Oral iron (e.g. ferrous gluconate or ferrous sulphate)	May cause gastrointestinal disturbance — constipation, diarrhoea, indigestion, black stools
	Parenteral preparations	Avoid in first trimester
Laxatives	e.g. **Lactulose, senna**	Considered safe in pregnancy and breastfeeding
Oxytocics		To aid uterine contractility, either in induction of labour or in augmentation of labour, or postpartum for prevention or treatment of uterine atony
	Syntocinon	In labour, generally given by intravenous infusion so the amount given can be titrated against its effect It takes 20–30 minutes for oxytocin to reach a steady state and the rate of infusion should therefore not be increased at time intervals of less than 30 minutes Should not be administered within 6 hours of vaginal prostaglandins For treatment and prevention of postpartum haemorrhage, larger doses can be given either by slow intravenous or intramuscular bolus or by intravenous infusion Can cause water retention and hyponatraemia
	Ergometrine	Treatment and prevention of postpartum haemorrhage

(Continued)

(Continued)

Class of drug	Drug	Use and risk/contraindications
Oxytocics		Can cause nausea, vomiting and hypertension Contraindicated in women with pre-eclampsia Can be given intramuscularly or intravenously Has a sustained action, up to 2–3 hours
	Syntometrine (oxytocin 5 IU/ml with ergometrine 0.5 mg)	Active management of the third stage of labour Given intramuscularly Has the advantage of the speed of action of oxytocin (within 3 minutes) and the sustained action of ergometrine The disadvantage is the side-effect profile of ergometrine
Prostaglandins	**Prostaglandin E$_2$** Dinoprostone	Induction of labour Given by the vaginal route in the form of gel or tablets Maximum dose gel = 3 mg (4 mg in primigravida with unfavourable cervix); maximum dose tablets = 6 mg (less in multipara) Oxytocin should not be given within at least 6 hours of prostaglandin because of the risk of uterine hyperstimulation
Tocolytics		To stop uterine activity
	Beta-sympathomimetics (e.g. ritodrine, terbutaline, salbutamol)	Associated with significant maternal side-effects, such as tachycardia, palpitations, tremor, nausea, vomiting, headaches, thirst, restlessness, chest pain and breathlessness Blood sugar levels may rise Great care should be taken when

Class of drug	Drug	Use and risk/ contraindications
		administering these drugs and the lowest possible dose should be given
	Calcium channel blockers (e.g. nifedipine)	These have the advantage of oral administration and fewer side-effects than some of the other agents Profound maternal hypotension is a risk
	Magnesium sulphate	Flushing, nausea, vomiting, palpitations and headaches are common maternal side-effects Magnesium levels need to be monitored
	NSAIDS (e.g. indometacin)	Maternal side-effects include gastrointestinal bleeding, peptic ulceration, thrombocytopenia, allergic reactions and impaired renal function Fetal side-effects when used in the long term include oligohydramnios, fetal renal impairment, premature closure of the ductus arteriosus, intraventricular haemorrhage and necrotising enterocolitis
	Oxytocin antagonists (e.g. atosiban)	A new class of drug that appears to have fewer side-effects

Appendix II

Normal Values in Pregnancy

Laboratory or physical measurements are presented as a range representing the average in a particular population. The physiological changes of pregnancy may affect what is considered 'normal' for the non-pregnant population. In addition, 'normal' values in pregnancy might be different at different gestations and hence care must be taken when deciding whether a test result(s) is actually abnormal for the woman/fetus concerned. A large sample of women having a straightforward physiological pregnancy is necessary to produce accurate pregnancy value ranges and hence there can be small variations from book to book.

Units of Measurement

Care needs to be taken in the interpretation of units of measurement as abbreviations are used and represent very different amounts. In addition, values might be expressed in SI or traditional units. For example:

g = grams   L = litres
mg = milligrams   dL = decilitres (N.B. prefix 'd' signifies 10^{-1})
mmol = millimoles

Weight Gain in Pregnancy

Average weight gain during pregnancy is about 12.5 kg; however this varies according to the woman's pre-pregnancy body mass index BMI (weight/height^2). Those with a low BMI are expected to gain more weight, whereas those women who are obese should gain less.

Category	Pre-pregnant BMI
Low (underweight)	<19.8
Normal	19.8–26.0
High (overweight)	26.1–29.0
Obese	>29.0

Biochemistry

Test/units	Non-pregnant Typical range	Pregnant Typical range	Comments
Alanine transaminase (ALT) u/L	6–40	No change	Raised levels indicate liver damage
Alkaline phosphatase IU/L	40–120	Doubled by late pregnancy	Usually elevated in third trimester due to placental production of enzyme
Bile acids (total) μmol/L	<9		Values of total bile acids ≥14 μmol/L are viewed as abnormal, indicating cholestasis
Bilirubin μmol/L	<17		Little change from non-pregnant range
Creatinine μmol/L	50–100	75 approx is upper limit of normal	Lower in mid-pregnancy but rises towards term
Potassium mmol/L	3.5–5.3	Unchanged	Unchanged in pregnancy
Albumin g/L	30–48	25–35	Total protein and albumin are both lower in pregnancy
Urea mmol/L	2–6.5	Usually ≤4.5	Lower in pregnancy
Uric acid μmol/L	150–350	Lowest values in second trimester, 10 × gestational age in weeks is approx upper limit of normal	Increases with gestation, although lower levels than non-pregnant

Haematology

Note: Pregnancy is a hypercoaguable state and prothrombin, partial thromboplastin and thrombin times are slightly faster than controls.

Test/units	Non-pregnant Typical range	Pregnant	Comments
Clotting time	12 min	8 min	Observe whether blood is clotting or oozing from venepuncture sites in high-risk groups
Fibrin degradation products $\mu g/ml$	Mean 1.04	High values in third trimester and especially around time of birth	
Fibrinogen g/L	1.7–4.1	By term 2.9–6.2	Marked increase in pregnancy, especially in third trimester and around time of birth
Haematocrit L/L	0.35–0.47	0.31–0.35	Lower in pregnancy
Haemoglobin g/dL	11.5–16.5	10.0–12.0 Should be ≥ 10 in third trimester	Good iron stores needed to maintain pregnancy levels. Fall in first trimester whether or not iron and folate taken
Platelets $\times 10^9 L$	150–400	Slight decrease in normal pregnancy Lower limit of 'normal' = 120	No functional significance
White cell count $\times 10^9 L$	4.0–11.0	9.0–15.0 Higher values up to 25.0 around time of birth	Normal increase in pregnancy. Rise in infections

Appendix III

Glossary of Terms and Definitions

Notification and Registration of Birth

It is the legal duty of the father or any other person in attendance or present within 6 hours after the birth, to notify the birth. This must be done within 36 hours of birth for any child born after 24 completed weeks of pregnancy, whether alive or dead. It is usual for the midwife to undertake this notification. In addition to biographical information about the mother and her baby, the midwife will record the period of gestation, any congenital malformation and factors that may put the baby at risk.

The purpose of notification is to enable the primary health care team to be aware of a baby's birth. Where appropriate, an entry for the 'at-risk' register is compiled from the details supplied; this is used for providing supervision of care for the children concerned. The birth information is also made available to the Registrar of Births and Deaths of the district in which the birth took place.

Registration of birth

Every birth must be registered in the district in which it took place. Births must be registered within 6 weeks (3 weeks in Scotland), although under certain circumstances that time might be extended by the Registrar of Births and Deaths. There is a statutory fine for those who fail to register.

The primary duty to register a birth rests with the mother of the child, although in the case of a married couple the father may attend to register. If a mother is unmarried and wishes the father's name and details to be included, the couple should attend together to give details to the Registrar. If this is not possible, the mother could register the baby with her details only, and then the couple could re-register the birth later, adding the father's particulars. An unmarried father may also attend alone to register if he takes with him a Statutory Declaration made by the mother that he is the father of the child, or certain other court orders. In the event of the parents being unable to register the birth, a number of other people, including a senior administrator at the hospital where the child was born or someone present at the birth, which could be the midwife, are qualified to register a birth.

Statistics

At the time of registration, the Registrar also collects further information that is not entered in the Register but is used for statistical purposes and passed to the Office of National Statistics.

Stillbirths

Definition of stillbirth

A 'still-born baby' means a baby that has issued forth from its mother after the 24th week of pregnancy and which did not at any time after being completely expelled from its mother, breathe or show any other signs of life.

Registration of stillbirths

In order to register a stillborn baby, the mother or other informant must have a Medical Certificate of Stillbirth issued by a medical practitioner or midwife who is present at the stillbirth or who examines the body of a stillborn baby. Informants who have responsibility to register a stillbirth are the same as those in the case of a live birth.

The Registrar will record the details in the Stillbirth Register and issue an authority for burial or cremation. If the baby is to be cremated, the Medical Certificate of Stillbirth must be signed by a registered medical practitioner.

The midwife responsible for the care of the woman and her baby must notify the Supervisor of Midwives of the stillbirth.

Registration of Death of a Baby

This is the responsibility of the family. They should notify the Registrar of any child who has died after having been born alive.

Birth and Death Rates

Vital statistics relate to life and death events, and specifically to the systematic collection of numerical data in order that they may be summarised and studied. In measuring health, there are difficulties in finding objective data to quantify; therefore it is pertinent to study the numbers of deaths occurring at different ages and their causes.

Figure 1 shows the periods relating to different types of death that are of special interest to midwives.

Definition of 'stillbirth rate'

To calculate the rate of stillbirth, the number of actual stillbirths in a year is compared with the number of total births (both live and still).

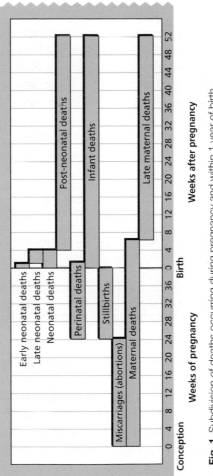

Fig. 1 Subdivision of deaths occurring during pregnancy and within 1 year of birth.

This ratio is then related to a group of 1000 of those total births. The mathematical formula is as follows:

$$\frac{\text{No. of still births}}{\text{No. of total births}} \times 1000 = \text{Stillbirth rate per 1000 total births}$$

Perinatal death

- *Perinatal death*. This is either a stillbirth or a death occurring in the 1st week of life (early neonatal death).
- *Perinatal death (or mortality) rate*. This is the number of stillbirths and early neonatal deaths per 1000 total births.

Neonatal death

- *Neonatal death*. This is a death occurring in the first 28 days of life. Neonatal deaths are divided into early neonatal deaths, which occur during the first 7 days of life, and later neonatal deaths, which occur during the next 21 days. The reason for this is that the causes of early death are more similar to those of stillbirth, whereas the causes of later deaths are different.
- *Neonatal death rate*. This is calculated per 1000 live births.

Infant death

- *Infant death*. This is a death occurring in the 1st year of life. This includes all neonatal deaths and those termed postneonatal deaths.
- *Infant mortality rate*. This is calculated per 1000 live births. This rate is taken as one of the best measures of a nation's health.

Maternal deaths

In 1952, major changes took place in the system for reviewing maternal deaths in England and Wales. The outcome was a series of triennial reports followed by similar systems in Northern Ireland in 1956 and Scotland in 1965. From 1985 all four countries in the UK worked together to produce a common report. The overall responsibility for collating data and producing the final triennial report lies with the Confidential Enquiry into Maternal and Child Health (CEMACH). Prior to 2000, maternal deaths were reported in the Confidential Enquiries into Maternal Deaths (CEMD).

- *Maternal death.* This is defined as 'the death of a woman while pregnant or within 42 days of termination of pregnancy, from any cause related to or aggravated by the pregnancy or its management, but not from accidental or incidental causes'.

- *Maternal mortality.* In the UK this is the number of deaths per 100 000 maternities.

- *International maternity mortality rate (MMR).* This is the number of deaths per 100 000 live births. This figure is useful for international comparisons but care is needed in its interpretation.

- *Direct maternal deaths.* These are classified as those resulting from complications of pregnancy, labour and the puerperium, from interventions, omissions or incorrect treatment, or from a chain of events resulting from any of these (e.g. thromboembolism, haemorrhage, pre-eclampsia and eclampsia, sepsis, anaesthesia, amniotic fluid embolism).

- *Indirect maternal deaths.* These result from previous existing disease or diseases that developed during pregnancy/the puerperium, where death was not due to direct obstetric causes but was aggravated by the physiological effects of pregnancy (e.g. cardiac disease, psychiatric illness).

- *Coincidental deaths* (referred to as fortuitous in the international classification). These are deaths from unrelated causes which happen to occur in pregnancy/the puerperium (e.g. domestic violence, although incidents might first arise in pregnancy).

- *Late deaths.* These occur between 42 days and 1 year after abortion, miscarriage or delivery, and are due to direct or indirect maternal causes of death.

Note. CEMACH gives details of deaths that are included/excluded from official statistics and those that are included in the triennial report. CEMACH also provides a 'Midwifery Summary and Key Findings' website: www.cemach.org.uk.

Common Definitions

Abortion
Termination of pregnancy before the fetus is viable, i.e. before 24 weeks' gestation in the UK.

Abruptio placentae
Premature separation of a normally situated placenta. Term normally used from viability (24 weeks).

Acardiac twin
One twin presents without a well-defined cardiac structure and is kept alive through the placental circulation of the viable twin.

Acridine orange
A stain used in fluorescence microscopy that causes bacteria to fluoresce green to red.

Aetiology
The science of the cause of disease.

Amenorrhoea
Absence of menstrual periods.

Amniotic fluid embolism
The escape of amniotic fluid through the wall of the uterus or placental site into the maternal circulation, triggering life-threatening anaphylactic shock in the mother. (The word 'embolism', denoting a clot, is a misnomer.)

Amniotomy
Artificial rupture of the amniotic sac.

Anterior obliquity of the uterus
Altered uterine axis. The uterus leans forward due to poor maternal abdominal muscles and a pendulous abdomen.

Antigen
A substance which stimulates the production of an antibody.

Anuria
Producing no urine.

Atresia
Closure or absence of a usual opening or canal.

Augmentation of labour
Intervention to correct slow progress in labour.

Bandl's ring
An exaggerated retraction ring seen as an oblique ridge above

the symphysis pubis between the upper and lower uterine segments, which is a sign of obstructed labour.

Basal body temperature
The temperature of the body when at rest. In natural family planning, it is taken as soon as the woman wakes from sleep and before any activity occurs or after a period of at least 1 hour's rest.

Bicornuate uterus
A structural abnormality of the uterus.

Bishops score
Rating system to assess suitability of the cervix for induction of labour.

Burns Marshall
A method of breech delivery involving traction to prevent the neck from bending backwards.

Calendar calculation
The fertile phase of the menstrual cycle is calculated in accordance with the length of the woman's 6–12 previous cycles.

Cardiotocograph
Measurement of the fetal heart rate and contractions on a machine that is able to provide a paper print of the information it records.

Central venous pressure line
An intravenous tube that measures the pressure in the right atrium or superior vena cava, indicating the volume of blood returning to the heart and, by implication, hypovolaemia.

Cephalopelvic disproportion
Disparity between the size of the woman's pelvis and the fetal head.

Cerclage
A non-absorbable suture inserted to keep the cervix closed.

Cervical ectropion
Physiological response by cervical cells to hormonal changes in pregnancy. Cells proliferate and cause the cervix to appear eroded.

Cervical intraepithelial neoplasm (CIN)
Progressive and abnormal growth of cervical cells.

Cervical ripening
The process by which the cervix changes and becomes more

susceptible to the effect of uterine contractions. Can be physiological or artificially produced.

Cervicitis
Inflammation of the cervix.

Choanal atresia
(Bilateral) membranous or bony obstruction of the nares; the baby is blue when sleeping and pink when crying.

Choroid plexus cyst
Collection of cerebrospinal fluid within the choroid plexi, from where cerebrospinal fluid is derived.

Coloboma
A malformation characterised by the absence of or a defect in the tissue of the eye; the pupil can appear keyhole-shaped. It may be associated with other anomalies.

Colposcopy
Visualisation of the cervix using a colposcope.

Commensal
Microorganisms adapted to grow on the skin or mucous surfaces of the host, forming part of the normal flora.

Conjoined twins
Identical twins in whom separation is incomplete so their bodies are joined together at some point.

Couvelaire uterus (uterine apoplexy)
Bruising and oedema of uterine tissue seen in placental abruption, when leaking blood is forced between muscle fibres because the margins of the placenta are still attached to the uterus.

Cryotherapy
Use of cold or freezing to destroy or remove tissue.

Deoxyribonucleic acid (DNA)
The substance containing genes. DNA can store and transmit information, can copy itself accurately and can occasionally mutate.

Diastasis symphysis pubis
A painful condition in which there is an abnormal relaxation of the ligaments supporting the pubic joint.

Dichorionic twins
Twins who have developed in their own separate chorionic sacs.

Diploid
Containing two sets of chromosomes.

Disseminated intravascular coagulation/coagulopathy
A condition secondary to a primary complication where there is inappropriate blood clotting in the blood vessels, followed by an inability of the blood to clot appropriately when all the clotting factors have been used up.

Dizygotic (dizygous)
Formed from two separate zygotes.

Doering rule
The first fertile day of the cycle is determined by a calculation based upon the earliest previous temperature shift. This is an effective double-check method to identify the onset of the fertile phase.

Dyspareunia
Painful or difficult intercourse experienced by the woman.

Echogenic bowel
Bright appearances of bowel, equivalent to the brightness of bone. Also associated with intra-amniotic bleeding and fetal swallowing of blood-stained liquor.

Echogenic foci in the heart
Bright echoes from calcium deposits in the fetal heart, often the left ventricle. These do not affect cardiac function.

Ectopic pregnancy
An abnormally situated pregnancy, most commonly in a Fallopian tube.

Embryo reduction (see Fetal reduction)

Endocervical
Relating to the internal canal of the cervix.

Epicanthic fold
A vertical fold of skin on either side of the nose, which covers the lacrimal caruncle. Can be common in Asian babies, but may indicate Down syndrome in other ethnic groups.

Erb's palsy
Paralysis of the arm due to the damage to cervical nerve roots five and six of the brachial plexus.

Erythema
Reddening of the skin.

Erythropoiesis
The process by which erythrocytes (red blood cells) are formed. After the 10th week of gestation, erythropoiesis rises and seems to be involved in red cell production in the bone marrow during the third trimester.

External cephalic version (ECV)
The use of external manipulation on the pregnant woman's abdomen to convert a breech to a cephalic presentation.

False-negative rate
The proportion of affected pregnancies that would not be identified as high-risk. Tests with a high false-negative rate have low sensitivity.

False-positive rate
The proportion of unaffected pregnancies with a high-risk classification. Tests with a high false-positive rate have low specificity.

Ferguson reflex
Surge of oxytocin, resulting in increased contractions, due to stimulation of the cervix and upper portion of the vagina.

Fetal reduction
The reduction in the number of viable fetuses/embryos in a multiple (usually higher multiple) pregnancy by medical intervention.

Fetofetal transfusion syndrome (twin-to-twin transfusion syndrome (TTTS))
Condition in which blood from one monozygotic twin fetus transfuses into the other via blood vessels in the placenta.

Fetus-in-fetu
Parts of a fetus may be lodged within another fetus. This can only happen in monozygotic twins.

Fetus papyraceous
A fetus that dies in the second trimester of the pregnancy and becomes compressed and parchment-like.

Fibroid
Firm, benign tumour of muscular and fibrous tissue.

Fraternal twins
Dizygotic (non-identical) twins.

Fundal height
The distance between the top part of the uterus (the fundus) and the top of the symphysis pubis (the junction between the pubic bones). Measurement of this is undertaken to assess the increasing size of the uterus antenatally and decreasing size postnatally.

Haematuria
Blood in the urine.

Haemostasis
The arrest of bleeding.

Haploid
Containing only one set of chromosomes.

HELLP syndrome
A condition of pregnancy characterised by haemolysis, elevated liver enzymes and low platelets.

Herpes gestationis
An autoimmune disease precipitated by pregnancy and characterised by an erythematous rash and blisters.

Homan's sign
Pain is felt in the calf when the foot is pulled upwards

(dorsiflexion). This is indicative of a venous thrombosis and further investigations should be undertaken to exclude or confirm this.

Homeostasis
The condition in which the body's internal environment remains relatively constant within physiological limits.

Hydatidiform mole
A gross malformation of the trophoblast in which the chorionic villi proliferate and become avascular.

Hydropic vesicles
Fluid-filled sacs, or blisters.

Hypercapnia
An abnormal increase in the amount of carbon dioxide in the blood.

Hyperemesis gravidarum
Protracted or excessive vomiting in pregnancy.

Hypertrophy
Overgrowth of tissue.

Hypovolaemia
Reduced circulating blood volume due to external loss of body

fluids or to loss of fluid into the tissues.

Hypoxia
Lack of oxygen.

Hysteroscope
An instrument used to access the uterus via the vagina.

Induction of labour
Intervention to stimulate uterine contractions before the onset of spontaneous labour.

Intraepithelial
Within the epithelium, or among epithelial cells.

Intrahepatic cholestasis of pregnancy (ICP)
An idiopathic condition of abnormal liver function.

LAM
A method of contraception based upon an algorithm of lactation, amenorrhoea and a 6-month time period.

Lanugo
Soft downy hair, which covers the fetus in utero and occasionally the neonate. It appears at around 20 weeks' gestation and covers the face and most of the body. It disappears by 40 weeks' gestation.

Løvset manœuvre
A manœuvre for the delivery of shoulders and extended arms in a breech.

Macrosomia
Large baby.

Malposition
A cephalic presentation other than normal anterior position of the fetal head, e.g. occipito-posterior.

Malpresentation
A presentation other than the vertex, i.e. face, brow, compound or shoulder. (Breech may be included in this category.)

Mauriceau–Smellie–Veit
A manœuvre to deliver a breech, which involves jaw flexion and shoulder traction.

McRobert's manœuvre
A manœuvre to rotate the angle of the symphysis pubis superiorly and release the impaction of the anterior shoulder in shoulder dystocia. The woman brings her knees up to her chest.

Monoamniotic twins
Twins who have developed in the same amniotic sac.

Monochorionic twins
Identical twins who have developed in the same chorionic sac.

Monozygotic (monozygous)
Formed from one zygote (identical twins).

Multifetal reduction (see Fetal reduction)

Naegele's rule
Method of calculating the expected date of delivery.

Neoplasia
Growth of new tissue.

Neutral thermal environment (NTE)
The range of environmental temperature over which heat production, oxygen consumption and nutritional requirements for growth are minimal, provided the body temperature is normal.

Nuchal fold >5 mm at 20 weeks' gestation
An increased thickness of fetal skin and fat at the back of the fetal neck. Subcutaneous fluid (nuchal translucency) cannot usually be visualised after 14 weeks.

Oedema
The effusion of body fluid into the tissues.

Oligohydramnios
Abnormally low amount of amniotic fluid in pregnancy.

Oliguria
The production of an abnormally small amount of urine.

$PaCO_2$
Measures the partial pressure of dissolved carbon dioxide. This dissolved CO_2 has moved out of the cell and into the bloodstream. The measure of $PaCO_2$ accurately reflects the alveolar ventilation.

PaO_2
Measures the partial pressure of oxygen in the arterial blood. It reflects how the lung is functioning but does not measure tissue oxygenation.

Paronychia
An inflamed swelling of the nail folds; acute paronychia is usually

caused by infection with
Staphylococcus aureus.

Pedunculated
Having a stem or stalk.

*Pemphigoid gestationis (see
Herpes gestationis)*

Perinatal
Surrounding labour and the first
7 days of life.

pH
A solution's acidity or alkalinity
is expressed on the pH scale,
which runs from 0 to 14. This
scale is based on the concentration of hydrogen ions in a
solution expressed in chemical
units called moles per litre.

Placenta accreta
Abnormally adherent placenta
into the muscle layer of the
uterus.

Placenta increta
Abnormally adherent placenta
into the perimetrium of the
uterus.

Placenta percreta
Abnormally adherent placenta
through the muscle layer of the
uterus.

Placenta praevia
A condition in which some or
all of the placenta is attached in
the lower segment of the uterus.

*Placental abruption (see
Abruptio placentae)*

Polyhydramnios
An excessive amount of amniotic fluid in pregnancy.

Polyp
Small growth.

Porphyria
An inherited condition of
abnormal red blood cell
formation.

Postpartum
After labour.

Pre-eclampsia
A condition peculiar to pregnancy, which is characterised by
hypertension, proteinuria and
systemic dysfunction.

*Primary postpartum
haemorrhage*
A blood loss in excess of 500 ml
or any amount which adversely
affects the condition of the
mother within the first 24 hours
of delivery.

Progestogen
Synthetic progesterone used in hormonal contraception.

Prostaglandins
Locally acting chemical compounds derived from fatty acids within cells. They ripen the cervix and cause the uterus to contract.

Proteinuria
Protein in the urine.

Pruritus
Itching.

Ptyalism
Excessive salivation.

Puerperal fever/pyrexia
A rise in temperature in the puerperium. This is poorly defined in the textbooks but is assumed to be based on the definition of pyrexia, which is a rise above the normal body temperature of 37.2°C. Where pyrexia is used as a clinical sign of importance, the elevation in temperature is generally taken as being 38°C and above.

Puerperal sepsis
Infection of the genital tract following childbirth; still a

major cause of maternal death where it is undetected and/or untreated.

Puerperium
A period after childbirth where the uterus and other organs and structures that have been affected by the pregnancy are returning to their non-gravid state. Usually described as a period of up to 6–8 weeks.

Quickening
Recognition of fetal movements by the woman in early pregnancy.

Retraction
Process by which the uterine muscle fibres shorten after a contraction. Unique to uterine muscle.

Rubin's manœuvre
A rotational manœuvre to relieve shoulder dystocia. Pressure is exerted over the fetal back to adduct and rotate the shoulders.

Sandal gap
Exaggerated gap between the first and second toes.

Secondary postpartum haemorrhage

An 'excessive' or 'prolonged' vaginal blood loss which is usually defined as occurring from 24 hours to 6 weeks after the birth.

Selective fetocide

The medical destruction of an abnormal twin fetus in a continuing pregnancy.

Sheehan syndrome

A condition where sudden or prolonged shock leads to irreversible pituitary necrosis, characterised by amenorrhoea, genital atrophy and premature senility.

Short femur

Shorter than average thigh bone, when compared with other fetal measurements.

Shoulder dystocia

Failure of the shoulders to traverse the pelvis spontaneously after delivery of the head. Incidence is around 0.3% of deliveries.

Siamese twins

Conjoined twins.

Speculum (vaginal)

An instrument used to open the vagina.

Subinvolution

The uterine size appears larger than anticipated for days postpartum, and may feel poorly contracted. Uterine tenderness may be present.

Superfecundation

Conception of twins as a result of sexual intercourse with two different partners in the same menstrual cycle.

Superfetation

Conception of twins as a result of two acts of sexual intercourse in different menstrual cycles.

Surfactant

Complex mixture of phospholipids and lipoproteins, produced by type 2 alveolar cells in the lungs, that decreases surface tension and prevents alveolar collapse at end-expiration.

Symphysiotomy

A surgical incision to separate the symphysis pubis and enlarge the pelvis to aid delivery.

Symphysis pubis dysfunction (see Diastasis symphysis pubis)

Talipes

A complex foot deformity, affecting 1 per 1000 live births and more common in males. The affected foot is held in a fixed flexion (equinus) and in-turned (varus) position. It can be differentiated from positional talipes because the deformity in true talipes cannot be passively corrected.

Teratogen
An agent believed to cause congenital abnormalities, e.g. thalidomide.

Torsion
Twisting.

Trizygotic
Formed from three separate zygotes.

Twin-to-twin transfusion syndrome (see Fetofetal transfusion syndrome)

Uniovular
Monozygotic.

Unstable lie
After 36 weeks' gestation, a lie that varies between longitudinal and oblique or transverse is said to be unstable.

Uterine involution
The physiological process that starts from the end of labour that results in a gradual reduction in the size of the uterus until it returns to its non-pregnant size and location in the pelvis.

Vanishing twin syndrome
The reabsorption of one twin fetus early in pregnancy (usually before 12 weeks).

Vasa praevia
A rare occurrence in which umbilical cord vessels pass through the placental membranes and lie across the cervical os.

Withdrawal bleed
Bleeding due to withdrawal of hormones.

Wood's manoeuvre
A rotational or screw manoeuvre to relieve shoulder dystocia. Pressure is exerted on the fetal chest to rotate and abduct the shoulders.

Zavanelli manoeuvre
Last choice of manoeuvre for shoulder dystocia. The head is returned to its pre-restitution position, then the head is flexed back into the vagina. Delivery is by caesarean section.

Zygosity
Describing the genetic make-up of children in a multiple birth.

Index

Please note that page references to Boxes, Figures or Tables situated away from the text will be in *italic* print.

M